DATE DUE FOR

UNIVERSITY LIE

Any b
is ca

D

A HISTORY OF NEUROPHYSIOLOGY IN THE 17TH AND 18TH CENTURIES
From Concept to Experiment

A History of Neurophysiology
in the
17th and 18th Centuries
From Concept to Experiment

Mary A. B. Brazier

Departments of Anatomy and Physiology
UCLA School of Medicine
Los Angeles, California

Raven Press ■ New York

Raven Press, 1140 Avenue of the Americas, New York, New York 10036

Made in the United States of America

Library of Congress Cataloging in Publication Data

Brazier, Mary Agnes Burniston, 1904-
  A history of neurophysiology in the 17th and 18th centuries.

  Includes bibliographical references and index.
  1. Neurophysiology—History—17th century.   2. Neurophysiology—History—18th century.   I. Title.
QP353.B73   1984   599′.0188   83-23106
ISBN 0-89004-553-4

Second Printing, November 1984

Preface

In this volume, the first of two designed to cover three centuries, I have attempted to extract from the wealth of material about the 17th and 18th centuries that which is germane to our present understanding of the nervous system, and to highlight the development in that era from age-old concepts to the modern one of experimentation.

The goal of these volumes is to acquaint the modern worker in the neural sciences with the gradual growth of knowledge about the fuctioning of our nervous systems. Taken for granted today is the fact that the agent that operates our nerves and muscles is electricity, but when the 17th century opened not even the differentiation between magnetism and electricity had yet been made. Once identified, this mysterious invisible agent continued to puzzle the world of physics and of physiology (a word not yet coined). In the final decade of the 18th century that world was rocked by the findings of Galvani, and the science of electrophysiology was born. It had an uphill fight for recognition and understanding in the 18th century, in which only two forms of electricity had received recognition, namely, "atmospheric" and "natural." To these now had to be added "animal electricity."

In the account that follows I have attempted to describe for the reader those original experiments whose results would replace old ideas with experimental proof. Where possible, the worker's own sketch of his experiment is reproduced—for this was a time that preceded the age of photography. Where actual quotations are given, the source will be found in a footnote. Reading lists are appended that include the writings of those great men that are germane to neurophysiology, together with selected studies of their works, which can guide the student who wishes to read more deeply in this field.

Important for the recognition of the transition from traditional methods to the new experimentation without constraints is an awareness of the age in which the experimenter was living—the intellectual environment, the political flavor of thought, and the freedom to disagree with ancient dogma. This background forms part of the central core of this work, which presents the historical breakthrough in thought and experiment about the nervous system in the 17th and 18th centuries.

MARY A. B. BRAZIER

Acknowledgments

To thank all the great number of individuals who helped me amass the large quantity of data that make up the content of this book is so impossible a task that some may unfortunately remained unnamed. Many scholars were generous in sending me materials including photographs, books, and manuscripts; I feel myself greatly indebted to the following: A. M. Luyendijk-Elshout, Leiden; the late P. Anokhin, Moscow; the late L. Belloni, Bologna; W. Berg, Halle; D. Biesold, Leipzig; C. D. Blakemore, Oxford; M. L. R. Bonelli, Florence; J. A. W. Brak, Amsterdam; W. F. Bynum, London; E. Clarke, London; the late E. Fadiga, Bologna; the late H. Fischgold, Paris; B. Flerkó, Pècs; the late E. Guttmann, Prague; A. M. Ivanitsky, Moscow; D. H. Ingvar, Lund; W. Kaiser, Halle; W. Kirsche, Berlin; P. G. Kostyuk, Kiev; the late V. Kruta, Prague; G. A. Lindeboom, Amsterdam; E. Lugaresi, Bologna; H. Matthies, Magdeburg; C. McC Brooks, New York; V. L. Merculov, Leningrad; G. Moruzzi, Pisa; C. Newman, London; A. Nicolai, Berlin-Karlshorst; the late C. D. O'Malley, Los Angeles; P. Passouant, Montpellier; the late G. Pupilli, Bologna; K. E. Rothschuh, Münster; J. Storm van Leeuwen, the Hague; W. Storm van Leeuwen, Utrecht; the late A. Tournay, Paris; D. B. Tower, Bethesda; G. Wiener, Leipzig.

Of the many libraries and museums that have eased my search, the staff of the following have been among the most patient: Académie des Sciences, Paris; Bibliothèque Nationale, Paris; Biblioteca Nazionale Centrale, Florence; Biblioteca Universitaria, Pisa; Bodleian Library, Oxford; British Library (British Museum), London; Conservatoire des Arts et Métiers, Paris; Countway Museum, Harvard Medical School; Deutsches Museum, Munich; Institut für Geschichte der Medizin der Universität, Vienna; Institute of Electrical Engineers, London; Musée Carnavalet, Paris; Museo di Storia della Scienza, Florence; Museum Boerhaave, Leiden; National Library of Medicine, Bethesda; Neidersachsische Landesbibliothek, Hannover; Royal Society, London; Sächsische Akademie der Wissenschaften zu Leipzig; Science Museum, South Kensington, London; Scola Normale Superiore, Pisa; Teylers Museum, Haarlem; University Museum, Utrecht; Wellcome Historical Library, London. I am greatly indebted to the librarians, curators, and directors.

The research for this book has been greatly facilitated by the excellent collection of historical books and manuscripts in the Biomedical Library of the University of California Los Angeles. The author is indebted to the National Library of Medicine, Bethesda, Maryland, for a grant to aid in this search.

The author also wishes to thank Mrs. Anna Venero for her patient typing of the many stages of the manuscript.

FORMAL ACKNOWLEDGMENT

This publication was supported in part by NIH Grant LMO 3462 from the National Library of Medicine.

MARY A. B. BRAZIER

Contents

List of Illustrations

PART I
Neurophysiology in the 17th Century—
From Concept to Experiment

Prologue

This historical account of the science of neurophysiology takes as its starting point the year 1600. Before that time, although there were great thinkers, there was little exact science of the nervous system. How the concepts of these thinkers came to influence the working scientists in the centuries to follow is traced, for the construction of this study is based on the scientist's recognized procedure: frame a working hypothesis and then design experiments to test it. Many of the discoveries in the field of neurophysiology are the outgrowths of ideas, the hypotheses of nonexperimentalists—philosophers, historians, and writers.

In contrast to medicine, a science demanding synthesis of observations, experimental physiology, with its reliance on analysis and laboratory findings, has little significant history before the 17th century. Leaders in medicine developed and practiced its therapies for many years before they felt the need to understand the nature and functions of the body's parts in any truly physiological sense and, when the urge for this knowledge first arose, it was to come as much from the philosophers as from the healers of the sick.

Neurophysiology (a term not to come into use until centuries later) had as a legacy from the ancients only their speculative inferences and their primitive neuroanatomy. Aristotle had confounded nerves with tendons and ligaments, and had thought the brain bloodless and the heart supreme—not only as a source of the nerves, but also as the seat of the soul. The function of the brain according to his views was to condense the hot vapors rising from the heart. Herophilos and Eresistratos had recognized the brain as the center of the nervous system and the nerves as concerned with both sensation and movement. However, preliminary to all disciplines was the development of the scientific method and in this Aristotle was a forerunner.[1] If Aristotle is to be evaluated as a scientist, it must be admitted that he was almost always wrong in every inference he made from his vast collections of natural history and numerous dissections; yet in spite of the stultifying effect of the immoderate worship given to him by generations to follow, he earns a position by his invention of a kind of formal logic. Although his system lacked what the modern scientist uses most, namely, hypotheses and induction, his was a first step toward the introduction of logic as a tool for the scientist. Unfortunately Aristotle did not use his logic for this purpose himself. As Francis Bacon, who was the outstanding opponent of Aristotelianism in the 17th century, wrote, Aristotle "did not consult experience in order to make right propositions and axioms, but when he had settled his system to his will, he twisted experience round, and made her bend to his system."

---

[1]The fragments of Aristotle's writings that exist (probably his lecture notes) were not collected until more than 200 years after his death. His *Opera* were among the early scientific works to be reproduced (in Latin, 1472) by the printing press invented in the West nearly 1800 years after his death. English translations *(The Works of Aristotle)* were published by the Clarendon Press, Oxford, in several volumes between 1909 and 1931, edited by J. A. Smith and W. A. Ross.

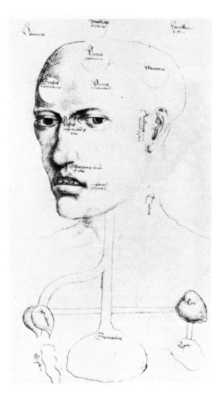 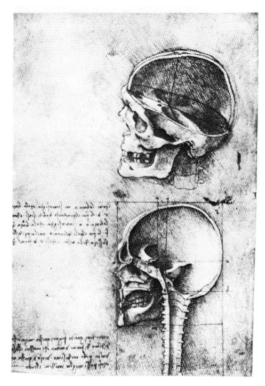

FIG. 1. In the 4th century A.D. and for several hundred years to follow, the faculties of the mind were thought to be housed in the ventricles of the brain.   **Left:** a 15th century illustration designed to illustrate the 1494 edition of Aristotle's *de Anima*. Four regions of the brain are labeled: *sensus communis, virtus cogitativa, virtus imaginativa,* and *memoria.* (Courtesy of the Incunabula Collection at the National Library of Medicine, Bethesda.)   **Right:** Leonardo's localization of the *sensus communis.* In the lower figure his own words state: "Where the line a–m is intersected by the line c–b there the meeting place of all the senses (senso commune) is made." (Courtesy of the Royal Library at Windsor Castle.)

    In terms of anatomy, although for many centuries the heart had reigned over the brain, some site in the brain for mental processes was sought even in the dark ages when, in fact, our various functions were assigned to the ventricles rather than to the solid tissue. Numerous illustrations of this idea came down to us, all devoid of scientific meaning and, all but a few, crude in execution—many being merely copies of earlier ones. What is striking, however, is that all of these depict a *sensus communis* and place it anteriorly. Figure 1 from the 15th century, an exception for its artistic beauty, is an example of this placement of the *sensus communis* and we notice more posterior sites for "virtus cogitativa," "virtus imaginativa," and "memoria."

    One great artist who, unlike the others, was also an experimentalist, gave us his exact stereotaxic coordinates for finding the *sensus communis.* Figure 1 depicts Leonardo's drawing of the skull; in his marginal notes in mirror writing he says (in translation) "Where the line a–m is intersected by the line c–b, there the meeting place of the senses *(senso commune)* is made." Elsewhere in his writings we find that he believed the *sensus communis* to be the site of the soul.

The aim of the following account is to trace the development of ideas as to how the nervous system works and the great progress that was made when dissatisfaction with traditional but unproven theories led to the testing of these concepts by experiment. In the 17th century for the first time the function of the nerves was scientifically explored and some very tentative attempts made to understand the brain. Their structure was better known than their function, for dissection has a much longer history than physiology; anatomy had flowered in the previous century with the great masters, da Vinci, Vesalius, and Estienne.

This study has been written around the major figures who made the first giant steps toward a rational science of what was then called natural philosophy, but, as they did not work in solitude, an effort has been made here to describe them within the historical settings of their times—political, artistic, literary, at peace or at war. These great men of the 17th century were not students only of the nervous system, although it is from this area of their work that material has been extracted here for description. Many actually achieved fame in other fields, but their contributions to neurophysiology are the milestones emphasized in the following chapters. As we read, we find speculation flowed freely, even if it was rarely in the form of a working hypothesis formulated for testing. But experiment won, marking this as a century of revolutionary knowledge about our nervous systems.

SUGGESTED READING

Butterfield, H. *The Origins of Modern Science 1300–1800*. Bell, London, 1949

Daumas, M. *Histoire de la Science. Encyclopédie de la Pléiade*. Presses Universitaires de France, Paris, 1957.

Hall, A. R. *The Scientific Revolution*. Longmans, London, 1954.

Michel, H. *Les Instruments des Sciences*. Société Française du Livre, Paris, 1968

Sarton, G. *Introduction to the History of Science*, 3 vols. Williams & Wilkins, Baltimore, 1927–1948.

Singer, C. *A Short History of Scientific Ideas to 1900*. Dover, New York, 1957.

Wolf, A. *A History of Science, Technology and Philosophy in the 16th and 17th Centuries*, 2 vols. Macmillan, London, 1950.

CHAPTER I

The Forerunners: Experimentation Challenges the Ancients

One critical problem overrides all others in the early history of neurophysiology—the nature of the nerve impulse. Every writer, whether physician, scientist, or philosopher, searched for the solution, and many gave up trying for a material explanation, granting the accolade to the soul. Not until the end of the 18th century was the agent identified as electricity. The very first step toward identifying this intangible force was the necessary differentiation of its powers from those of magnetism. This important discovery was made in 1600.

William Gilbert (1544–1603)

The opening year of the 17th century was marked by a tragic event—the burning of Giordano Bruno for his unorthodox philosophy—but it was also marked by a significant scientific event—the appearance of William Gilbert's classic book *De Magnete*, the culmination of 18 years of experiment. This work was a landmark for the future of the physical sciences and electrophysiology because of its dawning recognition of a difference between static electricity and magnetism (two powers thought at the time to belong to the occult). The first book to advocate empirical methods, it was therefore the first to urge the step from concept to experiment. More than unique, the book was revolutionary in its experimental approach. It appeared in an age when scholasticism was concerned with classification on qualitative lines, without measurement and without validation. Authoritative statements of the ancients were the guides, and induction from experiment was virtually unknown. Gilbert's

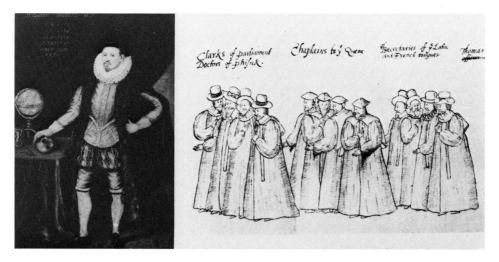

FIG. 2. William Gilbert. A portrait found by Sylvanus Thompson in an antiquary's shop. (Gift of Miss Helen Thompson.) **Right:** The funeral procession of Queen Elizabeth I, from the Camden Manuscript. Gilbert has been identified as the third from the left in the group labelled "Clarks of parliament Doctors of physick." (Courtesy of the British Museum.)

book makes a plea for "trustworthy experiments and demonstrated arguments" to replace "the probable guesses and opinions of the ordinary professor of philosophy."

In 1601 Gilbert was appointed one of the physicians to Queen Elizabeth (whom he survived only briefly), and a sketch identified as his portrait appears in the contemporary drawing (now in the British Museum) made by William Camden, Court Herald, of her funeral procession in 1603. For a man of such firm belief in scientific method as Gilbert, it cannot have been easy to be physician to the Queen, who was greatly under the influence of the famous Dr. John Dee, an alchemist and astrologer, who guided her by spirit messages at seances held in his house. Dee's crystal ball, together with his own record of these seances, his *Spiritual Diaries*, are still preserved in the British Museum. (A portrait of Dee, at the age of 67, painted by an unknown artist, is in the Ashmolean Museum in Oxford.)

The exact date of Gilbert's birth is uncertain, but it is known that he was born in his father's house in Colchester, East Anglia and lived part of his life there; a portion of the house still stands, having been carefully restored. There is a memorial tablet to him in the church at Colchester and a statue in the Chapel of St. John's College, Cambridge, where he studied for eleven years, receiving his degree in 1569. At the end of the 19th century, the English physicist Sylvanus Thompson undertook intensive research on Gilbert and founded the "Gilbert Club" to publish a new translation of *De Magnete*. Thompson's research revealed that a contemporary portrait by Cornelius Kettle, bearing the date 1591, had hung in the School Gallery adjoining the Bodleian Library in Oxford. In 1751 this portrait was declared decayed beyond repair, but not before an engraving had been made of it, which was published in Waldron's *Biographical Mirror* in 1796. By good fortune Thompson found another small portrait, very similar to the engraving but with Gilbert's hand, not on a terrella, but on a skull—the mark of the physician. The artist and date are unknown (Fig. 2, left).

What Gilbert achieved (and used as an example of the reward for the empirical approach) was clarification of the conditions in which iron can be magnetized and its relation to the naturally occurring magnetic iron ore known as the lodestone. This led him to suggest that

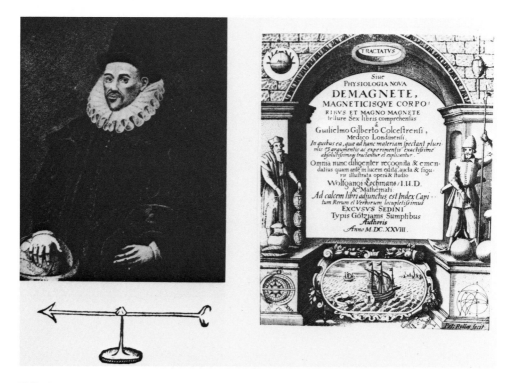

FIG. 3. **Left:** Engraving by Clamp of the portrait made by Cornelius Kettle in 1591 and now lost. Gilbert's hand is on a terrella. Below is Gilbert's drawing of his "versorium," the first electroscope. **Right:** Title page to the second edition (posthumous) of Gilbert's *De Magnete*, printed in Stettin in 1628. Logos at each of the four corners reproduce drawings from the original book. The sketch of the ship with the lodestone floating behind it was an added flight of fancy.

the earth itself is a magnet held together by magnetism, rotating daily on its axis—an explanation supporting the Copernican theory. Gilbert perceived this rotation to be imperative, for should the same half of our earth always face the sun: "in other parts, all things would verily be frightful and stark with extreme cold; whence all high places would be very rough, unfruitful, inaccessible, covered with a pall of perpetual shades and eternal night." And it is the sun, he said, that causes this rotation: "The Sun (the chief agent in nature) as he forwards the courses of the Wanderers, so does he prompt this turning about of the Earth by the diffusion of the virtues of his orbes, and of light."

Gilbert is even explicit about the more controversial feature of the Copernican theory, the heliocentric universe. This is his description of how our globe revolves: "The Earth, then, which by some great necessity, even by a virtue innate, evident, and conspicuous, is turned circularly about the Sun, revolves."[1]

Gilbert's views on gravitation are also expressed in relation to the sun and planets: "[Their] cohesion of parts and aggregation of matter [are due to the] same appetance as terrestrial things, which we call heavy, with the Earth." That the concept of the earth as a magnet would imply an explanation of gravity was apparently not repudiated by Galileo, who made frequent references to Gilbert after reading *De Magnete*.[2] Well into the 19th century, neurologists were searching for an organ in our heads necessary for the perception of gravity.

---

[1]William Gilbert. *De Magnete*, p. 224. Gilbert Club translation.

[2]Galileo. *Dialogues on the Two Chief Systems of the World*, p. 426. Translation by Salusbury, London, 1667. *Systema cosmicum*, p. 393. Strasburg, 1635.

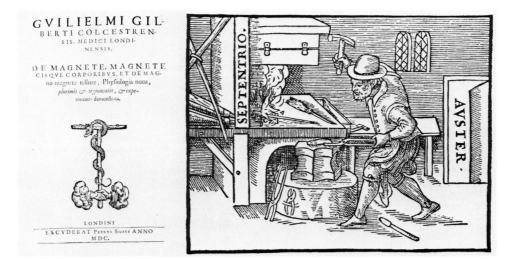

FIG. 4. Left: Title page of the first edition (1600) of *De Magnete*, which lists the great magnet of the earth and a new physiology demonstrated by many arguments and experiments. The colophon of the serpent coiled around a T-shaped support was a woodcut from the 16th century, lost in the Great Fire of London. **Right:** Woodcut from Gilbert's book, similar to a 16th-century design illustrating the making of a magnet by hammering, after lining it up in a north–south position (septentrio–auster). (From *De Magnete*, 1600.)

The different actions of lodestones and rubbed amber had been noted in the previous century but only bizarre explanations had been proposed. In the library of the Institution of Electrical Engineers in London there is a 16th-century treatise, *De Subtilitate*, written by Cardano, a physician and mathematician, describing the properties of lodestones and noting that their subtle attraction differed from that of rubbed amber.[3]

Gilbert, fully conversant with the magnetic needle of the mariners, designed and made a needle that was attracted to static electricity (and not to a magnet). This he named a versorium, since it "turned about" when brought near a piece of rubbed amber; unlike a magnet, it was independent of a north–south orientation. What he had invented was the first detector of electricity, the electroscope; it could not measure, but it could grade degrees of attraction.

Centuries were to pass before the all-important role of electricity in the nervous system was to receive recognition, but it was this 17th-century physician who first clearly differentiated it from magnetism. He devoted an entire chapter to "electrica" (the Latin name he coined from the Greek for amber), defining the attraction to amber and jet and the conditions under which objects are repelled. (Descartes was unwilling to accept such an apparently insubstantial force. Only centuries later were we to learn that, in the electromagnetic field that we inhabit, such a force is far from incorporeal.)

Gilbert proceeded to identify many substances other than amber that attract light objects when rubbed (his definition of an "electrick"), such as sulphur, glass, and wax—all of which would be used in the following years as sources of static electricity. It was the use of frictional electricity that led, nearly 200 years later, to the discovery of intrinsic electricity in our nerves.[4]

Gilbert died in 1603, having launched his appeal for the scientific method during the golden age of Elizabethan England; among his contemporaries were Shakespeare, Walter

[3]Giralamo Cardano (1501–1576). *De Subtilitate*, p. 158. Nuremberg, 1550, Basel, 1554.

[4]L. Galvani. *Commentarius. De Viribus Electricitatis in Motu Musculari*. Bologna, 1791.

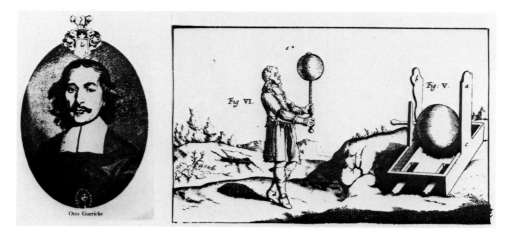

FIG. 5. Otto von Guericke (1602–1686), indefatigable experimenter of friction electricity and designer of a powerful air pump. The woodcut of his frictional machine shows, floating freely above his head, a feather that has been repulsed by the charged globe. (From Book III of *Experimenta nova Magdeburgica de vacuo spatio*. Amsterdam, 1672.)

Raleigh, Philip Sydney, John Donne, and Francis Bacon. After his death, a later poet, John Dryden, was to praise him in a famous couplet: "Gilbert shall live till lodestones cease to draw or British fleets the boundless Ocean awe." In his will, Gilbert wrote "I geve to the Colledge of Phisitons in London all my bookes in my librarye, my Gloves, and Instrumentes, and my Cabenet of myneralles." All were lost in 1666, in the Great Fire of London.

Otto von Guericke (1602–1686)

Gilbert had noted that objects were sometimes repelled by rubbed amber, but he did not offer an explanation; the concept of electric charge evaded him. A long time after his death the phenomenon was observed again by Otto von Guericke, the Burgomaster of Magdeburg, a town then in the Margravate of Brandenburg and not yet engulfed by Prussia. In 1672 he brought out a great book illustrating the frictional machine that he constructed from a sulphur ball. Gilbert had devised the first electroscope, but von Guericke's machine was the ancestor of those used by all future experimenters in the nervous system until it was replaced by the Leyden jar in the second half of the 18th century.

Von Guericke's interest was in the similarity between the attraction of objects to his globe and that of all objects to the earth. More than a century was to pass before Newton clarified the phenomenon of gravitation. Von Guericke's interpretation was that:

> From these experiments it must be seen that there exists in the earth for the preservation of itself a virtue of this sort, which also can be excited in an especially suitable body, namely, this globe, so that it acts more in it than in the earth itself (for whatever this globe attracts, it snatches it, as it were, or draws it away from the earth).

Not until 1831 was the relationship between electricity and magnetism so well understood that Michael Faraday could design an instrument operating by the induction of an electric current by a moving magnet (the basis of many of our electrophysiological instruments). Guericke, a correspondent of Leibniz, was interested in other scientific puzzles, one of which he shared with Pascal and with Descartes: Can a vacuum exist? He made what was effectively an air pump with which he conducted many experiments, the most notorious

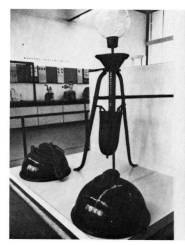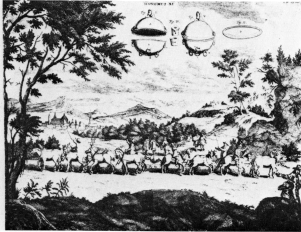

FIG. 6. Left: Von Guericke's air pump, preserved in the Deutsches Museum in Munich, and a contemporary depiction of the famous testing for the power of a vacuum. Eight horses were harnessed to each hemisphere, pulling in opposite directions, but they failed to break the vacuum. (From Book IV of *Experimenta Nova Magdeburgica de vacuo spatio*. Amsterdam, 1672.)

being the one in 1657 in which he evaculated two copper hemispheres and harnessed two teams of horses to try to pull them apart. The original hemispheres and Guericke's air pump (interesting for comparison with Boyle's) can be seen in the Deutsches Museum in Munich (Fig. 6).

Robert Boyle (1627–1691)

The air pumps of von Guericke were soon to be followed by other, modified designs, including the well-known one by Robert Boyle. The scientific world was still fascinated by what became known as the "Torricellian vacuum," the characteristics of which were to absorb Pascal (to whom Boyle refers) and lead eventually to the understanding of atmospheric pressure. Von Guericke had designed several pumps, each an improvement on the previous one. Boyle, too, was to embark on the design of air pumps and with his second we find the famous experiment on asphyxiating an animal by evacuating the air. As with the experimenters at the Accademia del Cimento, this was the closest he came to a biological experiment although all of Boyle's mechanical designs (such as barometers and thermometers) remain some of the basic technology of the life sciences. In many of these he was aided by Robert Hooke, who himself was to promote the technology of microscopy in his famous work, *Micrographia*.[5] As a consequence, Boyle had a great influence on the development of experimental science in the 17th century.

Born in 1627, the son of the Earl of Cork, Robert Boyle, "the father of chemistry," as tradition has it, was from his youth an ardent proponent of the goal to "increase natural knowledge by means of experiment." Schooled at Eton (where the science buildings are now named for him), he never went to college, but at Oxford he was created a "Doctor of Physic" in 1675. In Oxford, his companions and friends were to draw the century out of the dark ages: Christopher Wren, Thomas Willis, and Robert Hooke being those whose interests were to turn to the nervous system. Meeting in his house, and called by Boyle "the

[5]R. Hooke (1635–1703). *Micrographia*. Martyn & Allery, London, 1665.

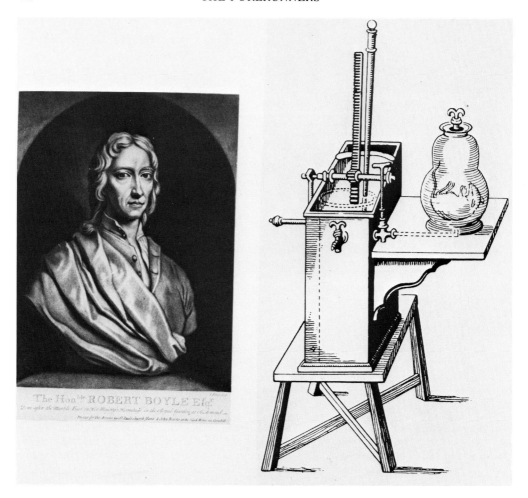

FIG. 7. **Left:** Posthumous bust of Boyle made by Rysbrack in 1734, one of a group, now at Kensington Palace, that includes Locke and Newton. (Courtesy of the Curator, Kensington Palace.) **Right:** Boyle's famous air pump, with his demonstration that "there is in the Air a little vital Quintessence." (From *The Spring and Weight of the Air*, 2nd edn, 1662.)

invisible college,"[6] the group was later to prove instrumental in the planning, after the Restoration of the Monarchy, for a Royal Society.

Boyle's first excursion into writing was *Seraphick Love*, a religious tract, but his first scientific book (1662) became a classic: *The Spring and Weight of the Air*. For physicists, the book is famous for his description (in the second edition in 1662) of Boyle's Law of gases, relating their volume to the reciprocal of the pressure, but for biologists we note that he was concerned with the role air played in life (Fig. 7). "Perhaps," he wrote, "there is some use of Air which we do not understand, that makes it so continually needful to the Life of Animals." He supposes that "there is in the Air a little vital Quintessence." Boyle was sufficiently averse to Aristotelianism to attack the dogma of four elements in the treatise called *The Sceptical Chymist* (written as a Socratic dialogue), and in his insistence on the

[6]Letter to his tutor, Marcombes, October 22, 1646. *The Works of the Honourable Robert Boyle*, edited by T. Birch. 5 vols. Millar, London, 1744.

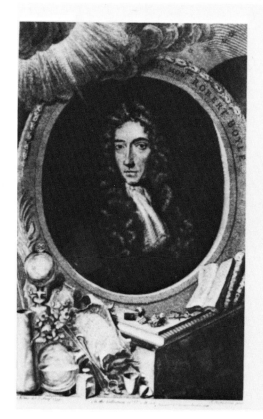

Experiments and Notes

ABOUT THE

MECHANICAL ORIGINE

O R

PRODUCTION

O F

Electricity.

By the Honourable
ROBERT BOYLE Efq;
Fellow of the *R. Society.*

L O N D O N,
Printed by *E. Flefber,* for *R. Davis*
Bookfeller in *Oxford.* 1675.

FIG. 8.   Robert Boyle and the title page of the small tract he wrote on electricity.

presence of some essential quality in the air we breathe, he opened the way for the work of Mayow.

All his life, Boyle was an intensely religious man, studying the Testaments in their original Hebrew and Greek. Following the colonization by the Pilgrims, he was appointed Governor of the Corporation for the Spread of the Gospel in New England from 1661 to 1689.

We find more interest in biology, or at least in medicine, in his two-volume treatise on *The Usefulness of Experimental Philosophy*, published in 1664. In a section in which he named the (then rarely used) word "physiological," he reported experiments on frogs, insects, and birds (although the experimenter was unnamed). There are some rather surprising passages under the heading "therapeutical." There are also notes at the Royal Society reporting Boyle joining in experiments in Oxford in which the effect of cutting the phrenic nerves in a dog was demonstrated. Although effects of such drastic surgery were noted, as was common at the time, no deeper search for the mechanism was made. Writing three-quarters of a century after Gilbert, Boyle published a tract on magnetism and one on electricity[7] but no inspired vision of the future revealed that the latter was the answer to the question this century was asking: How is the nerve impulse carried?

[7]R. Boyle, *Experiments and Notes about the Mechanical Origin of Electricity.* Fuller, London, 1675.

Francis Bacon (1561–1626)

The influence of Francis Bacon on the development of science in Europe in the 17th and 18th centuries cannot be exaggerated. Only secondarily an experimentalist (in the chemistry of minerals), he was nevertheless the most outstanding proponent of replacing speculation with observation.

Born in 1561, in an age of magic, alchemy, and astrology, Bacon's philosophical life was devoted to the infiltration of science into all three. "The aim of magic," he wrote, "is to recall natural philosophy from vanity of speculations to the importance of experiments."[8] The means by which knowledge was to progress was by collaborative effort of scientists working together in groups and societies for the exchange of information. This plea is his famous *New Atlantis*, published posthumously in Latin, but already outlined in an earlier essay *In Praise of Knowledge*,[9] and in his major work, *The Advancement of Learning*. His plan reads like a description of the centers of research we find today in all countries—centers where facilities, instrumentation, and libraries are shared by groups working on common problems.

Bacon developed this idea in the form of a fantasy, in which a group worked together in "Solomon's House" on the imaginary island of Bensalem. All kinds of explorations and experiments were to be made by collaborative research with communal instruments for work. The results were then reported for appraisal by three interpreters with whom lay the decision as to whether or not publication of the results was morally and soundly acceptable. With such a procedure made a reality, Bacon hoped that his achievement of proven axioms would emerge by induction from experiment.

Bacon's enduring influence lay in his opposition to Aristotelianism—still regnant in the universities. In his campaign for societies of scientists, freedom from this traditional restriction was one of his principal goals. His strongly worded views on how science should be freed of tradition were that knowledge should be based on logically designed experiments, not developing from a theoretical evaluation but from the experimental facts themselves. Axioms derived by induction from planned experiment should indicate the next experiment to be done before a generalization could be made. The ultimate goal was scientific certainty.

Born in the reign of Elizabeth, Bacon was trained to be a statesman, educated at Trinity College, Cambridge and, in law, at Gray's Inn. At the age of 23, he was elected to the House of Commons, serving throughout the period of war with Spain (and the Armada) and eventually becoming Lord Chancellor (Fig. 9). On his 60th birthday the king made him Viscount St. Albans.[10] He died in disgrace and poverty but left a magnificant legacy, alive to this day: recognition of the need for the expansion of science and its application for the benefit of mankind.

Bacon's philosophy of science bridges the passing of vitalism into mechanism. He believed in humors working in our bodies, but they were virtues derived from material substances. In his views about body and mind, Bacon was far ahead of his time, having reached the opinion as early as 1605 that, not only does the body affect the working of the mind, but also the mind affects the working of the body. In his words:

---

[8]F. Bacon, De dignitate et augmentis scientarum. In: *The Works of Francis Bacon*, 7 vols. (London, 1887–1892).

[9]Published in 1605, the same year as Cervantes' *Don Quixote*.

[10]John Aubrey tells us "He had a delicate, lively, hazel Eie; Dr. Harvey tolde me it was like the Eie of a viper." (O. L. Dick. *Aubrey's Brief Lives*. Secker & Warburg, London, 1949.)

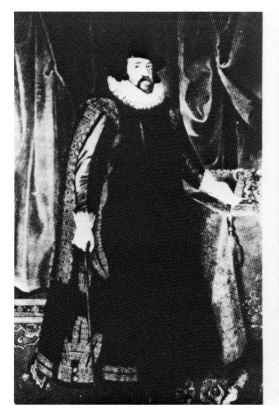 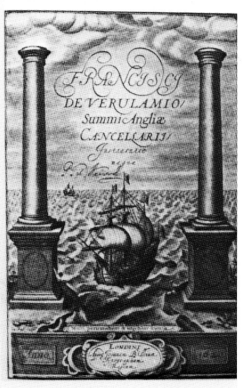

FIG. 9. Left: Francis Bacon in his robes as Lord Chancellor. (From the portrait in the National Portrait Gallery in London.) **Right:** Frontispiece to his *Great Instauration*, the first book of which is *Novum Organum*.

> For the consideration is double; either how, and how far the humours and temperament of the body, do alter or work upon the mind; or again, how and how far, the Passions and Apprehensions of the mind do alter or work upon the Body. The former of these we see sometimes handled in the Art of Physick; but the same hath by strange ways insinuated itself into Religion. For the Physician prescribes Remedies to cure the Maladies of the mind; as in the cures of Frenzies and Melancholy: they do also administer Physick to exhilerate the Mind.[11]

Bacon did not go so far as to identify what part of the body was involved—was it the Aristotelian heart? or the viscera? This issue was faced more openly by his contemporary, Robert Burton, the author of the great 17th century classic of psychiatry, *The Anatomy of Melancholy*.

Burton was a Galenist and believed in humors; he believed in natural spirits, in vital spirits, and in animal spirits: the first "begotten in the liver," the second "in the heart," and the third "in the nerves." And he accepted the vital presence of the soul. But when he came to see "the part affected" by melancholy, he wrote: "Some differences I find among writers, about the principal part affected in this disease, whether it be the brain, or heart, or some other member. Most are of the opinion that it is the brain. . . ."[12]

[11]From Wats' translation in 1674 of F. Bacon. *Of the Advancement and Proficiencie of Learning: of the Partitions of Science* (in Latin), 1605.

[12]Robert Burton (1577–1640). *The Anatomy of Melancholy*. 3 vols. Gripps, Oxford, 1621.

The 17th century can claim the first break from reliance on the occult, and from the acceptance of demons and magic as the cause of behavioral eccentricities and madness, and the dawning of recognition of the role of the brain.

BIBLIOGRAPHY

William Gilbert (1544–1603)

Selected Writings

De Magnete. Magnetisque corporibus; et de magno magnete tellure; Physiologica nova plurimis et argumentis et experimentis demonstrata. Peter Short, London, 1600. (English translation by P. F. Mottelay, with a biographical memoir. London, 1893. Available in paperback edition. Dover Press, New York, 1958. English translation by the Gilbert Club of London. Chiswick Press, London, 1900.)

De Magnete, 2nd and 3rd editions (in Latin) (with different plates), prepared by Wolfgang Lochmann of Pomerania. Published posthumously. Gotzianio, Stettin, 1628 and 1633.

Secondary Sources

Waldron, F. G. *The Biographical Mirror*. 2 vols. Harding, London, 1796.

Thompson, S. P. *Gilbert, Physician*: a note prepared for the three-hundredth anniversary of the death of William Gilbert. Privately printed, limited edition, 1903.

Otto von Guericke (1602–1686)

Experimenta nova Magdeburgica de vacuo spatio. Amsterdam, 1672.

Secondary Sources

Heathcote, N. H. de V. Guericke's sulphur glove. *Annals of Science*, 6:293–305 (1950).

Priestley, J. *The History and Present State of Electricity, with Original Experiments*. London, 1769.

Robert Boyle (1627–1691)

Selected Writings

Seraphick Love (Some Motives and Incentives to the Love of God).Herringman, London, 1659.

New Experiments Physico-mechanicall, Touching the Spring of the Air and its Effects. Hall, Oxford, 1660.

Certain Physiological Essays. Herringman, London, 1661.

The Sceptical Chymist. Henry Hall, London, 1661.

The Usefulness of Experimental Philosophy. 2 vols. Hall, London, 1664.

The Works of the Honourable Robert Boyle. 5 vols. Edited by T. Birch. Millar, London, 1744.

Secondary Sources

Birch, T. *The Life of the Honourable Robert Boyle. Clarendon Press, Oxford, 1744*.

Boas, M. *Robert Boyle and Seventeenth Century Chemistry*. Cambridge University Press, Cambridge, England, 1958.

Fulton, J. F. *A Bibliography of the Honourable Robert Boyle*. Clarendon Press, Oxford, 1961.

Fulton, J. F. Robert Boyle and his influence. *ISIS*, 18:17–102 (1932).

Gunther, R. T. *Early Science in Oxford*. 12 vols. Oxford University Press, Oxford, 1923–1945.

Wood, A. A. *Fasti Oxoniensis, or Annals of the University of Oxford, 1591–1691*. Parker, Oxford, 1820.

Francis Bacon (1561–1626)

Selected Writings

The Two Books of Francis Bacon. Of the Proficience and Advancement of Learning, Divine and Humane. Henrie Tomes, London, 1605.

Novum Organum (the first book of which is called the *Great Instauration*) (in Latin). Billium, London, 1620.

New Atlantis (published posthumously). Newcomb, London, 1627.

Of the Advancement and Proficiencie of Learning: of the Partitions of Sciences (in Latin), 1605. English translation by Gilbert Wats, 9 vols. London, 1674.

Secondary Sources

Anderson, F. H. *Philosophy of Francis Bacon*. University of Chicago Press, Chicago, 1948.

Crowther, J. G. *Francis Bacon. The First Statesman of Science*. Cresset Press, London, 1960.

Farrington, B. *Francis Bacon. Philosopher of Industrial Science*. Schumann, New York, 1949.

Luxembourg, L. K. *Francis Bacon and Denis Diderot. Philosophers of Science*. Humanities Press, New York, 1967.

Rossi, P. *Francesco Bacone: Della magia alla scienza*. Laterza, Bari, 1957. English translation by S. Rabinovitch. *Francis Bacon: From Magic to Science*. University of Chicago Press, Chicago, 1968.

Sortais, G. *La Philosophie Moderne depuis Bacon jusqu'a Leibniz*, 2 vols. Lethielleux, Paris, 1929.

Spedding, J., Ellis, R. L., and Heath, D. D. (eds.). *The Works of Francis Bacon*, 7 vols. London, 1887–1892.

CHAPTER II

The Mechanistic Revolution Opens

René Descartes (1596–1650)

For scholars of the seventeenth century concerned with the workings of the brain, nerves, and muscles, 1664 was an *annus mirabilis*. That year saw Steno's work on muscles and glands, Croone's anonymously written theory of muscle contraction, Willis' *Cerebri Anatome*, and the treatise that was to have the most lasting interest for all physiologists, philosophers, and psychologists: *Traité de l'Homme*, by Descartes. In its field, the most influential book of that century, it only became known to its readers (in a Latin translation) 12 years after the death of the writer, and another two years passed before it could be read in his original French. English readers had to wait much longer for a full translation. Of Descartes' prolific work, this is the one germane to the history of the nervous system.

Descartes' views in other fields—geometry, meteorology, and optics—were well known in his lifetime and had already evoked considerable attention and controversy. His *Discours de la Méthode* and *Les Passions de l'Ame* had stirred wide interest, so that when the *Traité de l'Homme* appeared, readers were prepared for his mechanistic approach.

This great man, bred in the gentle landscape of Touraine, was to devote his life to a search for truth, seeking for himself a quiet environment for free thinking, according to his early biographer, Borel.[1] He wrote a text that was to influence all scientists who worked with experimental methods, his *Discours de la Méthode*. In it, he discusses not experimental method, but his own method of thought and his theory of knowledge. Scientists had just begun to observe nature and turn their backs on statements made by the ancients, as they advanced to meet a new and brilliant challenge; mathematics and mechanics were the tools

---

[1] "...sibique solitarius in villula per 25 annos remansit, admirandaque multa meditatione sua detexit." Pierre Borel (1620–1689). *Renati Cartesii Vita Eodem*. Sigismund, Frankfurt, 1660.

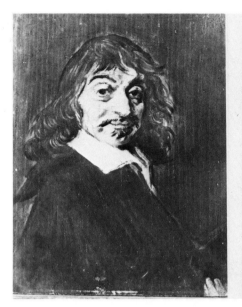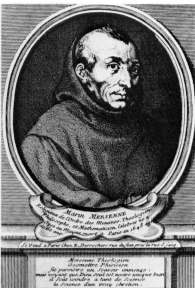

FIG. 10. Left: Portrait of Descartes by Frans Hals, the original of the famous copy in the Louvre. (Statens Museum for Kunst, Copenhagen.) **Right:** Marin Mersenne, priest in the order of Minimes in Paris, who corresponded with the philosophically minded scientists of his day and made his convent their meeting place. Dubbed "l'Académie Mersenne," it stood from 1611 in the street named for it, la Rue des Minimes" (close to what is now the Place des Vosges). The convent was closed by the Revolution.

they were to use. These tools would not only elucidate the scientific experiment but also provide the basis for an all-embracing theory of science, including biology and cosmology.

For psychologists and philosophers the most quoted tenet of Descartes is his conviction of his existence being derived from the fact that he could think. Originally expressed in French ("je pense, donc je suis"), it is usually quoted in Latin: "Cogito ergo sum." For the experimental scientist the more important phrase in *Discours* concerns Descartes' insistence that he must have no doubts before he can believe—he sought "quelquechose en ma créance, qui fust entièrement indubitable."[2]

It is fortunate that Descartes was a frequent letter writer and that he preserved copies of his letters, for in them one can follow the development of his thinking. A great number were written to Father Marin Mersenne in Paris, correspondent of many contemporary scientists (Fig. 10); other papers were found after his death in Stockholm. From these we learn how Descartes intended a theory unifying cosmology and the physiology of man, to be developed in an overall treatise to be called *Le Monde*, and we find that he had begun to write down his thoughts as early as 1629.

Descartes withheld his *Traité de l'Homme* during his lifetime for fear of retribution from the Catholic Church, which he was unwilling to oppose (although his cosmology rested on that of Copernicus). As he wrote in 1633 in a letter to Father Mersenne concerning the movement of the earth, "Je confesse que s'il est faux, tous les fondemens de ma philosophie le sont aussi." At this time, the censure and trial by inquisition of Galileo for his espousal of the Copernican heliocentric world was of fundamental distress to all scientists. Formal

[2]*Discours de la Méthode.*

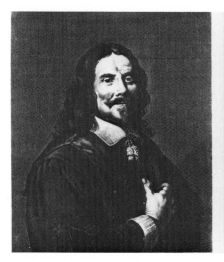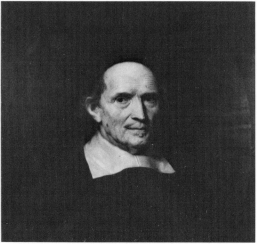

FIG. 11. Two eminent Dutchmen concerned with the teaching of Cartesianism in Utrecht. **Left:** Regius (Henri le Roy), Professor of Medicine at the University of Utrecht, who enthusiastically taught the views of Descartes. **Right:** Paul Voetius, Professor of Metaphysics at the University of Utrecht, who persuaded the magistrates of the city to ban Descartes' writings.

forgiveness has not to this day been granted to Galileo, but a carefully worded partial apology ("Il eut beaucoup à souffrir.") was made by Pope John Paul II[3] in 1979 to a scientific meeting in honor of Einstein at the Pontifical Academy in Rome.

But it was not only the Church that was antagonistic to Descartes' ideas. At a time when he had moved to Holland for quiet and meditation, Descartes' unorthodox ideas about the soul and his concept of automatism were already known through his *Discours de la Méthode*, published in French in 1637. These were very disturbing to the traditionalists in philosophy, one of whom, Paul Voetius, had in 1641 become professor of metaphysics at the University of Utrecht and in 1642 succeeded in persuading the magistrates of the city to ban Descartes' book. This was less punishment than Voetius (an opponent of a heliocentric universe) desired. He had hoped to have Regius (Henri le Roy, professor of medicine at the University of Utrecht, who was teaching Descartes' theories to his students) dismissed from his chair as a heretic. Regius was, however, restricted to lecturing only in physics and medicine, and later he was to lose Descartes' support on grounds of disagreement and plagiarism. Regius, perhaps enthralled by Harvey's work on circulation, had embroidered on Descartes' ideas of animal spirits flowing down the nerves from the brain; he envisaged them mingling with the blood and circulating back through the heart to the brain.[4] The whole affair is described in Descartes' correspondence[5] with the Dutchman Regius, using Latin as their common language, and in his letters to Father Mersenne.

This shameful episode no doubt influenced Descartes' decision not to publish *Traité de l'Homme* in his lifetime, for his letters reveal anxiety to avoid controversy, some of which involved his theories of geometry and dioptrics. When his letters were published posthumously, the volumes were reviewed in England by Oldenburg, who remarked that "Disputes

[3]"Les concordances diverses que j'ai rappelées ne resolvent pas seules tous les problèmes de l'affaire Galilée, mais elles contribuent a créer un point de depart favorable a leur solution honorable. . . ." Pope John Paul II, 1979.

[4]H. Regius. *Fundamenta physices*. Elsevier, Amsterdam, 1646.

[5]C. E. Adam and P. Tannery. *Oeuvres de Descartes*, Vol. 3. pp. 369–375, 454–464, 485–586, 491–494.

[had] no place in Geometry, since all proofs are there, as are many demonstrations; yet M. Des-Cartes hath had several scufles touching that Science.[6]

With the French edition of *Traité de l'Homme* was published his description of the human body, renamed by the editor, Clerselier, *La Formation du Foetus*. Also included was *Le Monde ou Traité de la Lumière*, the latter a portion of Descartes' original plan for the overall treatise: *Le Monde*. His earlier writings had prepared his readers for a mechanistic approach but, nevertheless, any suggestion that the operation of man's body could be likened to an automaton was clearly disturbing. Although Descartes, schooled by the Jesuits, was a confirmed dualist and a believer in a deity, he proclaims this belief in the opening phrase of *Traité de l'Homme*: "Ces hommes seront composez comme nous, d'une Ame et d'un Corps. . . ." He is writing here of "these men," his models, who "like ourselves" have a soul. The model he has conceived of the animal body is comprehensible in terms of automata, but it is, as he insists, made by the hands of God ("être faites des mains de Dieu"). These statements may have been inserted to be protective, but there is no reason to distrust the belief that he had declared very explicitly in Part 4 of his *Discours de la Méthode*.

Extracting from the treatise on the physiology of man, Descartes' model of the nervous system incorporates some traces of the ancients, though these were overshadowed by novel proposals. Discarding Galen's doctrine of humors (but accepting the concept of hollow canal-like nerves), he believed in the ultimate fractionation of body fluids into minute particles ("petites parties") always in motion, a variant of the Epicurean theory of the atomists as embraced by Gassendi and Charleton. He held that some of these particles (the motion of which is "God-given") are filtered out of the blood as it passes through the various organs, only the finest, the most rarified distillate, remaining to reach the pineal. It is these, "les plus vives, les plus fortes, et les plus subtiles parties de ce sang," that bring sensation to the cavities of the brain where they produce "un vent très subtil, ou plutôt une flamme très vive et très pure, qu'on nomme les Esprits Animaux." These subtle spirits, to which he gives only an efferent role, are the masters of the nervous system (their name being derived from the Latin for a current of air, and in no way denoting feral). The spirits gather in the pineal body, the tiny organ that later in the development of Descartes' treatise is found to be (only in man) the seat of the soul. Pictured many times by the illustrators of the various editions of Descartes' treatise, this gland is represented incorrectly as standing on the floor of the ventricle. As almost none of the plentiful illustrations were drawn (or even seen) by Descartes, being pictorial renderings of the illustrators' interpretations, he should not be held responsible for this anatomical error, and, in fact, he himself describes the pineal as suspended between the ventricles that contain the animal spirits.[7] The pineal arises in the midline as a neuroectodermal process from the roof of the diencephalon.

There is direct evidence from his letters that Descartes, when in Amsterdam, visited slaughter houses to examine brains, and his sketches and notes found after his death are now in the Leibniz collection in the Niedersächsische Landesbibliothek in Hannover. They include a rough drawing of the underside of a sheep brain (Fig. 12) which he dissected in great detail.[8] In describing his findings, he noted the structural relationships of the choroid plexus, the ventricles, and the tissues, including those that surround the pineal body. He described how the ascending spirits derived from the blood reach the pineal by the infun-

[6]*Phil. Trans. roy. Soc.*, 2:392–394, 1667.

[7]"Adjoustons icy que la petite glande qui est le principal siège de l'âme est tellement suspendue entre les cavitez qui contienent ces esprits. . . ." Descartes, Article 34 in *Les Passions de l'Ame*. 1649.

[8]C. E. Adam and P. Tannery. Pars. III excerptorum Anatomicorum ex M. Cartesii. In: *Oeuvres de Descartes*. Vol. 11, pp. 579–583. 1909.

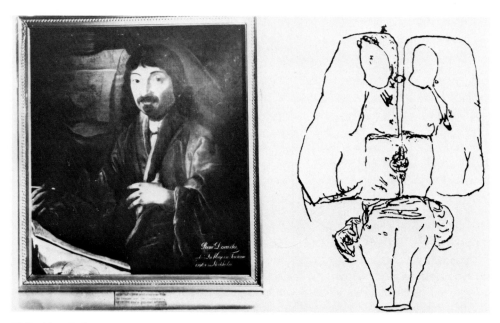

FIG. 12.   Left: Portrait of Descartes from the Museum of Art in Yakutsk, East Siberia. The portrait was painted in Stockholm and shows him at the end of his life. (Gift of V. Merkulov, former Director of the Pavlov Museum in Leningrad.)   **Right:** Sketch of underside of sheep's brain made by Descartes in an Amsterdam slaughterhouse. (Leibniz collection in the Niedersachsiche Landesbibliothek, Hannover.)

dibulum and the gland "they call the pituitary." Only the finest particles can reach the pineal for its blood is supplied by the narrowest arteries. The larger particles move to the cortical surface where they act as a nutrient ("ou elles servent de nourriture à sa substance").

Clerselier, Descartes' friend, literary executor, and editor of the French edition of *Traité de l'Homme*, took, almost unchanged, the illustrations he had contracted to have made by Louis La Forge and the Dutchman, Gerard van Gutschoven. We are told that the initials of these artists, "F" or "G," indicate illustrations where disagreement had occurred, the initial representing the source of the one chosen for publication. By far the greater number of illustrations showing the pineal protruding into the ventricle and ruling the disposition of the animal spirits were based on the interpretations of Clerselier and van Gutschoven. That both these men should repeat so frequently this anatomical error seems strange, for the pineal is clearly pictured in the works of Casserius[9] and Vesalius,[10] the famous Paduans of the previous century. But it was the proposed role, rather than the anatomy of the pineal, that was important to Descartes. It is of some interest that he had looked for the pineal at the autopsy of a woman but had been unable to identify it.[11]

It is perhaps of secondary interest that at the autopsy of a distinguished Oxford physician, the surgeon's report reads that "[the pineal was] harder than ordinary (and talking to a Gentleman then present of Des Cartes [sic] his Opinion, that it was the Seat of the Soul) I prest it ... and kept it as a great Raritie ... ,[12]—a soul for the cabinet of curiosities.

[9]Giulio Casserio (d. 1616). *Tabulae anatomicae.* Deuchinus, Venice, 1627.

[10]A. Vesalius (1514–1564). *De Humani corporis fabrica.* Oporinus, Basel, 1543.

[11]C. E. Adam and P. Tannery. Letter to Mersenne. 1 April, 1640. *Oeuvres de Descartes,* Vol. 3, p. 45.

[12]*Phil. Trans. roy. Soc.,* 16:228–231, 1686.

Only the finest and most rarefied of the spirits enter the pineal body (which Descartes called "une petite glande"), where they map the sensory impressions, for this is the control tower for the complete nervous system. The pineal is pictured as moving on its base, so that it can direct the flow of spirits to appropriate pores in the wall of the ventricle, opening them to let spirits flow out down the nerves, these being envisioned as hollow canals. When the spirits reach the muscles they force a change in their shape and by this means effect muscular movements ("et par ce moyen de faire mouvoir tous les membres").

It is in this description of a physical flow causing a mechanical movement that Descartes speaks of the toys—the automata so popular in his day—and of the automated grottoes and fountains designed by Francini for Henri IV (relics of which can still be found by those willing to explore the wilder regions of St. Germain-en-Laye). And here we learn of the rational soul—"l'âme raisonnable"—which must be situated in the brain, where it can control the flow as the "fontenier" controls the water pressure in the "gardens of our Kings." The rational soul is put in the brain by God ("Dieu unira une Ame Raisonnable à cette machine").

In addition to the age-old concept of hollow nerve canals with spirits flowing through them, Descartes added a "marrow" within the nerve composed of delicate threads reaching up to the ventricles of the brain to act as sensors. They share the same canal with the animal spirits but have no motor function ("Les esprits animaux sont portés par les mêmes tuyaux depuis le cerveau jusques aux muscles"). Nowhere does he propose a dual system differentiating sensory and motor nerves.

It is in *Les Passions de l'Ame* and *Meditationes*, published during his lifetime, that we read about Descartes' choice of the pineal as the seat of the soul. He is insistent that the soul must be part of the body ("Il est certain que l'âme doit être jointe à quelque partie du cors."). He chose the pineal because it is single and midline and, since all other organs as well as the limbs are double, it can be the sole receiver, unifier, and controller of impressions.[13] It seemed to Descartes that the heart could not play this role because it is the source of heat. This heat, held to be due to the rapid interaction of the particles in the blood and so important for life, is a fire without light—"un feu sans lumière."

The identification of the powers of the soul with the pineal drew many criticisms. Some of these came in letters to Father Mersenne who forwarded them to Descartes at his retreat in Holland. The pineal body is similar in shape to a pine cone and is frequently referred to in this correspondence as the "conarium." Descartes, in replies to Mersenne, defended his choice. It must be a single organ, he said: "I cannot find such a part in the whole brain except this gland." The soul must be joined to some part of the body[14] and it must be moveable,[15] so as to receive all impressions and to direct appropriate outflow. The concept of valve-like properties for the pineal was not unique to Descartes, proposals of this kind having come from Fernel, the philosopher–physician of the previous century.[16]

Nor was the assigning of the soul to the pineal an original idea of Descartes'. Some of the Greeks had already chosen it for this role but theologians were never happy with it. Even Bishop Berkeley, when he read Descartes, felt impelled to deride the idea, writing

[13]"La raison que me persuade que l'âme ne peut avoir en tout le corps aucun autre lieu que cette glande, où elle exerce immédiatement ses fonctions, est que je considère que les autres parties de notre cerveau sont doubles." *Les Passions de l'Ame.* Article XXXII.

[14]C. E. Adam and P. Tannery. *Oeuvres de Descartes*, Vol. 3, pp. 119–123.

[15]Ibid. "Letter to Mersenne, 21 April, 1641."

[16]C. Sherrington, *The Endeavour of Jean Fernel.* Cambridge University Press, Cambridge, England 1946.

two essays to refute it.[17] Three centuries passed before this little organ was to enter the world of hormones, led by the discovery of melatonin and its role in circadian rhythms.

In the same book, *Les Passions de l'Ame*, Descartes writes of involuntary movements—passages interpreted by some to suggest reflexes—but is concerned with his philosophy rather than his physiology, the text being about love, hate, joy, and fear—what are read today as psychological qualities. We learn little from it about the mechanisms of neuro-muscular action. These we find in the posthumous *Traité de l'Homme* and in *La Description du Corps Humain* bound with it in the same volume.

In describing the pineal as the seat of the rational soul, Descartes makes it clear that it acts as a controller and not as the pump that forces the animal spirits down the nerves. It plays this same role in the lower animals who have no rational soul. In this he differed from Borelli for whom (although he made no attempt to locate it) the soul was nevertheless a motivating force.

In the text of 1648, *La Description du Corps Humain*, Descartes makes this distinction even clearer:

> C'est pourquoi je tacherai ici de prover, et d'expliquer tellement toute la Machine de notre Corps, que nous n'aurons pas plus le sujet de penser que c'est notre Ame qui excite en lui les movements que nous n'expérimentons point être conduits par notre volonté que nous avons de juger qu'il y a une Ame dans une horloge, que fait qu'elle montre les heures. (p.101)

It is largely this exposition of his insistence that some of the body's organs can work without the action of the soul that led some readers to equate such movements with reflex action, although they are more accurately involuntary movements, such as respiration.

In *Traité de l'Homme*, Descartes makes a clear distinction between the particles carried to the pineal by the blood and sensory messages reaching it from the periphery. The latter are operated by little strings ("petit filets") pictured explicitly in Clerselier's illustrations and described by Descartes: "as by pulling at one end of the rope one rings a bell at the other." Often presented in secondary sources as the original design of a reflex (a noun he did not use),[18] this arrangement of strings, coming from the receptors including those for smell, taste, and hearing, to a control center housing the soul, which then directs the release of spirits brought by the blood, is far from the physiological concept of a nervous reflex. More than a century passed before interaction between sensory and motor systems was demonstrated at the spinal level.

In terms of the strongly contrasting Pavlovian concept of a conditioned response, Descartes voiced a preliminary understanding when he was engrossed in his studies of memory. In a letter to Father Mersenne in 1630, Descartes said: "If you whipped a dog five or six times to the sound of a violin, he would begin to howl and run away as soon as he heard that music again."[19] He refers again to this type of behavior in *Les Passions de l'Ame*. The mechanism he proposed for memory was an increase in size of the pores in the wall of the ventricle through repeated use.

The Russian Sechenov, working two centuries later and anticipating Pavlov by several years, was to develop his concept of mental activity as being carried out by reflexes in the brain.[20] All higher brain function was held by Sechenov to be a material reflex, and he

---

[17]A. C. Fraser. *The Works of George Berkeley*. Clarendon Press, Oxford, 1871.

[18]In a much quoted passage from *Les Passions de l'Ame* there appears on one occasion only the word "reflechis," to describe the *process* of bending within the gland of spirits toward appropriate openings in the ventricular wall.

[19]Adam and Tannery, Vol. 1, p. 128.

[20]Ivan Michailovich Sechenov (1829–1905). *Reflexes of the Brain* (in Russian). Medizinsky Vestnik, 1863. English translation in *Sechenov's Selected Works*. State Publishing House, Moscow, 1935.

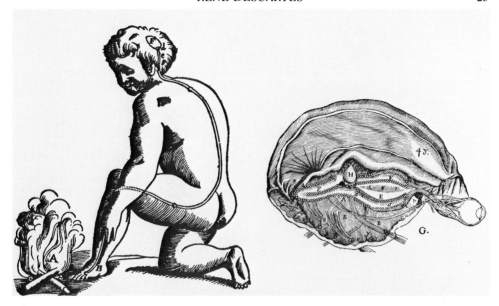

FIG. 13. Left: Illustration in *Traité de l'Homme* of Descartes' concept, by which the movement of particles caused by the flame irritates the foot at *B*, pulling on the threads *c-c* to the brain, to open pores and discharge animal spirits down to many muscles that turn the body and withdraw the foot. **Right:** Van Gutschoven's drawing in *Traité de l'Homme* depicting the pores in the fibrous walls of the ventricle and the conelike pineal, placed centrally, where it can direct outflow of animal spirits to muscles to affect movement.

postulated that the memory trace of a past sensory experience could be evoked by the recurrence of any fraction of it, even if this fraction were quite insignificant and unrelated in its apparent meaning.

In his theory of muscle contraction being dependent on the inflow of animal spirits, Descartes recognized the need to explain how, in a muscle group, the contraction of one muscle must necessarily be accompanied by the relaxation of its opponent. The antagonist muscles that he chose as his example of reciprocal action were those that turn the eyeball; in this case, we have one of the rare sketches drawn by Descartes, the origin of the more stylized illustration of his publishers.[21] The opposing muscles were envisioned as each with its own inflow of spirits and each with a shunt, operated by a valve, through which the spirits from the contracting muscle could oppose the flow down to the antagonist.

We are fortunate that Descartes was such a prolific letter writer for many of his ideas were described in more detail to his correspondents than in his published works. The recipients of these letters included men of the Church and members of the aristocracy, the two privileged groups of the 17th century who were educated. Among them was the poet Constantijn Huygens, father of a famous scientific son, who was attracted by Descartes' methods and wrote from the Hague to support him in his arguments with the Jesuits.[22] From the letters of this period, with the exception of those to Father Mersenne, we learn little more about Descartes' concepts of nervous activity; most were in response to correspondents interested in his philosophical ideas—one of them was Princess Elizabeth of Bohemia.

[21]*De Homine Figuris, et Latinitate Donatus Forentio Schuyl*, p. 25. (This illustration is not included in the French *Traité de l'Homme*.)

[22]Constantijn Huygens (1596–1687). Letter to Descartes, 25.5.1642. *The Correspondence of Descartes and Constantyn Huygens, 1635–1647*. Clarendon Press, Oxford, 1926.

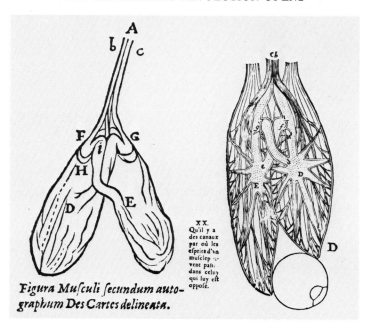

FIG. 14. Left: Original sketch by Descartes illustrating "the canals by which the spirits of one muscle can pass into that which opposes it." Valves in the canals, "*i*," can open or shut as required for reciprocal innervation. (From *De Homine*.)   **Right:** Illustration from the French edition of Descartes' *Traité de l'Homme, Treatise*, interpreting his text and showing more clearly the valves (*f* and *g*) acting to shunt the spirits into the appropriate muscle.

Elizabeth's mother, the daughter of James I of England, had married Frederick, Elector Palatine and "Winter King" of Bohemia (Shakespeare's *Tempest* was performed at their wedding). But disaster was to follow in a crushing defeat in 1620 by the Hapsburg armies determined to uproot the hold of the Reformation on Bohemia. The royal house fled from Prague, and Bohemia disappeared as an autonomous kingdom from the map of Europe. It was therefore from exile that Elizabeth pursued her correspondence with Descartes.

His other royal correspondent was the reigning Queen Christina of Sweden. Christina's call to him to come as her tutor and principal consultant in her plan to establish an Academy in Stockholm uprooted him from his Dutch retreat in a move to the Swedish winter to which his health succumbed.

Christina was at this time only 24, having succeeded, at the age of 6, her famous father Gustavus Adolphus, who was killed during the Thirty Years' War at the Battle of Lützen. Ardent in her pursuit of knowledge, not only for herself but also for her country, she gave outstanding support to its major university at Uppsala. She was indeed a patron of learning and a great entrepreneur. During his brief four months in Stockholm fulfilling her scholastic demands, Descartes also found time to indulge his lifelong interest in music by writing the libretto for a ballet: "La Naissance de la Paix,"[23] performed two months before he died. He took this opportunity to express his deep loathing of war.

Christina outlived him by 39 years. She left Sweden after renouncing the throne and the Lutheran religion of her native country and converting to the Catholic faith in 1655, a move that was to win her a tomb in St. Peters. She continued her interest in scholarly works and,

---

[23]Descartes' verses and their Swedish translation by Georg Stiernhielm are preserved in the Universitetsbiblioteket in Uppsala.

at her own expense, had Borelli's now famous *De motu animalium* published after his death. Her great library of manuscripts,[24] which she took with her on leaving Sweden, found a home in the Vatican Library, but disappointingly contains no writing by Descartes. When, in 1981, the Vatican's Secret Archives were opened to scholars, the proclamation of Christina's abdication was one of the documents shown. Another, more disquieting, was Galileo's retraction of his belief in the Copernican theory.

Descartes died early in 1650, and his body was sent to France after initial interment in Stockholm.[25] Controversy surrounds the story of this circuitous shipment, and the eventual destination of his remains is uncertain. For some years a skull, labeled as that of Descartes, was exhibited at the Musée de l'Homme in Paris. So tiny as to be even smaller than any yet measured, and covered by graffiti, this unconvincing object was eventually removed from display. A memorial tablet was erected in the church of Saint Germain des Près in Paris but it is uncertain that any such distinguished bones lie buried there. (The inscription proclaims Descartes to be the first "a renovatis in Europa Bonarum literarum studiis rationis humanae.")

His manuscripts in Stockholm suffered similar vicissitudes before reaching France, including the sinking in the Seine of the boat that carried them. His contemporary biographer, Pierre Borel,[26] listed those original works that were found, including Descartes' essay on music written in 1618 and printed posthumously in Holland.[27]

For future generations the influence of Descartes was to persist among the philosophers and those students of man who were to concern themselves with the struggle between vitalism and materialism. For the neurophysiologist, he left anatomical observations but no experimentally established findings. His strength was in identifying what must be sought: how the brain can sense the outside world, how the nerve can cause the muscle to contract, and how the contraction of one muscle group must necessarily be accompanied by the relaxation of its opponent. This was the first time scholars were alerted to this physiological necessity, and it heralded the concept of reciprocal innervation, a mechanism that had to wait more than two hundred years for its experimental resolution. His legacy in every case was a mechanically operating model.

Descartes' ideas about the nervous system failed the crucial test of experimental proof. But what survived with immense power was his conviction that the animal body was governed by the same physical laws as the rest of the phenomena of the universe. Two more centuries passed before this view received general acceptance. In the second half of the 20th century, familiar with a particulate view of the universe and all that it contains, one remembers with awe this 17th-century genius who proposed it as the model for our nervous systems.

Any account of Descartes in the context of the sciences of the nervous system, as presented here, must of necessity skim over his intense interest in mathematics. This led him to a wide interchange of correspondence including a letter published in Hooke's *Philosophical Collections*[28] in which he writes of the need for a compendium of mathematics, including its theory. Descartes was the inventor of coordinate geometry, and vitally concerned with the laws of motion, including the motion of the planets. He defined linear inertia-less motion

[24]A copy of the catalogue is in the Bodleian Library, Oxford.

[25]A. Baillet. *La Vie de Monsieur Des-Cartes*, 2 vols. Horthhemels, Paris, 1691. Abridged translation by "S. R." Simpson, London, 1693.

[26]Pierre Borel. *Vita Renati Cartesii. Summi Philosophi.* Sigismund, Frankfurt, 1670.

[27]Descartes, *Musicum Compendium*, 1618, published 1650. Translation by W. Robert, American Institute of Musicology. Vol. 8, 1921.

[28]Robert Hooke. *Philosophical Collections*, Vol. 5, pp. 144–145. London, 1680.

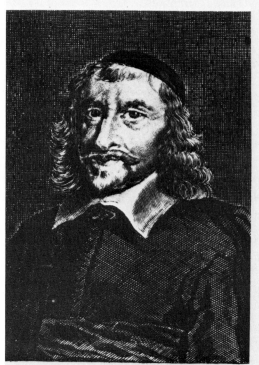

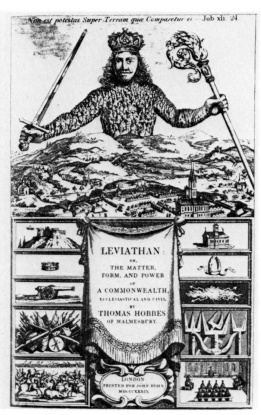

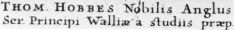

FIG. 15.   **Left:** Portrait of Thomas Hobbes made while he was in exile in Paris. Publication was forbidden by him because the inscription described him as tutor to the Prince of Wales. (From the Cabinet des Estampes in the Bibliothèque Nationale, Paris.)   **Right:** Title page of Hobbes' most famous work, published in 1651.

and postulated a centrifugal force for revolving bodies. In 1644, Descartes produced a detailed theory of the formation of the earth developing from its central heat "as if it were only a machine in which there is nothing whatever to be considered but the shape and movement of its parts."[29] Opposition from the Church was to be expected, but opposition to his mathematics was also developing.

CONTEMPORARY CRITICS OF DESCARTES' MATHEMATICS

Thomas Hobbes (1588–1679)

Descartes' propositions and his mathematics were disturbing to philosophers. In England, one of the early entrants into the discussions was Thomas Hobbes, according to whom matter and motion explained not only the body but also the workings of the mind. An empiricist, he was entranced by mathematics and was thus drawn to the writings of his contemporary. He was extremely critical of Descartes' *Dioptrique* and conveyed his comments to Father Mersenne who, as middleman, forwarded them to Descartes in Holland. This was the start

[29]*Principia Philosophiae*. Part 4, 1644.

of a correspondence, always through Mersenne, that was essentially mathematical in detail even though later Hobbes was also to criticize Descartes' philosophical *Meditations*. This correspondence began while Hobbes was still in England and continued after his exile to Paris. There he lived for eleven years, becoming personally acquainted with Mersenne and Gassendi. He refused to meet Descartes when he came to Paris in 1645,[30] although they met several years later and were apparently partially reconciled.[31]

Hobbes was profoundly influenced by the challenge of Galileo, whom he visited in 1636. Hobbes' writings touch on the nervous system in his best known work *Leviathan* (1651), essentially a political text arguing for controlled government. His interaction with Cartesians and those studying the human brain led him to open his tract with a materialistic commentary on how we receive sensations, and whether or not our thinking and our imagination are under our control. Hobbes proposed an entirely materialistic view of nature—all behavior being subject to physical laws (a theory that, needless to say, caused a great outcry from the Church). An intimate glimpse of Hobbes is to be found in John Aubrey's *Brief Lives*, which tells us that Hobbes lived to a great age even though he was greatly impaired by the syndrome now known as Parkinson's disease.

During Descartes' lifetime not all of his critics were as ungracious as Hobbes. One who met with him was Pascal although the reports of their discussions are not of the nervous system but of atmospheric pressure, a subject in which Pascal was then engrossed.

Blaise Pascal (1623–1662)

Even after his death, Descartes was derided for likening man's body to a machine. One of his younger contemporaries faced the same accusation—specifically about the brain. At the age of 19, Blaise Pascal, born in France of scientific parents, had designed the first automatic adding machine, the forerunner of today's computers. After developing many improvements, he was able to obtain a legal patent for its manufacture. (Seven of the original machines are still in existence.[32]) In the next three years he was to design 50 different models, one of which he presented to Queen Christina of Sweden in 1652 with a long and eloquent letter that gives no hint of the change to come in his life.[33] The first adding machine was not designed for science but to help his father, a tax collector at the Cours des Aides, which is why a few of his instruments calculate sols and deniers, complicating the usual decimal addition since there were twelve deniers to a sol. (It was Napoleon who later established a decimal currency in France.)

Pascal was proud and assertive about his invention, replying to the critics' claim that his design needed to be less complex that had they given as much thought as he had, and had tried as many lines of development to reach his end, they would realize that a less complex machine could not accomplish the same results.[34] He also wrote angrily about potential copyists.

Pascal's designs caught on immediately, for automatic adding and subtracting were attractive accomplishments. Two hundred years passed before anyone achieved automatic multiplication and division, and three hundred before the adoption of the binary system,

[30]Letter from Hobbes' patron, Charles Cavendish, to John Pell, May 11, 1645. In: *Correspondence du P. Marin Marsenne*, Vol. 13. Editions du CNRS, Paris, 1979.

[31]Letter from Cavendish to John Pell, August 2, 1648. Birch Manuscript, British Museum.

[32]Three models can be seen in the Conservatoire des Arts et Métiers in Paris.

[33]This letter has been reproduced in: M. Arland. *Pascal. Éditions à l'enfant poète*. Paris, 1946.

[34]"Avis necessaire a ceux qui auront curiosité de voir la machine arithmétique et de s'en servir." 1645.

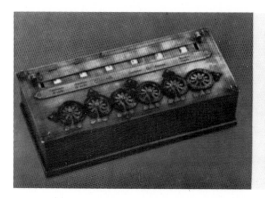 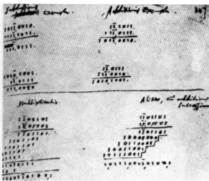

FIG. 16.   Left: One of the surviving mechanical calculators designed by Blaise Pascal. (Courtesy of the Conservatoire des Arts et Métiers.)   **Right:** The binary system of numbering, now used in all computers, first designed by Thomas Heriot (1560–1621). Above, two examples are labeled as "subductions" and two are additions. Below the line are two examples of multiplication. (Manuscript by courtesy of the British Museum.)

although, in fact, a binary system for adding, subtracting, and multiplying had been designed by Thomas Heriot before Pascal was born.[35] Heriot was the brilliant young mathematician from Oxford who navigated for Sir Walter Raleigh on his voyage to the new world in 1585 to establish a colony on Roanoke Island, Virginia. Heriot later wrote an account of their explorations, *A briefe and true report of the New Found Land of Virginia* (published in London in 1588).

Pascal was unhappy that his machine was frequently called a mechanical brain (just as today the same comment is made about the modern computer).[36] He made it clear that his machine merely did what it was told and did not initiate a mental process. He pointed out that it surpassed the lower animals in being able to effect calculations but fell short of them by its lack of operations of the will: "La machine arithmétique fait des effets qui approches plus de la pensée que toute ce que font les animaux; mais elle ne fait rien qui puisse faire dire qu'elle a de la volonté, comme les animaux." Cartesians would question that even the animals had "will."

Pascal and his father Étienne, were friends of Father Mersenne, Descartes' correspondent. Mersenne shared the young man's interest in geometry, and several of his own writings on this subject have been preserved.[37] Before he was 20, Pascal, too, was writing about analytic geometry,[38] and continued to do so for the rest of his brief life. His *Essai pour les coniques* was widely read, and was later to draw criticism from Leibniz.

This was a time when savants were especially drawn to Torricelli's work on atmospheric pressure and the properties of the vacuum. An experiment was needed to test whether or not a vacuum existed in nature. In 1648, encouraged by his science-oriented father, Pascal initiated an expedition to Puy-de-Dôme, a high hill in his native province of Auvergne, to test Torricelli's work on atmospheric pressure, experiments he himself had previously attempted on the high tower of Saint-Jacques in Paris (a tower restored and still standing with

[35]Thomas Heriot.MSS 6786, Folio 347, British Museum.

[36]*Pensées*, No. 340 in the Brunschweig edition. Garnier Fréres, Paris, 1961.

[37]For example, *L'Universe géometrie Synopsis* (1644) at the Bibliothèque Nationale in Paris, where a fine collection of Mersenne's manuscripts is preserved.

[38]*Essai pour les coniques*. Paris, 1640.

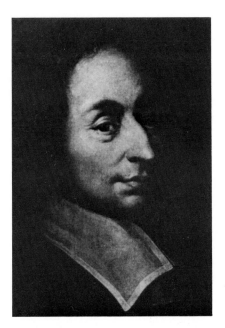 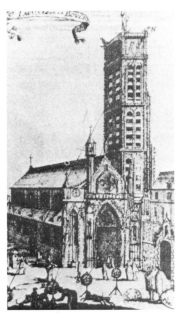

FIG. 17. Left: Blaise Pascal, from the portrait by Quesnel made after his death. **Right:** The Church of Saint-Jacques-de-la-Boucherie in Paris, from the tower of which he made his experiments on atmospheric pressure. Today the tower stands alone, with a statue of Pascal at its base.

a statue of Pascal at its feet). The tests on the mountain consisted of observing the drop in height of a mercury column as it was carried up the hill, a second column having been left at ground level to act as a "control" for diurnal changes in air pressure. From this truly well-designed experiment, several publications on the vacuum resulted and caused Pascal to deny the much quoted phrase that nature abhors a vacuum.[39] These efforts to explain atmospheric pressure antedated Boyle's work on "the Spring of the Air"[40] but no one foresaw that the findings could provide barometric prediction of the weather.

The previous year, Pascal had met twice with Descartes (with whom he was in marked disagreement), and one wishes that some record of their conversations had survived. They had much in common beyond their interest in these physical phenomena. Pascal emphasized that man, although "a weak reed," was, as Descartes had declared, a thinking animal ("L'homme n'est qu'un roseau le plus faible de la nature; mais c'est un roseau pensant").

Primarily a scientist, Pascal continued to work to perfect his calculating machine and to solve geometric problems. His health was failing and a change was imminent. He had converted to Janssenism and, after a short retreat to the Abbey of Port Royal, he wrote a defense of the Janssenists in their altercations with the Jesuits, essays entitled *Lettres provinciales*, published anonymously and quickly put on the Papal Index. Although drawn more and more to the contemplation of religious contentions, Pascal resisted entering Port Royal permanently and continued to work on arithmetic theorems, including how to win at the gaming tables. His health finally failed, and he died in Paris in 1662 at the age of 39.

---

[39]La Nature n'a aucune repugnance pour la vide. *Traité du Vide*. Paris, 1663.

[40]R. Boyle (1627–1691). *New Experiments Physico-Mechanicall, Touching the Spring of the Air and its Effects.* W. Hall, Oxford, 1660.

After his death many notes handwritten by Pascal (now in the Bibliothèque Nationale) were found and published by the Janssenists of Port Royal as the *Pensées de M. Pascal, sur la religion et sur quelques autres sujets*. The majority of these "thoughts" are indeed about theological quarrels, but among them we find his opposition to Descartes' view of the nervous system as a machine,[41] an attack on Oliver Cromwell for his Protestantism, and his own protest against his calculating machines being considered to have thoughts.

Pascal's *Pensées* have become part of classic literature, and since their posthumous publication have evoked criticism from theologians and free thinkers alike. Some of the most pungent comments come, as one would expect, from Voltaire who analyzed them "thought by thought."[42] He had an admiration for Pascal and felt that wrong was done him by the publication of everysmall note found after his death. Surely, he argued, Pascal intended to edit them. ("J'ai toujours cru, que Pascal n'avait jetté des idées sur le papier que pour les revoir et en rejetter une partie."[43])

Voltaire attributes the melancholy of Pascal's thoughts to the ill health that plagued him in the last year of his life, calling it not astonishing that, in a man of so delicate a temperament, the organs of his brain became deranged by his illness ("... soit parvenus à déranger les organes de son cerveau"). He lived, Voltaire says, seeing an abyss beside his chair. Leibniz also attributed *Pensées* to a melancholia suffered by Pascal.

To philosophers and theologians, Pascal was immediately recognizable as one of their own, but although a deep thinker—carrying the logic of his mathematics into his theological concepts—he was also a truly practical man. For example, Pascal held the patent for the first public transportation system in Paris, inaugurated in 1662. These horse-drawn omnibuses ran for six years and were known as "carrosses-à-cinq-sous" (the cost of a ride). The first route was Porte–St. Antoine–Luxembourg, starting at the Bastille, and it opened before he died in 1662. Two years after his death, a mechanical arithmetic machine was designed by Samuel Morland in London, apparently without knowledge of the several designs of Pascal. An original is in the Museum of the History of Science in Florence.

BIBLIOGRAPHY

René Descartes (1596–1650)

Selected Writings

Discours de la Méthode pour bien Conduire la Raison, et Chercher la Verité dans les Sciences. (Published together with *La Dioptrique, les Météores et la Géometrie.*) Maire, Leyden, 1637. Translated by Thomas Newcombe. John Holden, London, 1649.

Meditationes de Prima Philosophia. Soly, Paris 1642.

Principia Philosophiae. Elzevir, Amsterdam, 1644.

Les Passions de l'Ame. Le Gras, Paris, 1649.

De Homine Figuris, et Latinitate Donatus Forentio Schuyl. Moyardum and Leffen, Leyden, 1662.

Traité de l'Homme. (Including *La Formation du Foetus.*) Edited by Clerselier, Le Gras, Paris, 1664. Translated by T. S. Hall. Harvard University Press, Cambridge, Mass., 1972.

[41]"Je ne puis pardonner Descartes; il aurait bien voulu, dans sa philosophie, pourvoir se passer de Dieu."

[42]F. M. A. Voltaire, *Remarques sur les pensées de M. Pascal.* Garnier, Paris, 1743.

[43]Voltaire, Letter to Gravesande, Professor of Mathematics in Leyden, 1 June, 1741. *Mélange de philosophie avec des figures.* 1757.

Primary Sources

Adam, C. E., and Tannery, P. *Oeuvres de Descartes*. 12 vols. Cerf, Paris, 1896–1910.

Adam, C. E., and Tannery, P. (eds.). *Oeuvres Inédites de Descartes*, 2 vols. Foucher de Carile. Durand, Paris, 1859 and 1860.

Secondary Sources

Baillet, A. *La Vie de Monsieur des-Cartes*. 2 vols. Horthhemels, Paris, 1691.

Borel, P. *Renati Cartesii Vita Eodem*. In: *Historiarum et Observationum Medicophysicarium Centuriae IV*. Sigismund, Frankfurt, 1660.

Haldane, E. S. *Descartes, His Life and Times*. Murray, London, 1905.

Hall, T. S. *Treatise of Man, René Descartes. A Translation*. Harvard University Press, Cambridge, Mass., 1972.

Hall, T. S., Descartes' physiological method; position, principles, examples. *J. Hist. Biol.*, 3:53–79, 1970.

Kemp Smith, N. *Descartes' Philosophical Writings* (with translations.) Macmillan, London, 1952

Kenny, A. *Descartes. Philosophical Letters*. Clarendon Press, Oxford, 1970.

Lenoble, R. *Mersenne ou la naissance du mechanisme*. Vrin, Paris, 1943.

Blaise Pascal (1623–1662)

Selected Writings

Traité de l'équilibre des Liquides et de la Pesanteur de la Masse de l'Air   (Published posthumously). Gauthier-Villars, Paris, 1663.

Avis Necessaire à Ceux qui Auront Curiosité de Voir la Machine Arithmétique et de s'en Servir. Paris, 1645.

Expériences Nouvelles Touchant la Vide. Paris, 1647.

Récit de la Grande Expérience de l'Équilibre des Liqueurs. Paris, 1648.

Traité du Vide (1651). Paris, 1663.

Géometrie du Hasard. (Address to the Academie Parisienne de Mathematiques.) Paris, 1654.

Traité de Triangle Arithmétique (1654). Paris, 1665

Éléments de Géometrie (1657).

Lettres Provinciales (Anonymous) (1656–1657).

Pensées de M. Pascal. Desprée, Paris, 1669.

Oeuvres de Blaise Pascal, 5 vols, edited by C. Bossut. The Hague, 1779.

L'Oeuvre Scientifique de Pascal. Presses Universitaires de France, Paris, 1964.

Secondary Sources

Arland, M. *Pascal. Éditions à l'Enfant Poete*. Paris, 1946.

Beguin, A. *Pascal par Lui-mème*. Écrivains de toujours, Paris, 1967.

Humbert, P. *L'oeuvre Scientifique de Pascal*. 1947.

Humbert, P. *Cet Éffrayant Génie*. Paris, 1957.

Taton, R. Sur l'invention de la machine arithmétique. *Rev. Hist. Sci.* 16:139–160 (1963).

CHAPTER III

A New Technique Comes to Neural Science

Antoni van Leeuwenhoek (1632–1723)

In the mid-17th century a new opportunity developed for sceptics of Galen's concept of pipe-like channels within the nerves bearing animal spirits to the muscles. This was the technical step from the single magnifying glass to the primitive microscope. During the first half of the century, several scientists had been experimenting with biconvex lenses, but the outstanding contribution was that of Leeuwenhoek who proceeded to apply the technique to multiple explorations of nature.

Antoni van Leeuwenhoek was born in 1632 in Delft, the city of Vermeer, in the same decade that saw the births of Swammerdam and Steno (with both of whom he corresponded). Unlike them, he had no university education but worked in various trades, gaining success and eventually entering into town affairs; on Vermeer's early death at the age of 43, he was appointed guardian of the insolvent estate.

Leeuwenhoek had been experimenting with lenses, but had he not attracted the attention of his fellow townsman, the physician Regnier de Graaf, a corresponding member of the Royal Society, history might never have known of his achievements. Two professional sources for scientific publication had been established in 1665: the *Philosophical Transactions of the Royal Society* and the *Journal des Sçavans* of the Académie des Sciences, but they were closed to nonmembers. An amateur could submit a paper only after introduction by a member. At that time a foreigner could be elected a member, but not a Fellow, of the Royal Society. De Graaf offered to introduce Leeuwenhoek, urging him to write of his findings to Oldenburg, then Secretary of the Royal Society. This introduction resulted in a long series of letters beginning in August 1673 and continuing for many years, mostly describing the microscopic structure of insects, seeds, and "animalculi" that he could see in ditchwater, sweat, and spittle. His descriptions of "animalculi" were not received without skepticism—the Society requested Robert Hooke "to make a microscope" able to check Leeuwenhoek's claims. This accomplished, Hooke reported full confirmation of "seeing great numbers of exceedingly small animals swimming to and fro."[1] Leeuwenhoek also described the corpuscles in blood and identified spermatozoa in man, discoveries about which he wrote many letters, some unpublished, but all preserved by the Royal Society.

For the history of neural anatomy, the letters of interest are those that describe the optic nerves, the structure of muscles, the spinal marrow, and the pia mater of the brain. Most of these observations were from the anatomy of cows, which he obtained from the local slaughter house.

In a letter to Oldenburg, written on 7 September 1674,[2] Leeuwenhoek declared that he "could find no hollowness" in the optic nerves of cows in which he was searching for anatomical evidence for or against the Galenist theory; nor was he more successful with the vagus nerve. This was to become the first of a long series of letters on this subject, but only three months later in a second letter a less definitive statement was forwarded to Oldenburg.[3] He explained that, "Having acquainted Dr. Schravesande, that I could perceive no cavity in the Optic Nerve, he told me that Galen had on a clear Sun-shiny day seen a hollowness therein, encouraging me to view that Nerve again with more attention." He wrote:

> I took therefore, afresh, eight distinct Optic Nerves, and observed that after those nerves had been but a little while cut off from the Eye, the filaments, of which they are made up did shrink up, which shrinking cannot be so much on the external surface or coat of the Nerve, as t'is of the filaments that lie within the same: And upon this shrinking up, a little pit comes to appear about the middle of the Nerve; and t'is this pit in all probability, that Galen took for a cavity.

Was this "pit" indeed evidence for a canal within the nerve? Leeuwenhoek goes on, in the same letter, to describe a transverse section in more detail: "Having then dried such a Nerve, and made a transverse segment thereof, I not only saw in it a hole, but very many, which made it resemble a Leathern Sive. . . ."

His comment that this was a "dried" nerve gives us some clue to the technical difficulties of microscopy in the days before techniques for hardening and staining had been developed. Leeuwenhoek, in all his accounts, whether of nerves or muscle or brain, describes seeing "globules," and one necessarily wonders whether or not these were optical effects introduced by his biconvex lens, which, of necessity, was neither achromatic nor devoid of spherical aberration. To view his specimens we are told, by a contemporary curator at the Royal Society, that:[4]

> Mr. Leeuwenhoek fixed his objects, if they were solid, to a silver point, with glew; and when they were fluid, or of such a nature as not to be commodiously viewed unless spread on glass, he first fitted them on a little plate of talc, or excessively thin-blown glass, which he afterwards glewed to the needle.

Having thus "fixed" his specimen and adjusted its position by a movable screw, Leeuwenhoek viewed it through a pinhole in one of the plates between which lay the biconvex lens of his "microscope." These lenses were ground by Leeuwenhoek himself, and tests of the few remaining examples indicate a magnifying power of at least 175 times. There was, of course, no possibility of seeing the nerve cell.

The use of biconvex lenses was not new to Leeuwenhoek. A picture of a simple microscope, very similar to his, and thought to have been designed by Torricelli in 1644, was

[1]T. Birch. *The History of the Royal Society of London, 1756–1757*, p. 352. Millar, London.

[2]*Phil. Trans. roy. Soc.*, 9, 178–182, 1674.

[3]*Phil. Trans. roy. Soc.*, 10:378–385, 1675.

[4]A. Schierbeck, *Measuring the Invisible World: The Life and Work of Antoni van Leeuwenhoek, F.R.S.* Abelard-Schuman, London, 1959.

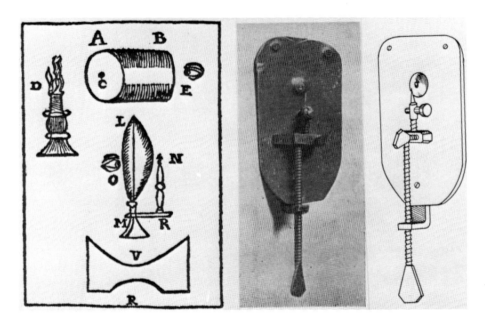

FIG. 18. **Left:** Torricelli's microscope, showing the eye *(O)* peering through the biconvex lens to see the object *(N)*. (From A. Kircher, *Ars Magna Luces et Umbrae in Mundo*, 1646.) **Center:** One of the few remaining original microscopes made by Leeuwenhoek. The two metal plates holding the lens are made of brass. (Museum of the University of Utrecht. Courtesy of the Director, Dr. P. H. Kylstra.) **Right:** A sketch of the microscope showing the silver point on which the specimen was mounted and the adjustable screw to bring it in position.

published by the Jesuit, Athanasius Kircher.[5] Among his diverse interests was astronomy, which led him to the use of lenses. In one of his several works, *Ars Magna Lucis et Umbrae in Mundo*, which appeared in 1646, the use of the pinhole and biconvex lens is illustrated. It is clear from *Scrutinium physico-medicum*, published in 1658, that he used double-lens microscopes of this type himself—"Nonnulli utuntur duabus lentibus."

A crude sketch of a cross section of optic nerve had been published by Leeuwenhoek in a letter to the Royal Society in 1675.[6] It is not in the *Transactions*, however, but in a letter, written when he was 84, to a citizen of Delft that we find the now famous rendering of a cross section of peripheral nerve, which Leeuwenhoek had comissioned by an artist (Fig. 19).[7] Unfortunately, the text of the accompanying letter (published in Latin) is equivocal as to the presence of canals, which he hoped to find in the nerves:

> Often, and not without delight, I have observed the structure of the nerves to be composed of very slender vessels of indescribable fineness, running lengthwise to form a nerve. The diameter of the vessels is such that, if it is compared with its canal, it is a third larger than the canal.
> I have been unfortunate in this procedure for I have been unable to display these cavities to anyone, for no sooner did I move them to my eyes for examination than almost immediately, in less than a minute, they dried out and contracted so that this astonishing sight wholely vanished beyond recall.

The letter continues to describe more experiments in which he was convinced he "very distinctly recognized the canals" and remarked that in cross sections, on drying out, "little

[5]Athanasius Kircher (1602–1680). *Ars Magna Lucis et Umbrae in Mundo*. Rome, 1646.
[6]*Phil. Trans. roy. Soc.*, *10*:378–385 (1675).
[7]*Epistolae physiologicae*, No. 32.

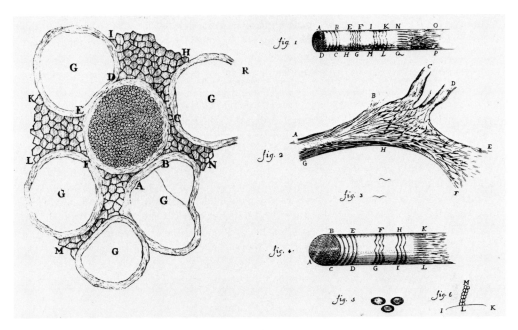

FIG. 19. Left: The drawing Leeuwenhoek had made by an artist to depict in cross section what he described as "very slender vessels of indescribable fineness, running lengthwise to form the nerve." (*Epistolae physiologicae*, No. 32.) **Right:** Leeuwenhoek's drawings of muscles. His *fig. 1*, from an ox's tongue, shows the circular "rimples," which he conceived as giving elasticity to the muscle "string"; *fig. 2* shows the filaments he saw when he flattened a muscle string; *fig. 3*, of "animalculi" is used to indicate degree of magnification; *fig. 4* is from a codfish, showing "rimples" of various forms; *fig. 5* shows blood corpuscles; *fig. 6*, lamination of an oyster shell. [*Philosophical Collections*, 2:152–159 (1677)].

hills [were] raised on them." His interpretation was that: "what humor was in them is driven out and rises up like little hills." The letter ends with the credo of a convinced Galenist:

> What material is that was enclosed in them I was never able to determine with certainty, although I believe that it was a very fluid humor which passed off as vapor.

Thus the first use of microscopy to settle this question failed. One hundred years later this issue was still unresolved. Although differently named, there was in Leeuwenhoek's letters what has been proposed to be the first description of axons within a myelinated fiber.[8] He wrote: "... after those nerves had been but a little while cut off from the eye, the filaments, of which they are made up, did shrink up, which shrinking cannot be so much on the external surface or coat of the Nerve, as t'is of the filaments that lie within the same."

In the context of the physiology of nerve and muscle, Leeuwenhoek used his microscope to examine the structure of muscle. He found what he described as muscular strings, some lying tightly together and enclosed by a membrane, and thus constituting what he called "a muscular chord."[9] What impressed him was the presence of apparent rings or "rimples" around them (see his fig. 1 in Fig. 19), which he conceived of as giving some elasticity to the muscle strings:

> I conjectured also, That this might give a reason of the motion of our Limbs, or rather of the stretching out and contracting of our Muscles, namely that when the Muscle is extended, these Muscular strings are without rimples, but when the muscle is contracted, each Muscular string is full of them.

[8]*Phil. Trans. roy. Soc.*, *10*:378–385 (1675).

[9]*Philosophical Collections*, 2:152–161 (1677).

Not only were the muscular chords made up of a great many muscular strings, but the strings themselves were also composed of fine filaments. Leeuwenhoek was struck by the delicacy of these components, measuring their widths under his microscope in comparison with a hair from his peruke or one from his beard. He found his calculations of the number of these fine components in any full muscle awesome. One should not be surprised, for with the exception perhaps of Robert Hooke's experiments, this was the first time they had been seen in such detail. It was a revelation of a microworld, previously unsuspected. Leeuwenhoek had enough vision to hazard that even his explorations might not have reached the end of the story, for he said "...We yet find that our furthest discoveries come short of seeing the utmost curiosity of Nature, and that wonderful fabrick which the Almighty Creator hath made use of in his Creatures."

Once again he described and criticized his technique, for, as in the case of nerves, he found that these muscle strings dried up very quickly under his microscope. This led him to put aside the muscles he had been using from ox and hare and move to the fish (fig. 4 in Fig. 19). He was astonished to find even more "filaments" within a muscle string. His preference for examining fish muscle was for the technical advantage of their wetness; he examined a great many different kinds and eventually worked up to the examination of muscles from a whale[10] (although it is not clear that he realized it was a mammal). In order to see the muscle strings in small insects more clearly, he soaked his specimen in brandy containing yellow saffron, a procedural ancestor of modern histologic staining methods. (This report, unfortunately, was not published in English.) Unlike Swammerdam, Leuwenhoek did not question how the nerve activated the muscle.

In his old age, Leeuwenhoek revised his views on the inner structure of muscles. He tells us he was in "the Autumn of [his] life being arriv'd to the age of 88¼ Years."[11] What he had previously thought to be fine fibers when seen in cross section, he now concluded were vessels. He based these views on old specimens he had "in a drawer...which had lain there some Years"; one necessarily wonders about their state of preservation. Several more letters on this topic followed during the next six years, the Royal Society choosing to translate them into Latin, a language Leeuwenhoek did not know.

Leeuwenhoek went on to study the brain in birds, sheep, and oxen, and detected blood vessels the size of which he measured by a hair of his head.[12] He followed the deposition of "blood globules" into the capillaries and drew a sketch[13] to send to the Royal Society (Fig. 20), but he thought that blood that reached the cortex was consumed for nourishment and that it did not return from there in the veins. The difficulties of this kind of study before hardening and staining must have been immense. With his microscope he was able to detect spermatozoa "swimming briskly" in the uterus of a bitch, thus destroying the opinion of many (including Harvey and De Graaf) that "the Semen Masculum never comes to the Uterus"[14]—another triumph for his microscope.

Leeuwenhoek was prolific in his construction of "microscopes" and bequeathed a collection (now unfortunately lost) to the Royal Society, of which he had been elected a member in 1680. These instruments were, however, catalogued when received on the death of Leeuwenhoek in 1723, and were reported by Martin Folkes,[15] the vice-president of the Royal Society, to consist of a small cabinet containing twenty-six microscopes, each supplied with an object to be viewed, some of which had broken off during the journey. All twenty-six

[10]*Phil. Trans. roy. Soc.*, *29*:55–58 (1714).

[11]*Phil. Trans. roy. Soc.*, *31*:129–141; 190–199 (1720).

[12]*Phil. Trans. roy. Soc.*, 15:875–895 (1685).

[13]*Phil. Trans. roy. Soc.*, 15:1120–1134 (1685).

[14]*Phil. Trans. roy. Soc.*, 22:552–560 (1700).

[15]*Phil. Trans. roy. Soc.*, *32*: 446–453 (1723).

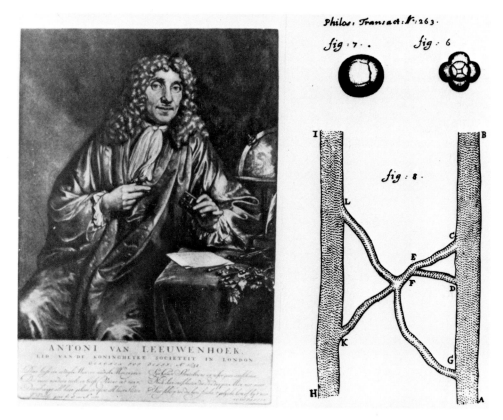

FIG. 20. **Left:** There are many portraits of Leeuwenhoek, but in this one, by Verkolje, he is shown holding one of his microscopes, and it records his membership in the Royal Society. **Right:** Leeuwenhoek's drawing of his concept of capillaries, which he had first described in a letter to the Royal Society, September 7, 1688. The sketch followed with a letter dated July 1, 1700. [From *Phil. Trans. roy. Soc.*, 22:552–560 (1700).]

were listed by Folkes, the ones most germane to this field being No. 18, noted as "Flesh of the Codfish (Cabeljaeuw) showing how the Fibres lie oblique to the Membranes," and No. 25, "An exceedingly thin Membrane, being that which cover'd a very small Muscle."

Seventeen years later the collection was reviewed again.[16] By this time the specimens had decayed even more but the lenses had survived, and a member of the Royal Society (Henry Baker) measured them for magnifying power. The greatest he found was 160 times, from which he concluded that some of Leeuwenhoek's findings must have been made with lenses of higher power than those in the Society's collection. After three centuries, the collection of Leeuwenhoek's material preserved at the Royal Society was examined again.[17] Nine little packets of specimens, some sectioned by hand, were found with carefully preserved files of his letters. One packet contained transverse sections of the optic nerve of a cow and was included with his letter of 1 June 1674. This, for the neurophysiologist, was the critical material he used for testing whether or not there were canals in nerves.

One of the few remaining original instruments, preserved at the University of Utrecht is shown in Fig. 18. It has a magnifying power of 175. There are many portraits of Leeuwenhoek but the one reproduced here (Fig. 20) was chosen because it shows his pride in membership

[16]*Phil. Trans. roy. Soc.*, *41*: 503–519 (1740).

[17]B. J. Ford. *Notes and Records of the Royal Society of London*, 36 (1), 1981.

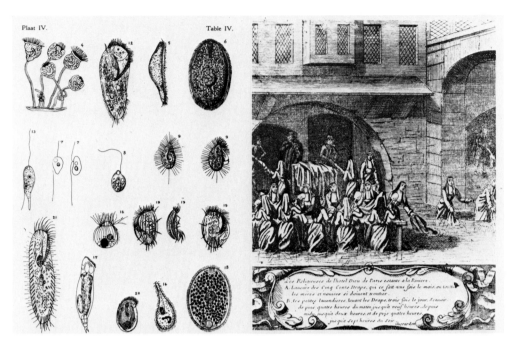

FIG. 21. Left: Leeuwenhoek's drawing of the "little animals" he found in ditchwater.   **Right:** Nuns from the Hôtel Dieu hospital in Paris washing the patients' sheets in the river Seine. (Courtesty of the Hôtel Dieu.)

of the Royal Society and has been said to depict his microscope, although the instrument he holds is unlike, and larger than, the few remaining examples of his craft.

In his own day, Leeuwenhoek's finding of "animalculi" stirred the most interest. It was so unthinkable that "little animals" could inhabit even river water, that the sheets from the beds of the patients in the hospital of the Hôtel Dieu were still being washed in the Seine by the religieuses.

It is not to our knowledge of the nerve that this industrious experimenter made his most critical contribution, but to opening the eyes of scientists to the swarming life that could be seen through his primitive microscope, for the science of microbiology was as yet unborn. For another two centuries scientists had to rely on the artists for what could be seen through the microscope. The first microphotographs were achieved by Alfred Donné in 1840.

Jan Swammerdam (1637–1680)

In the same period, and also in the Netherlands, the first truly experimental approach was being made to the problem of neuromuscular transmission. The Dutch naturalist, Jan Swammerdam, born in 1637, was the son of an apothecary who had taken the family name from a village on a tributary of the Rhine near Leyden, the city with a university that was an outstanding leader in science. The house where Swammerdam lived stood until recently (oude Schaus 18) with a tablet mounted in 1880, which says (in Dutch), "His research of nature remains an example forever." Swammerdam attended the Faculty of Medicine in Leyden from 1661–1663; among his teachers was Franciscus de le Boe Sylvius, the distinguished anatomist, and the originator of the famous Dutch gin, which he concocted as disinfectant and all-round "medicine for the poor." For the subject of his thesis, Swammerdam chose respiration, writing a text that wavers between the iatrochemical concepts of his teacher,

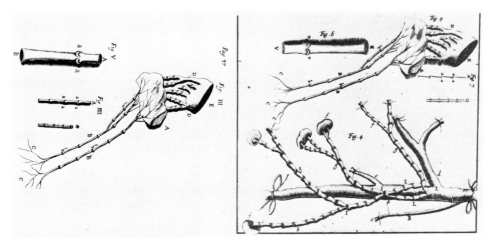

FIG. 22. The discovery of valves in the lymphatics. Dissections and drawings by Swammerdam, published with acknowledgment by Blasius (**right**) , also published by Ruysch and claimed as his own (**left**).

Sylvius, and a preview of iatromechanical studies of the movements of breathing. It is clear that he had read Descartes, but it was too early for the influence of Borelli.

He turned to the techniques of injection to define vessels anatomically, research that led him to the demonstration of valves in the lymphatics, a discovery he felt was claimed unfairly by Frederik Ruysch, another of Sylvius' students. Swammerdam's drawings were published by Blasius in his *Anatome animalium*,[18] with explicit identification of Swammerdam as the preparer and artist, but the material had been used by Ruysch without acknowledgment for his own tract, *Delucidatio valvularium*.[19] Ruysch, who became praelector of anatomy in Amsterdam, went on to develop this injection technique into the most extraordinary displays, some of which caught the eye of Peter the Great on his visit to the Netherlands. A whole room of Ruysch's preparations can be seen in the Academy of Sciences that Peter built on the banks of the Neva in St. Petersburg.

This was not the only occasion when Swammerdam experienced claims by others for discoveries he considered his own. With his injection technique Swammerdam had revealed the intimate anatomy of the female reproductive organs—the existence of ova and their passage down the Fallopian tubes to the uterus.[20] He gave his artistic skill to a fine drawing, which he dedicated to Nicolas Tulp. During this time De Graaf,[21] also an excellent anatomist, was making many similar discoveries, such as that of the Graafian follicles (which he thought were ova) and the corpora lutea. A dispute about priority developed, which was to end the friendship with Swammerdam.

Having earned the degree of Doctor of Physics from Leyden, Swammerdam began extensive research into entomology, which sparked his interest in comparative anatomy. These studies led him to the experimentation that proved so important for the understanding of the physiology of neuromuscular action. Swammerdam was a skilled dissector even to the

[18]Gerard Blasius (1626–1682). *Anatome animalium*. Amsterdam, 1661.

[19]F. Ruysch. *Delucidatio valvularium in vasis lymphaticus et lacteis*. The Hague, 1665.

[20]*Miraculum Naturae, sive uteri muliebris fabrica*. Severinus, Leyden, 1672.

[21]R. de Graaf (1641–1673). *De mulierum organis generatione inservientibus*, 1672.

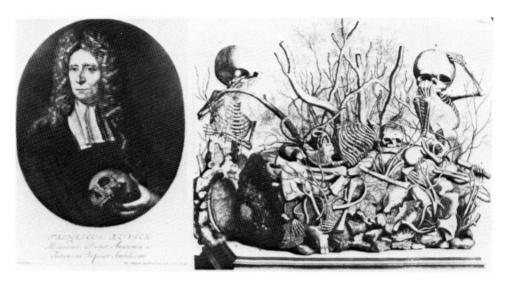

FIG 23.   Frederick Ruysch, from the portrait in Amsterdam, and one of his preparations prepared by injection. (Courtesy of the Academy of Sciences, Leningrad.)

minutiae of small insects, using magnifying glasses[22] and his own primitive microscope, not unlike the now famous early microscope of Leeuwenhoek, who had demonstrated it to him in Delft. He published widely in other branches of physiology, inventing new techniques that were soon adopted by others, and gathered together a great collection of specimens, adding to the "cabinet" that his father had established.

Swammerdam was one of the earliest biologists to work extensively with the frog, which became the almost universally chosen animal for class work. In addition to his experiments in neuromuscular action with his primitive microscope, he had searched for and found the capillary connection between the arterial and venous systems, a link not detected by Harvey. In the course of these studies, he found and described the red corpuscles in the blood of the frog:

> In the blood I perceived the serum in which floated an immense number of rounded particles, possessing the shape of as it were a flat oval but nevertheless wholly regular.

This note, dated 1658, was found after his death among the papers collected and published by Boerhaave, and thus antidates the similar observations of Malpighi (1661, in a letter to Borelli) and Leeuwenhoek (1674).

Using the frog as his experimental model, Swammerdam demonstrated many times, as had others, that irritation of the nerve caused the muscle to contract—"When the nerves are cut or touched with a knife, quite pronounced motions arise in the muscles to which they belong." Moreover, he had also shown that stimulation of the spinal marrow (the fibers of which he traced to the brain) caused contraction of the limbs. Singled out here from his many experiments is one that was designed to prove that, whatever the "animal spirits" were that caused a contraction, they did not inflate the muscle as pictured, for example, by Croone,[23] and as he had been taught in the lectures by Sylvius. He was convinced there were no cavities in nerve fibers.

---

[22]"Nowadays, I believe the magnifying glasses are in perfection, and so are the instruments that one has to use. And I found a very easy way to make all that myself, and I could teach it to another person in a quarter of an hour." (From: Letters to M. Thévenot, dated January 1678. Translated from the Dutch by G. A. Lindeboom.)

[23]William Croone (1663–1684). *De Ratione Motus Musculorum.* Hayes, London, 1664.

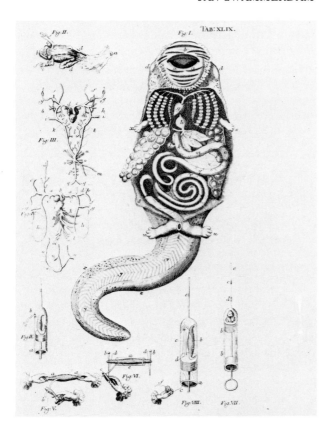

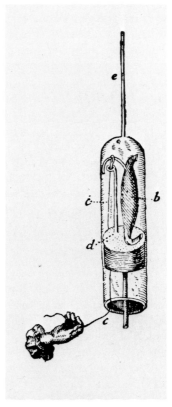

FIG. 24. **Left:** Page from *Biblia Naturae* illustrating Swammerdam's many experiments, including those to show contraction of frog muscle upon stimulation. The large dissection is of a tadpole. **Right:**Enlargement of Swammerdam's *Fig. VIII*, the first empirical test made to determine whether or not a muscle increased in volume on contraction or merely changed shape. The nerve muscle preparation is in a closed glass container sealed from the air by a bubble *(e)* in the fine pipe leading from it. A pull on the wire *(c)* stimulated the nerve mechanically. (From *Biblia Naturae*.)

The critical experiment by which he proved this is illustrated in Fig. 24, extracted from the original full page in which it is rather dwarfed by a dissection of a tadpole. The experiment was carried out in a vessel with a thin glass tube projecting from it, closed from the air by a very small drop of water. He introduced a silver wire by which he could pull on the nerve, mechanically stimulating it to cause a contraction of the muscle. The observation that the drop of water in the glass tube did not rise, although the muscle visibly swelled on contracting, convinced Swammerdam that whatever the "subtle matter" was that flowed from the nerve, it did not inflate the muscle to an increased size, only changing its shape, contracting longitudinally and expanding transversely. In fact, the movement of the drop of water indicated a slight decrease in volume (presumably due to the venous return). In his report of this experiment (published posthumously) Swammerdam concluded:[24]

> ...a muscle at the time of its contraction, undergoes no inflation or tumefaction, from the afflux or effervescence of the supposed animal spirits; but that, on the contrary, it in this state becomes smaller, or collapses; or, to express my meaning more clearly, it takes up less room than before.

Swammerdam reached important conclusions from the experiments, for example: "...no matter of sensible or comprehensible bulk flows through the nerves into the muscles" and

---

[24]From Floyd's translation of *Biblia Naturae*. London, 1758.

that there was no evidence for "imaginary fermentation between the spirits and blood." His experiments on the result of irritating the nerve in a nerve–muscle preparation led him to suggest that "the nerves are constantly and perpetually irritated to give motion to every muscle in the body." He was well ahead of his time in recognizing muscle tonus.

The fact that the stimulating wire was made of silver (filium argenteum) and the loop of copper (filium aeneum) has led some to credit Swammerdam with the use of bimetallic electricity as a stimulus to nerve. If this were an element of the stimulus it was used unwittingly by Swammerdam and this electrical phenomenon was to remain unknown for nearly 150 years.

Swammerdam, a true conceptualist, knew what must be demonstrated to prove the relationship of the nerve to the muscle and, writing like an anatomist, he said:[25]

> In the construction and motion of the muscle it is of particular interest to note in what manner the nerve is actually joined to the muscle; how it is constructed in the muscle; what its course, entrance, middle, distribution and end is; as also how it communicates with the moving fibre, and what effect it produces in it; also what that very subtle matter properly is which is undoubtedly conveyed to the muscle through the nerve.

This is an outstanding example of a reasoned concept anticipating its proof for lack of the necessary technology. Swammerdam's primitive microscope could not enable him to see the neuromuscular ending so familiar to us today, but he knew it must be there.

Although Swammerdam published many entomological studies during his lifetime, this critical experiment on nervous action was among the unpublished papers[26] he willed to his patron, Thévenot, the director of the Royal Library of Louis XIV.

That Swammerdam had at one time intended to publish the experiments on muscle and nerve was made clear by the finding after his death of 52 prepared copper plates made from his own drawings. But toward the end of his short life he had withdrawn into a religious mysticism and, as we are told by an early historian: "Intense application of his work made Swammerdam a hypochondriac and unfit for society and he plunged into the depths of mysticism. . . . He so injured his constitution by mortification, that he died in 1680, at the age of 43."[27] He was the third of his contemporaries to turn from science to religious contemplation. Pascal (who turned to the Janssenists) and his own friend Steno (who turned to the Jesuits) had made similar retreats from the world of science; in Swammerdam's case, it was a mystic Protestant cult that claimed him.

However, in his case, the escape was not final, for he returned to microscopy for the last four years of his life. Recent research by Lindeboom[28] shows that Swammerdam, using the simple microscopes he made himself, returned to study the inner structure of insects as well as red blood cells and spermatozoa in mammals.

After his death in 1680, Swammerdam's papers changed hands several times until finally purchased for 2,000 guilders (then a very large sum) by Boerhaave, and published by him 58 years after the death of the author. The book was printed in parallel columns of the original Dutch and a Latin translation by Jerome David Gaub. To this volume Boerhaave gave the title *Bÿbel der Natuure* or *Biblia Naturae*, prefacing it with a biographical sketch of Swammerdam. Within 20 years this book was translated into English and later into German.

[25]From Floyd's translation of *Biblia Naturae*. London, 1758.

[26]Preserved at the Museum Boerhaave in Leyden.

[27]William Hamilton. *History of Medicine*, 2 vols. Bentley, London, 1831.

[28]G. A. Lindeboom. Jan Swammerdam als microscopist. *Tijdschrift voor des Geschiedenis der Geneeskunde, Natuurwetenschappen, Wiskunde en Techniek*, 4:87–110 (1981).

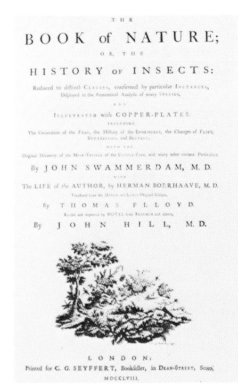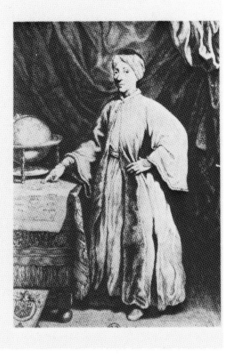

FIG. 25. **Left:** Title page of the English edition (1758) of *Biblia Naturae*, edited by Boerhaave, and published posthumously. **Right:** Melchisedec Thévenot, Parisian friend and correspondent of Swammerdam, and first receiver of his papers when he died. An intrepid traveller in Eastern countries, Thévenot had his portrait painted in oriental robes. He was a member of the Cours Municipal, and a clearer portrait of him is in the group painted by Georges Lallemant (at the Musée Carnavalet in Paris).

Swammerdam was an excellent artist and illustrated his works profusely, as well as contributing many drawings to the publication of his teacher, Blasius,[29] with whom he had studied in Amsterdam. These copper plates are lost, but those from Boerhaave's *Biblia Naturae* can be seen in the Museum Boerhaave in Leyden and his letters to Thévenot in the Library of the University of Göttingen.

No known portrait of Swammerdam exists. In the 19th century, a publisher took one of the heads from Rembrandt's famous picture of Nicholas Tulp's *Anatomy Lesson* and distributed a lithograph that he labeled with Swammerdam's name. Swammerdam was a schoolboy at the time Tulp was teaching, so this was a stroke of imagination rather than fact.

Nicolaus Steno (1638–1686)

The puzzle of how muscle contracted was approached from another angle by a friend and fellow student of Swammerdam, Niels Stensen. Stensen was born in Copenhagen in 1638 and educated there for three years, going on to Amsterdam and then to the famous University of Leyden, founded in 1575 as a Protestant center for the seven northern provinces of the Spanish Netherlands. (The University was extremely influential in the eventual break from the rule and the religion of Spain.) Stensen's student days had not been entirely peaceful—

---

[29]G. Blasius, *Anatome Animalium*. Amsterdam, 1661.

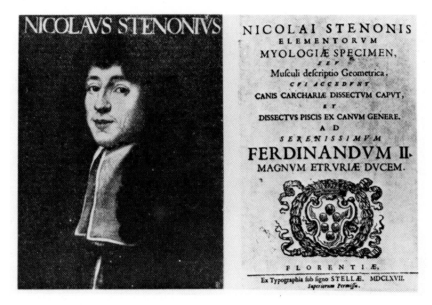

FIG. 26. Portrait of Steno from the Uffizzi Gallery in Florence and the title page of his *Elementorum myologiae*, one of the most influential treatises to unseat the concept of animal spirits.

in 1658 Copenhagen, then a walled city, was beseiged by the Swedish forces of Charles Gustavus. During this time Stensen enrolled in a student regiment and played a part in the successful defense of his native city, although it was to be attacked again in the struggle for dominance over navigation through the Sound between the two countries.

Stensen (who, on leaving Denmark, was to become better known as Nicolaus Steno) came from a strongly Lutheran family and received his initial scientific education from Thomas Bartolin, a member of the famous Danish family that contributed so much to the medical sciences. Manuscripts of Stensen's student notes and excerpts he made from his omniverous reading (a collection he named *Chaos*) are still preserved in the Biblioteca Nazionale in Florence. Bartolin made a major contribution in unraveling the anatomy and physiology of the lymphatic system,[30] and no doubt it was this interest that led to Steno's own discovery[31] (when he was working with Gerard Blasius at Amsterdam) of the duct that now bears his name: the duct of the parotid salivary gland. Rather disgracefully, Blasius tried to claim this discovery for himself when confusion lay in the differentiation of glands for secretion from those of the lymphatics.[32] Anticipating Lower, Steno clearly proved that tears come not from the brain but from the lachrymal glands.[33]

From his study of the lymphatics Steno's interest turned to the heart, which, in contradiction to earlier opinions, he showed to be purely muscular in construction. This finding caused dismay to those who still accepted the ancient dictum that the heart was the site of innate heat. But Steno's finding was soon established beyond doubt by Richard Lower in his *Tractatus de corde*,[34] using Steno's illustration as his Plate 4.

[30]Thomas Bartolin (1616–1680). *Vasa lymphatica nuper hafniae in animalibus inventa et hepatis exsequiae.* Copenhagen, 1654.

[31]*Disputatio anatomica de glandulis oris.* Leiden, 1662.

[32]G. Blasius (1626–1682). *Medicina generalis*, Chapter 13. Amsterdam, 1661.

[33]*Observationes Anatomicae.* Leiden, 1662.

[34]Richard Lower (1631–1681). *Tractatus de corde.* Allestry, London, 1669.

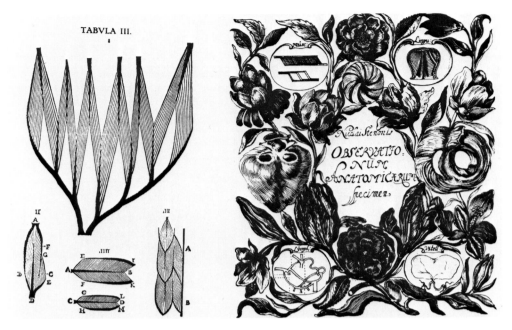

FIG. 27. Steno's geometric design of muscle fibers and their reorientation during contraction. The frontispiece of his treatise, published in 1662, includes a vignette of his purely mechanical concept of muscle contraction.

Steno moved his investigations from the heart to the problem of skeletal muscle. With his knowledge of the fluid function of the lymphatics, he became extremely critical of still-existing concepts of animal spirits. He wrote:[35]

> Concerning the fluid of muscles how uncertain, or rather how wholly wanting, is our knowledge. Fluid certainly exists in the fibrillae of which the motor fibres are composed and between the fibrillae, also between the motor fibres themselves, in the membranous fibrillae, and between the membranous fibrillae; but in truth it is by no means clear whether these fluids are all of one kind or whether, just as they are distinct in the seats which they occupy, so they differ in material properties. Nor is it known whether any of these fluids are really like any one of the fluids so far known to us. Animal spirits, the more subtle part of the blood, the vapour of blood, and the juice of the nerves, these are names used by many, *but they are mere words, meaning nothing.*

Here is one of the first challenges of the 17th century to Galen's dictum, persisting from the first century A.D., that muscular contraction is caused by animal spirits flowing down the nerve from the brain to inflate the muscle.

Of the many works by this industrious scientist, those of principal interest for the history of the physiology of muscular motion are his studies of skeletal muscle. Steno, with a great interest in mechanics and a realization that any concept of function must recognize structure, approached contraction from the viewpoint of the fibers, connective tissue, and tendons. Like Walter Charleton[36] before him, Steno established that it is not the tendons that contract; he held that they merely alter the angle they form with the longitudinal muscle fibers. The

[35]N. Steno. *Discours sur l'Anatomie du Cerveau.* Robert de Ninville, Paris, 1669. Steno's own words for this historic declaration were: "Spiritus animales, subtiliorem sanguinis partem, vaporem ejus, et nervorum succum multi nominant, sed verba haec sunt, nihil experimentia."

[36]Walter Charleton (1619–1707). *Exercitationes physico-anatomicae sive oeconomia animalis novis in medicina hypothesibus superstructurae.* London, 1658.

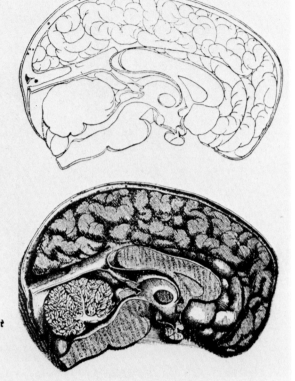

DISCOVRS

DE

MONSIEVR STENON,

SVR

L'ANATOMIE

DV CERVEAV.

A

MESSIEVRS DE
l'Assemblée, qui se fait chez
Monsieur Theuenot.

A PARIS,
Chez ROBERT DE NINVILLE, au bout du Pont
S. Michel, au coin de la ruë de la Huchette,
à l'Escu de France & de Nauarre.

M DC. LXIX.
AVEC PRIVILEGE DV ROY.

FIG. 28. Steno's lecture in Paris in 1665 on the anatomy of the brain was not published until four years later, and then as a small pocket-sized text. The several illustrations of transections of the brain made after total removal illustrate Steno's tenet that cross sections, necessitating sawing through the skull, distorted the soft tissue of the brain—a criticism he made of Willis' horizontal sections. *(Discours sur l'Anatomie du Cerveau. Paris, 1669.)*

length or width of the body of the muscle thus changes with the angle of pull from the tendons. He designed a scheme by which the fasciculi of muscle fibers worked on the principle of parallelograms, which he illustrated for several kinds of muscles, including the gastrocnemius, biceps semimembranosus, and semitendinosus. (His illustration for the deltoid is seen in Fig. 27.) A vignette of this design for muscle is reproduced on the title page of his book on anatomy.[37] One wonders whether Steno's studies in crystallography suggested this scheme. Steno shared his friend Swammerdam's disbelief in the "balloon" concept of muscular contraction but, unlike Swammerdam, he was unable to design an experiment to refute it. Instead, his concept, geometrical in form, was based on his anatomical demonstration of the difference between tendons and muscle fibers and the important demonstration that the tendons did not alter in length.

In 1664 Steno visited with Thévenot, Swammerdam's patron in Paris, and it was there, in the following year, that he gave his sole contribution to the study of the brain—in a lecture that was to become famous. In the reign of the Sun King, Paris was a center of activity attracting men from many fields. Here Steno met Swammerdam and Ole Borch,[38]

---

[37]*Observationes anatomicae.* 1662.

[38]Ole Borch (1626–1690). *Conventus eruditorum.* (Manuscript in the Royal Library, Copenhagen.)

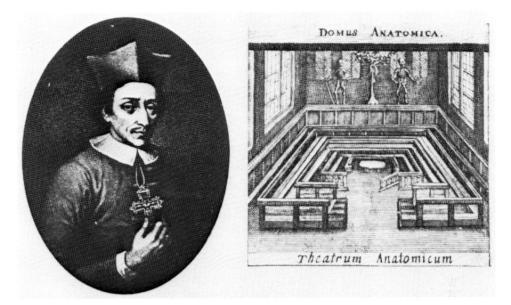

FIG. 29. Left: Steno in his closing years after his appointment as titular bishop to northern Europe. (From the portrait in the Institute of Anatomy at Copenhagen.) **Right:** The old anatomical theatre in which he had been educated and to which he returned to give a religously oriented lecture. This famous Domus Anatomicae in Copenhagen was destroyed by fire in 1728. (From: Thomas Bartolin, *Cista medica*, 1662.)

the Danish chemist (and recorder of these meetings that took place at Thévenot's). In the arts, that same year saw Racine's first play on the Paris stage *(La Thébaïde)*. The group that gathered at the house of Melchisedec Thévenot (later a member of the Académie Royale des Sciences founded in 1666) represented, in the main, those philosophers and scientists in France who were drawn to Cartesian concepts. Descartes had died in 1650, but the posthumous publication of his *Traité de l'Homme* was gaining ground against the Janssenism that had attracted Pascal away from science. (Two years earlier, the Church had put Descartes on the Index.) In his lecture, although critical of Descartes' anatomy, Steno praised him as surpassing all other philosophers.

In the period before his lecture, Steno had devoted himself to anatomy, and there are reports of his demonstrations to medical students.[39] When he delivered the lecture to the group at Thévenot's, he did not have plans for its publication, but four years later, it was printed in French.[40] By then, Steno had left Paris for Tuscany, but the stir that it caused reached him there. He had not hesitated in his lecture to be critical of others in the field for accepting the words of the ancients too readily and for speculating too freely on the function of the structures they dissected. He was especially critical of Thomas Willis whose *Cerebri anatome* had been published the same year, and it must be conceded that Willis did speculate freely, defending his methods as follows: "Anatomy may be sweetened with those kind of more pleasant speculations, as it were cloathing the Skeleton with flesh."[41]

It was not only such speculative writing by Willis to which Steno objected; he also made specific criticisms of his anatomical illustrations, suggesting that some errors might have been introduced by the technique (common to anatomists, including Willis) of horizontal

[39]*Journal des Sçavans.* March 25, 1665.

[40]*Discours sur l'anatomie du cerveau.* Robert de Ninville, Paris, 1669.

[41]Thomas Willis. *Cerebri anatome.* Martyn & Allestry, London, 1664.

sectioning of the brain while it still rested on the base of the skull. He wished that there were some way of dissolving the bone, and Steno's own illustrations for his lecture are from vertical cuts. In the days before hardening techniques had been developed for dissection, the brain substance was so soft that following the destination of the nerves was difficult.

Steno opened his lecture, entitled "On the Anatomy of the Brain," with the disarming statement (in "a sincere and public confession") that he knew nothing of the subject. And, in fact, there is little that he added to the general understanding of cerebral anatomy. He used the presence of the distinguished group to emphasize the still lingering error that animal spirits were housed in the ventricles, although he admitted to his failure to identify their nature. He declared:[42]

> We are still more uncertain about what relates to the Animal Spirits. Are they Blood, or a particular Substance separated from the Chyle by the Glands of the Mesentery? Or may they not be derived from a Lymphatic Serum? Some compare them to Spirit of Wine, and it may be doubted whether they are not the Matter of Light. Our common Dissections cannot clear up any of these difficulties.

Steno accepted that the soul resided in the brain, but, although he praised Descartes for explaining all human actions mechanically, he was extremely critical of Descartes' anatomy of the pineal gland (misjudging this partly from the illustrator's misconceptions of Descartes' own views). It is of interest that anatomy rather than function of the pineal received Steno's criticisms.

By the time his lecture was published, Steno was living in Tuscany. He was undergoing a rejection of his Lutheran upbringing and the Protestantism of his homeland, and was turning to Catholicism, a faith to which he converted in 1667, culminating in priesthood. Steno was eventually appointed by Pope Innocent XI as titular bishop, first in Greece and then in northern Europe. While remaining intensely religious, for a few years he continued to show interest in anatomical dissection, geology, and paleontology, returning to lecture at the famous Domus Anatomica in Copenhagen, but gradually matters of the Church took precedence. Steno died in Schwerin, in the Duchy of Mecklenburg, in 1686. His body was brought to Florence and buried in the crypt of the Basilica of San Lorenzo. (In 1953, when his remains were unearthed and moved to a more distinguished place in the chapel that is now named for him, his head was discovered to be missing.)

It is ironic that Steno, who had had an argument with Croone as to whether or not gall stones were "natural occurrences," should in the end have died from them.

BIBLIOGRAPHY

Antoni van Leeuwenhoek (1632–1723)

Selected Writings

More microscopical observations made by the same Mr. Leeuwenhoeck [sic] and promised in Number 97 of these Tracts communicated in his letters of August 15, 1673 and of April 7, 1674. *Phil. Trans. roy. Soc.*, 9:23–35 (1674).

More observations from Mr. Leeuwenhook [sic] in a letter of September 7, 1674 sent to the Publisher. *Phil. Trans. roy. Soc.*, 9:178–182 (1674).

Microscopical observations of Mr. Leeuwenhoeck [sic] concerning the optic nerve in a letter of December 7, 1674. *Phil. Trans. roy. Soc.*, 10:378–385 (1675).

---

[42]From the English translation by G. Douglas of Winslow's republication, in 1732, of the original French.

An account of several very curious Discoveries about the internal texture of the flesh of Muscles. *Philosophical Collections*, 2:152–161 (1677).

An extract of a letter from Mr. Anthony van Leeuwenhoek to the Royal Society containing his observations of the optic nerves. *Phil. Trans. roy. Soc.*, 17:949–960 (1693).

An extract of a Letter from Mr. Anthony van Leeuwenhoek, F.R.S. Dated October 12th 1713 Concerning the Fibres of the Muscles, etc. *Phil. Trans. roy. Soc.*, 29:55–58 (1714).

Epistolae physiologicae super compluribus naturae arcanis. (Letter No. 32 in Latin addressed to Domino Abrahamo van Bleiswyk. March 2, 1717.) Beman, Delft, 1719.

Brieven door Antoni van Leeuwenhoek, 4 vols. Hendrik von Krooneveld, 1697–1698.

Secondary Sources

Cole, F. J. Leeuwenhoek's zoological researches. *Ann. Sci.*, 2:1–46, 185–235 (1937).

Dobell, C. *Antony van Leeuwenhoek and His "Little Animals."* Harcourt-Brace, New York, 1932.

Hoole, Samuel. *The Select Works of Anthony van Leeuwenhoek, containing his microscopical discoveries in many of the works of nature* (translation). London, 1798.

Schierbeek, A. (Ed.). *The Collected Letters of A. v. Leeuwenhoek*, 2 vols. Swets and Zeitlinger, Amsterdam, 1939–1967.

Scheirbeek, A. *Measuring the Invisible World: The Life and Works of Antoni van Leeuwenhoek, F.R.S..* Abelard-Schumann, London, 1959.

Jan Swammerdam (1637–1680)

Selected Writings

Tractatus Physico-anatomico-medicus de Respiratione usuque Pulmonum. Gaasbeek, Leyden, 1667.

Historiae Generalis Insectorum, Pars prima. Ultrajecti, A. Van Dreunen, Utrecht, 1669.

Miraculum Naturae sive Uteri Muliebris Fabrica. Severinus, Leyden, 1672. (*Nova methodus cavitates corporis praeparandi*, added to 2nd edition, 1672.)

Biblia Naturae, 2 vols, edited by Boerhaave. Severinus, Amsterdam, 1737 and 1738. (English translation by Th. Floyd. London, 1758.) (Facsimile edition, G. Lindeboom, 1982.)

Secondary Sources

Birch, T. *The History of the Royal Society.* Millar, London, 1756, 1757.

Blasius, G. *Anatome Animalium.* Amsterdam, 1661.

Commelin, C. J. *Swammerdam.* Observationum Anatomicarum Collegii Privati, Amsterdam, 1667.

Hamilton, W. *History of Medicine*, 2 vols. Bentley, London, 1831.

Lindeboom, G. A. (Ed). *The letters of Jan Swammerdam to Melchisedec Thévenot*, 1678.

Schierbeek, A. *Jan Swammerdam (1637–1680). His Life and Works.* Swets and Zeitlinger, Amsterdam, 1967.

Stirling, W. *Some Apostles of Physiology.* Waterlow, London, 1902.

Nicolaus Steno (1638–1686)

Selected Writings

Disputatio anatomica de glandulis oris. Leyden, 1661.

Observationum Anatomicarum. Leyden, 1662.

Apologia prodromus, quo demonstratur, judicem. Blasium et rei anatomicae imperatum esse, et affectuum suorum servum. Leyden, 1663. In: *Opera Philosophica*, Vol. 1, edited by Maar Vilheim, pp. 143–154. Copenhagen, 1910.

De musculis et glandulis observationum specimen: cum duabus epistolis anatomicus. Copenhagen, 1664.

Elementorum myologiae specimen, sui musculi descriptio geometrica (translated by Foster). Florence, 1666–7.

Discours sur l'Anatomie du Cerveau. Robert De Ninville, Paris, 1669.

The Chaos Manuscript. Biblioteca Nazionale Galileiana, Florence.

Secondary Sources

Anatomical Observations of the Glands of the Eye and Their New Vessels Thereby Revealing the True Source of Tears, edited by E. Gotfredsen. Copenhagen, 1951.

Bastholm, E. The history of muscle physiology. *Acta Hist. Sci. Nat. Med.*, 7:178–189 (1950).

Bastholm, E. Niels Stensen's mycology. *Analecta Medico-Historica*, 3:147–153 (1968).

Rome, D. R. Nicolas Stenon et la "Royal Society of London." *Osiris*, 12:244–267 (1956).

Scherz, G. *Nicolaus Steno and His Indice.* Munksgaard, Copenhagen, 1958.

Stirling, W. *Some apostles of physiology, being an account of their lives and labours. Labours that have contributed to the advancement of the healing art as well as the prevention of disease.* Waterlow, London, 1902.

CHAPTER IV

Transition in the English Schools

The mid-17th century saw a developing trend in natural philosophy that was essentially a resurgence of the old theories of 5th century Greek atomists, who held that all matter, including the human body, was composed of particles, indestructible and always in motion. This was, in essence, a kind of determinism. With the movement away from explanation derived from argument and logic that came with recognition of experimental testing of hypotheses, atomism appealed to 17th century explorers now seeking a mechanistic explanation of the nervous system. For those studying the human brain, this was part of the move away from Aristotelian teachings and the belief that the brain played only a secondary role, functioning merely to condense the hot vapors coming from the heart.

The outstanding advocates of atomism were Democritus and Epicurus, whose views were wholly mechanistic. Even the soul was held to be composed of atoms and, for them, thought was a purely physical process. To 17th century scholars concerned with the brain and our nervous system, the omission in this theory of a "Creator" was disturbing. The first prominent challenger was Gassendi, a Catholic whose religious faith caused his objections.

Pierre Gassendi (1592–1655)

Pierre Gassendi, born just before the opening of the 17th century, was a gifted, multifaceted son of Provence, with a doctorate from Avignon, educated in philosophy, religion, and astronomy. He was a professor of mathematics and astronomy at the Collège Royal, and corresponded with Galileo. In the 17th century astronomers were struggling to separate their science from astrology, and those concerned with man's body and soul were seeking a place for him in cosmology.

Gassendi (described by Willis as "a most Skilful and Cause-Expressing Man") was labeled a freethinker by his contemporaries because he published attacks (in 1624) on Aristotle and (in 1630) on the occult beliefs of Robert Fludd. Quarrels with Descartes (provoked by Father

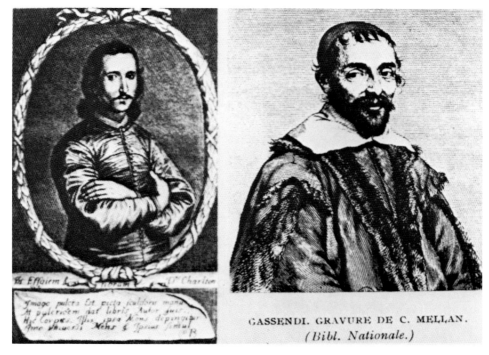

FIG. 30.   Walter Charleton (1619–1707) and Pierre Gassendi (1592–1656), champions of Atomism in their views of nervous action. The portrait of Charleton is from his *Physiologia Epicuro* (1654) and that of Gassendi from the Bibliothèque Nationale.

Mersenne) were to come later. During Gassendi's professorship in Paris, in 1642 and 1643, he held private teaching sessions in his home. Among the pupils was a young student of law named Jean Baptiste Poquelin, who was to have far more long-lasting fame than his teacher. He took the name of Molière and became the master of satire, sparing least of all the medical profession.[1]

Gassendi, although rejecting Aristotelianism, retained from it a belief in the unity of all nature and included this concept when he embraced the skeleton of Epicurean atomism. A Religious, having taken holy orders at Aix, he rejected the atheism inherent in atomism by declaring God as Creator of the atoms and their movements, and he removed the human soul from the main concept by declaring it to be immaterial. His ideas, transmitted to Descartes by their mutual correspondent, Father Mersenne, provoked an argument even before publication. Gassendi's major exposition of his views (in *Animadversiones*, in 1649) crossed the channel to upset puritan England. In the second (posthumous) edition (1658) an appendix was added specifically embracing the fundamental corpuscular theory but insisting on its divine origin.[2] Matter, according to Gassendi, was not inert but was composed of atoms perpetually in motion, indivisible, and indestructible. God created the atoms and directed their motion. Our ideas, he proposed, came to us through the movement of atoms in our senses leaving traces in the brain. Anticipating John Locke, Gassendi held that every idea that exists in the mind originates in the senses.

[1]Molière (1622–1673). *La Malade imaginaire*. Paris.

[2]Appendix to *Animadversiones*. 1649.

Walter Charleton (1619–1707)

Gassendi's works reached England during the period of the Cromwellian protectorate, a difficult time for Royalists. One of them, a young physician, Walter Charleton, born in Somerset in 1619, emerged as the major exponent of Gassendi's ideas. A prolific writer and a confirmed Epicurean atomist, Charleton was intent on presenting Gassendi's concepts more widely. This task flowered in 1654 in his large book of 2 volumes on natural philosophy, *Physiologia Epicuro–Gassendo–Charltoniana*. On the title page he states that the "Hypothesis of Atoms" was "founded" by Epicurus, "repaired" by Gassendi, and "augmented" by himself. Unusual for its period, the book was written, not in Latin, but in English.

It is in the second of these prolix books that Charleton, among a plethora of other topics, discusses the atomic theory of Epicurus. In the third book of Volume 2 he brings this theory into the context of the nervous system with an explanation of the sense of vision, assigned to the motion of atoms (thus defending the ideas of Gassendi). The wave theory of light lay far in the future. The other senses all received their (theoretical) explanations—hearing, smelling, tasting, as well as physical properties such as heat and cold, hardness and ductility, and what Charleton calls the "occult qualities"; these included electricity and magnetism. It was 54 years after Gilbert's magnificent *De Magnete*.

The words Charleton used for the receipt by our brains of sensory impressions foreshadow our vocabulary of the nerve impulse:

> ...we can have no other cognizance of the conditions or qualities of sensible objects but what results from our perception of Impulses made upon the organs of our senses by their species thither transmitted: assuredly the Physiologist is highly concerned to make the contemplation of Motion its Causes, Kinds and Universal Laws the First Link in the Chain of all his Natural Theorems.

The author felt some need to apologize for the enormous size of his work: "Ingenious Reader," he wrote, "I have kept you long at Sea, I confess, and (such was the Unskilfulness of my Pen, though steered, for the most part, according to the lines drawn on those excellent Charts of *Epicurus* and Gassendus) often shipwreck your Patience."

What emerges from all Charleton's many writings was his firm belief in the role of the Deity. The theological implications of the mechanical philosophy of atoms was as disturbing to him as to Gassendi, whom he admired. The atoms he believed in so strongly were, he said, created by God. Two of his many publications witness to his belief: *The Darkness of Atheism Dispelled by the Light of Nature* and *The Immortality of the Human Soul, Demonstrated by the Light of Nature*. But, unlike Glisson and Harvey, Charleton was not an Aristotelian—he believed in a separate soul animating the body in a mechanistic way.

In terms of the history of nerve and muscle, however, Charleton's importance can be demonstrated more readily from his earlier book, *Natural History of Nutrition, Life and Voluntary Motion*, rather than from his large memorial volume to Gassendi. He did not accept the presence of canals within the nerves and by geometrical reasoning came to doubt that muscles increased in volume on contraction (although he did not test this experimentally). As had Steno, he became convinced that it was not the tendons that contracted but the muscle fibers and he emphasized the importance of the blood supply.

As a Royalist, Charleton's standing rose after the Restoration in 1660. He had moved from Oxford to London ten years earlier, building his medical practice; he remained loyal to the absent monarch. Charleton introduced protests against England's civil war by commenting on the achievements of Harvey and Glisson. How could all of these be achieved, he asked, "in a land yet wet and reeking with blood...in a Nation so lately opprest by the Tyranny of Mars, and scarce yet free from the distractions of a horrid Civil War?" He was

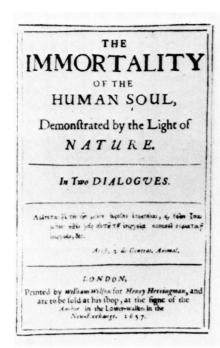

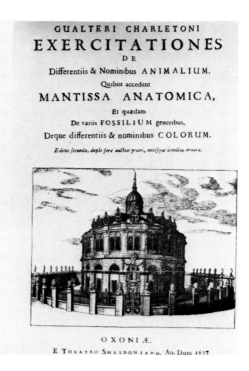

FIG. 31. Two title pages from Walter Charleton's works on theology in which he discusses the work of Harvey and of Glisson. On the right is a picture is of the Sheldonian theatre, where a printing press had been established to circumvent the strict licensing laws for publishing. The building, with its quaint surround of busts, was designed by Christopher Wren.

a founding member of the Royal Society and became a member and eventually President of the Royal College of Physicians.

Charleton's views on the importance in muscle contraction of the blood supply, although not his adherence to atomism, were shared by his famous contemporary, Thomas Willis. Birch tells us that they did not always agree, for at a meeting of the Royal Society on June 8, 1664, Charleton read a report showing differences between the brains of animals and man. Willis was informed because the results impugned Willis's *Cerebre anatome*. The Royal Society then declared that: "It is ordered likewise, that what shall pass between those two doctors upon this occasion shall not be made public without their consent."

Among those who attended Charleton's lectures was a much-travelled student of anatomy whose name has come down to us as the great diarist of the 17th century.

John Evelyn, remembered for the insight he gave into the thought and actions of his times, had a great interest in the nervous system. During a year of study in Padua he attended dissections of human cadavers in the famous anatomical theatre and received permission to take with him four preparations: a human spinal cord with nerves, a dissected specimen of the vagi and sympathetic nerves, an aorta with arteries, and veins. He gave these to the Royal Society whose museum was at that time housed in Gresham College. Later he recorded this gift:[3]

> I made ye Royal Society a present of ye tables of veins, arteries, and nerves which great
> curiosity I had caused to be made in Italy, out of ye Natural Human Bodies, by a learned

---

[3]John Evelyn (1620–1706). Entry dated October 31, 1667. *The Diary of John Evelyn.* edited by E. S. de Beer, 6 vols. Oxford, 1955.

physician, and the help of Veslingius[4] (Professor of Padua) from whence I brought them in 1646.

Evelyn realized the importance of these specimens; the dissection of human cadavers was frowned upon in England at that time, and he described his specimens as "being the first of that kind that had been seen there and, for aught I know in the world, though afterwards there were others." After an interim stay in the British Museum they were transferred at the beginning of this century to the museum of the Royal College of Surgeons where they can now be examined in the Hunterian Museum.

Francis Glisson (1597–1677)

During this time one of the most powerful English thinkers in the field of medicine was Francis Glisson, born just before the turn of the century in the West of England. Cambridge educated, and a Royalist, he was appointed in 1636 to the Regius Professorship in Physic, the only science-related chair of the five created by Henry VIII. His intensive studies of rickets, the liver, stomach, and intestines led him inevitably to a consideration of the nervous system. Essentially a vitalist, strongly opposed to his contemporary, Descartes, Glisson thought of a nutritive liquid secreted in the brain from elements brought by the blood and derived from the food we eat. He held that, during digestion this "succus nutritivus" spreads to the brain and spinal cord, inducing postprandial sleepiness. In sleep the brain and spinal cord contract and the "flux" then goes to other parts of the body to nourish them and to produce saliva, nasal mucosa, and tears.

For Glisson, this flux seemed initially an afferent one, and he was puzzled that the same nerves could carry nutrients to, as well as from, the brain. He concluded that there must be several channels within the nerve so that liquids could pass without mixing.

What emerges from Glisson's descriptions is that he contemplated the reverse of the procedure that concerned his contemporaries. He postulated that it is the movement of the muscle that puts the flow of the liquid up the nerve. The nerve is irritated into vibration by this muscle movement as it is irritated also by sensation and by appetite, this irritation becoming exaggerated in sickness. He acknowledged that no trace of this liquid was found at autopsy, but declared this the effect of death.

Glisson accepted Steno's design for the structure of muscle, but theorized that three factors were at work within it: an intrinsic stability, somewhat resembling the later theories of tonus; life-giving support from the blood (*influxus vitalis*); and an activating principle coming to it from the nerve (*influxus animalis*).

Glisson thought irritability was a biological property of all tissues, not only of muscle and nerve, and it is the term he used to describe the ability to react and then recover. His concept of an indwelling spirit (*spiritus insitus*) in all tissues seems to have first come to him when studying rickets, and was developed further in his work on the liver and the secretion of bile, as described in *Tractatus de Anatomia Hepatis* (1654).

The idea was elaborated even further in *Tractatus de Ventriculo et Intestinis* (1677) when he confronted the problem of the efferent role of nerves.[5] Unable to conceive of a single explanation to account for all the characteristics of the body's universal irritability, Glisson proposed three: an intrinsic one that was not necessarily conscious (*motus naturalis*), one provoked by external stimili (*motus sensitivus externus*), and one initiated by the soul (*motus*

---

[4]Johann Vesling (1598–1649), originally from Westphalia, was appointed professor of anatomy at Padua in 1632. His *Syntagma Anatomicum* (Pavia, 1641) was the outstanding anatomical text at the time of Evelyn's visit.

[5]*Tractatus de Ventriculo et Intestinis.* Brome, London, 1677.

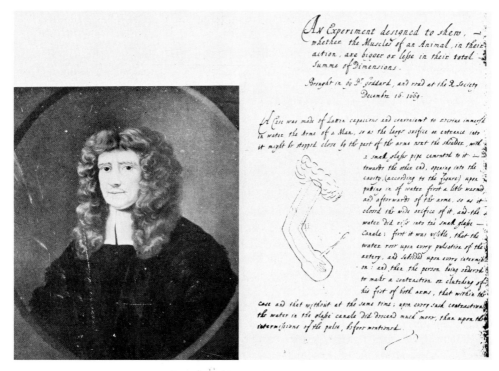

FIG. 32.   Left: Francis Glisson (1597–1677). The famous Bodleian portrait, now in the Radcliffe Scientific Library, Oxford.   **Right**: Jonathan Goddard's experiment before the Royal Society in 1669 to show that a man's arm does not increase in volume on contraction. (Registry of the Royal Society, by courtesy of the Librarian.)

sensitivus internus). To Glisson, the vitalist, the last of the three best explained our voluntary movements. Glisson was also an Aristotelian and fundamentally a theorist; nowhere in his writings does he suggest an experimental test of his own proposals although he was well aware of the conflicting theories of contemporaries. He quotes (without acknowledgment) Goddard's experiment to show that a man's arm does not increase in volume on contraction. Glisson used Goddard's experimental finding to argue that it was irritability, not inflation, that caused the muscle to contract. (See Figure 32.)

Despite Glisson's anatomical theories, his hypotheses produced no scientific data to add to the existing knowledge of nerve or muscle. But his elaborate concepts intrigued other workers and laid the ground for the development by Haller, in the next century, of a far more physiological theory of irritability, one that he confined to the muscle fiber and that heralded the modern concept of excitability.

A prolific writer, Glisson was elected a member of the Royal College of Physicians and of the newly formed Royal Society. Successful in the practice of medicine, he became personal physician to the powerful Lord Shaftesbury, as had another philosophically minded doctor, John Locke. He died at the age of 80 in 1677 leaving many unpublished manuscripts, which are now in the Sloane Collection of the British Museum.

In the following century, publication of *The History of the Royal Society* revealed the name of the experimenter who made the actual test of muscle contraction. The test was conducted before the Council of the Royal Society; the report was made on April 1, 1669; the member, Dr. Jonathan Goddard.

The *Proceedings* read:

> There was described an experiment, proposed by Dr. Goddard, to find, whether muscles in their contraction grew bigger upon the whole, or not? The experiment was by inserting a man's arm into an artificial arm made of tin, having a glass-pipe fitted and erected in the hand of it, so as being filled with water, and the hand of the fleshy arm clutched, the water in the pipe subsided; but being relaxed and opened, the water rose: which seemed to shew, that in contraction the muscles, upon the whole, were brought into less dimensions than in their dilation.

The audience was evidently sceptical for they asked Goddard "to bring a full account of this experiment in writing." Eight months later he delivered a very similar account, to which he added that the level of the water in the glass pipe rose and fell with the arterial pulse, but when the fist was clutched "upon each such contraction, the water in the glass canal did descend much more . . . than between the intermissions of the pulse before mentioned."[6]

Still skeptical, one of the most distinguished Fellows present, Robert Hooke, reverted to arguing the old concept of nervous transmission, saying, "there must be a very subtle volatile spirit, that enters into the muscles; and the same must very quickly be discharged again to cause the contraction and expansion of muscles."

In the Royal Society Register of that date there is a drawing of a man's arm closed in a vessel with a small tube attached. The drawing is crude but, as Goddard noted, the experimental design was sensitive enough to register the rise and fall of the arterial pulse and, as Swammerdam had found with his experiment on the frog, there was a decrease in volume when the man made "a contraction of clutching of his fist," presumably expelling the venous return.

Jonathan Goddard (1617–1665) was educated both at Oxford and later Cambridge, where he obtained his medical degree. Unlike most of his contemporaries at Oxford he was not a Royalist and, being a competent physician, was much sought after by the Parliamentary cause, becoming Physician-in-Chief to the Parliamentary army and eventually to Cromwell himself. During the interregnum, he was appointed Warden of Merton College, Oxford, a position he had to relinquish in 1660 upon the restoration of the monarchy.

The troubles brought by the Civil War did not, however, detract from Goddard's scientific reputation and, appointed by Cromwell as professor of physic at Gresham College in London, he held the position after the return of the King. There he was instrumental in the organization of the founding of the Royal Society under a Royal Charter from Charles II in 1662. He was an active experimenter, and kept a room in his house as a laboratory.

William Croone (1633–1684)

In England, a solution to the puzzle of the mechanics of muscular contraction was just as compelling as it was to Swammerdam and Steno across the Channel. The first to put forward a truly mechanical explanation and to make some tentative experiment to support it was William Croone, professor of rhetoric at Gresham College in London, Fellow of the Royal College of Physicians, and a distinguished founding member of the Royal Society in 1662. Two other professors at Gresham proved to have interests in the nervous system— Christopher Wren, in astronomy, and John Goddard in the chair of physic.

In 1664 Croone published an anonymous treatise, *De Ratione Motus Musculorum*, but his authorship was no mystery, for he himself presented a copy to the Royal Society that same year. Ten years later, he gave his discourse on "An Hypothesis of the Structure of a

[6]*Register Book of the Royal Society*, Vol. iv, p. 95.

Muscle" at the Surgeon's Hall, where he had been appointed lecturer on muscles in 1670 (the year of his marriage), having had to resign from Gresham College because of its rule of celibacy.[7]

The basis of Croone's theory of the conditions necessary for muscular contraction was centuries-old. Two kinds of spirits had to interact: one, a "spiritous liquid," derived from the nerve and the other, "the nourishing juice of the muscle," supplied by the blood; both were entirely material. On meeting, these two substances effervesced, causing the muscle to swell "like a bladder blown up." This explanation was popular and, in various forms, was basic to those proposed later by Thomas Willis and John Mayow at Oxford.

The published works of Descartes were read at Gresham College and at Oxford, although Willis ignored him. (They were not yet read at Cambridge.) Croone quoted Descartes' *De Homine* and criticized the Cartesian concept of the animal spirits, like "a very subtle wind." He insisted that the nervous influence, coming from the brain, must be a liquid, albeit a "most subtle, active and highly volatile liquor of the nerves, in the same way as we speak of spirit of wine or salt or others of this kind (cum spiritum vini, aut salis)."[8]

Croone made some rather simple experiments to this end by cutting nerves between a muscle and the brain and demonstrating the loss of contraction, an experiment that had, in fact, been made by Galen in the 2nd century.

As to the intimate structure of the muscle, Croone essentially accepted Galen's concept of fibers continuous with the tendons, with "flesh" filling the spaces between them. Of the proposal that nonmaterial spirits were involved, Croone said "that it is utterly unintelligible to me." Although he used the word "spirits," he insisted that they were material in the sense of volatile spirits of wine. "For this reason," he said, "I have clearly shown that those spirits in the nerves, called Animal, are nothing else than a rectified and enriched juice of this kind."

In order to support an entirely mechanical and chemical explanation, Croone separated the mind from the living body, which he considered[9]

> . . .to be nothing but a kind of machine or automaton and the Mind which is in us, we may move meanwhile by its own thought, or at least we may arrange to sit in the brain merely as a spectator of this play (corporis scena) which is acted out in the scene of the body.

Having convinced himself that a liquid came down the nerve, Croone questioned what impelled it to move. He pictured the nerve as composed of fine fibers and claimed to have demonstrated their presence in the spinal marrow. He conceived of a certain tonus in these cord-like nerves, similar to tension in the vibrating string of a musical instrument. The concept of vibration in nerves carrying an impulse is one that occurred to Borelli but reached its zenith in the following century in the philosophical writings of David Hartley.[10]

Like Swammerdam, Croone did not attempt a direct experimental proof of his theory but designed some diagrams from which he derived calculations to support his ideas. In his illustration, reproduced here (Fig. 33), he described the outline of the muscle before contraction (ABCD in his Fig. 1) and depicted by broken line the contour when contracted. EFG shows the route by which the animal spirits reach the muscle from the brain (marked H) via the medulla spinalis (SE). IKO denotes the arterial supply of the muscle, with LMN marking the venous return. Croone was insistent on the importance of the role of the blood.

[7]An outcome of this marriage was one of the Royal Society's most distinguished lectureships, the Croonian Lectures, founded by his widow on his death.

[8]*De Ratione Motus Musculorum*, Section 13.

[9]*De Ratione Motus Musculorum*, Section 26.

[10]David Hartley (1705–1757). *Observations on Man, his Frame, his Duty, and his Expectations.* Johnson, London, 1749.

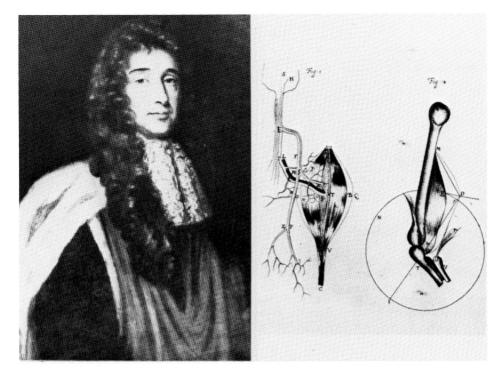

FIG. 33. **Left**: William Croone (1663–1684), from the portrait in the Royal College of Physicians. **Right**: Croone's diagram depicting the route (EFG) by which nervous fluid flows from the brain (H) to little bladders which inflate the muscle to expand from contour ABCD (*solid line*) to AQV (*dotted line*). On the right is a diagram of the direction of forces when bending the elbow. (From: *De ratione motus musculorum*, 1664.)

His description is vivid:

> For at the same time as the fibrils of the taut nerve HEG are struck in the brain, immediately these droplets of liquor exude from all its branchlets . . . this liquor creates an effervescence in the blood in an instant. And at the same instant blood flows through the artery IKO like water from an opened pipe. No sooner does the muscle begin to swell at its boundary than are the fibres also contracted, and so everything occurs at one and the same time in the twinkling of an eye. However that effervescence, as I have said, ceases almost immediately and the very active spirits are dissipated through the membranes of the muscle nearly in an instant and unless a new impulse arrives at once, the muscle is immediately pulled back and made flaccid by the inequality of the circulation of the blood through the fibres of the antagonist, and the blood flows out in greater quantity through the vein LMN.

Croone, a Londoner, fled the city at the outbreak of the plague in 1665 and traveled on the continent; in Montpelier, he met and had "considerable intercourse" with Steno. Here, almost certainly, he learned of the experiments of Steno's friend Swammerdam, proving that the volume of a muscle does not increase on contraction, for on his return to London he modified his own theory to one of a number of small bladders for each muscle fiber. Four years later he may have noted the experiment made before the Royal Society by his fellow member from Gresham College, Jonathan Goddard, which produced the same result.[11]

Croone attempted an experiment to show that when an artificial bladder changed its shape, shortening in length and expanding in width as water was poured into it, it was able to lift

[11]T. Birch. *The History of the Royal Society,* 4 vols. Millar, London, 1756–1757.

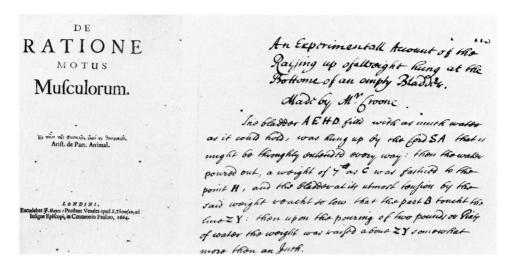

FIG. 34.   Left: Title page of Croone's work on the movement of muscles, first published anonymously in 1664.   **Right**: Notes in Croone's handwriting of an experiment in which he demonstrated to the Royal Society that, when water was poured into an empty bladder from which a weight was suspended, the bladder changed shape and lifted the weight. Croone maintained that this proved his concept of muscle contraction. (From the Register Book of the Royal Society, by courtesy of the Librarian.)

a weight attached to it. This he attributed to the pressure of the water against the sides of the bladder—the explanation that he was using for the strength of a contracted muscle. A report of Croone's experiment was submitted to the Royal Society[12] in 1661; and 10 years later, it was taught in his lectures to the Barber Surgeons (published in the English language in 1681 by the Royal Society). Each muscle fiber was thought to have "an infinite number of very small *Globules*, or little Bladders . . . all opening into one another." The mechanism of effervescence was essentially the same as in the original thesis. Time had passed and not only had the idea of a total volume increase on contraction to be jettisoned, but the findings of the early microscopists on the structure of muscle fibers needed reconsideration. Croone concluded that these confirmed his concept of "globules" on the fibers and he was pleased to read Borelli's posthumous work, which, although far more mathematical than Croone's, had developed along similar lines of hypothesis.

Although Croone's design of "bladders blown up" was not to endure, his concept of an effervescence in the muscle was close to the teaching of his contemporary, Thomas Willis, at Oxford, although Willis clung to a vitalistic explanation of the brain he so splendidly dissected. Neither Croone nor Willis faced up to the problem defined by Steno, namely, that the (muscular) heart continued to beat when taken out of the body, cut off from its nerves and blood supply (and from the soul).

Croone died in London in 1684, having left his mark on the arguments about nerves and muscle contraction. All his proposals were mechanistic in nature; his insistence on denying the action of spirits led him to his proposals of vibratory impulses in nerves and chemical reactions in muscles. It is for his application of physics and mathematics that he is remembered in the history of exploration of the nervous system as a significant figure in the 17th century.

[12]*The Register of the Royal Society*, 1:109 (Novemb. 6, 1661).

Thomas Willis (1621–1675)

Thomas Willis, the outstanding figure of the Oxford group, began his career in difficult times. The country was torn for 14 years by the Civil War, the end of which was marked by the fall of Oxford to the Parliamentary army and the surrender of the University's Royalist Legion in which Willis had enlisted as a soldier. During this stormy period Willis was in training in medicine at Oxford,[13] and it was not until after the Restoration in 1660 that his star began to rise. The University recognized him by appointing him, in 1660, Sedleian Professor of Natural Philosophy and, with his reputation as a Royalist and his increasing skill as a clinician, he was consulted by the King. In his burgeoning Oxford practice he frequently conferred with Richard Lower, who at that time was not medically qualified. Willis had been an early member of the "Invisible College," the group of brilliant minds whose meetings preceded the founding of the Royal Society, of which Willis became a member in 1663.

Willis did not accept the "indivisible" atoms of Gassendi and Charleton, although he believed in particulate elements, judging all matter to be made of five of these—"Spirit, Sulphur, Salt, Water and Earth." Spirits were of two kinds: the animal spirits, "endued with very active Particles which perpetually flow, though but in a very small quantity, through the passages of the Nerves from the Brain and Cerebel," and "the other slow and softer, which being every where laid aside through the Arteries from the bloody mass, is rendered more plentifully."

The role of the blood was immensely important to Willis. Essential to the action of the animal spirits was "nourishment" from the blood:[14]

> ...a double humor, viz. one spiritous and highly active, which flows altogether from the Brain and Cerebel, and being thence derived into the whole nervous stock, bestows upon them the sensitive and moving Faculties; and the other humor softer and more oily and sulphurous, which being supplied from the blood, and assused[15] immediately on every part, is the Author of their Heat and vegitation. Both these Juyces agree among themselves, and being every where joyned together and married, they are as it were a masculine and feminine seed mixed together; and so they impart to all parts both sense and motion, and all the powers of life and growth.

This fine anatomist used not only dissection but occasionally physiological experiment to support his insistence on the importance of the part played by the blood:

> ...and because, if the Spirit of Wine, tinctured with Ink, be put into an artery belonging to any Muscle, the Vein in the same time being tyed close, the superficies of all the fleshy fibres and transverse fibrils are dyed with blackness, the Tendons being then scarcely at all changed in their colour: it appears from hence, that the blood doth everywhere outwardly water all the flesh or fleshy fibres and only those.

This was the technique by which Willis established the anatomy of the anastomosis at the base of the brain that carries his name and is incorrectly called a "circle."

In his earlier work, Willis pictured the meeting of these two "spirits" as evoking a fermentation, as had others before him. Later, when he came to write his famous book on the anatomy of the brain, he had shifted his belief from the concept of fermentation to one of explosion (a suggestion that had been made also by Gassendi). Willis wrote:[16]

[13]One of his notebooks from this period has been preserved at the Wellcome Historical Museum.

[14]*Cerebri Anatome*, Chapter IX. Pordage translation, 1681.

[15]i.e., poured forth.

[16]*Cerebri Anatome*. Pordage translation, 1681.

> It is like the explosion of gunpowder and also the same spirits being continually consumed
> within the muscles more profusely than in the membranes and other parts, are in some
> measure restored by the nutritous blood; since the arterial juice joins more plentifully with
> the nervous juice . . . it may well be thought, that it also lays upon the spirits, brought thither
> with it, as it were certain nitro-sulphureous particles, and ultimately fixes them on them;
> and so, by reason of this copula, highly flatuous and apt to be rarified, the spirits themselves
> become more active, so that in every motive action, whereby the muscle is suddenly intu-
> mified, they, as if inkindled, are exploded.

In an age when a laudatory preface was expected for every book, Willis dedicated *Cerebri Anatome*, so brillantly illustrated by Christopher Wren, to the head of the Anglican church. The wording is that of a deeply religious man who approaches, as he says, "to unlock the secret places of Man's mind, and to look into the living and breathing Chapel of the Deity." This dedication may have eased the publication of the book through the licensing commission, for censorship was still powerful.

One of his pupils, John Locke, took notes during Willis' lectures and they have been published in an English translation.[17] From them, we learn what Willis taught about fibers, which he said ended in the muscles.

> These are not extensions of offshoots of the nerves as they are far too numerous; and, hence
> it follows that although the animal spirits continuously flow through the tubules of the nerves,
> they do not perpetually flow into and inflate the fibres. That great efflux of humours which
> sometimes accumulates from wounded tendons is not the succus carried by the nerves but
> a specific succus of the fibres. For the humour hidden in these fibres does not appear to
> consist of succus nervosus and animal spirits but partly of vital spirits carried through the
> arteries. The fibres seem to be replenished with this spirituous matter as much from the
> nerves as from the arteries, and seems to be the humidum primigenium. The spirits lying in
> these fibres are quiet until aroused by a command from the brain brought through the nerves,
> when they then perform their functions. The nerves, therefore, are a kind of channel through
> which animal spirits continuously flow whereas the fibres are lakes where they stagnate and
> are at rest.

In spite of Willis' great success in exploring the structure of the brain and nerves, he made little lasting contribution to the underlying mechanisms of their function. Willis held beliefs about the soul that forced him to consider his anatomical findings in the light of how they serviced the soul, and inevitably this colored his views of the animal spirits. These he held to "perform the offices of Sense and Motion" and to be "procreated wholly in the Cortical or Barky substance of the Brain and Cerebel." Strangely, for an anatomist, he accepted the presence of "narrow channels of the nerves," and still retained a belief that animal spirits seeped down the nerves, and that the role of the ventricles was to serve as reservoirs for this "nervous juice." "Further, we shewed that those Spirits, the Authors of either function, not only within the narrow Channels of the Nerves, but also in the large meeting places or Emporium of the Head. . . ."[18]

Recognized as a great anatomist, Willis was a powerful influence working against the growing revolt from Aristotelianism and must be held responsible for some delay in the acceptance of scientific study of the brain. He did not hesitate to speculate in assigning to anatomical structures such qualities as common sense (in the corpus striatum), imagination (in the corpus callosum), and memory (in the cerebral cortex). Memory, he likened to "a regurgitation or flowing back of the Spirit from the exterior compass of the Brain towards the middle." Animal spirits were responsible also for our appetites, which they evoked by

---

[17]K. Dewhurst. *Thomas Willis's Oxford Lectures*. Sandford, Oxford, 1980.

[18]*De Anima Brutorum*. 1672.

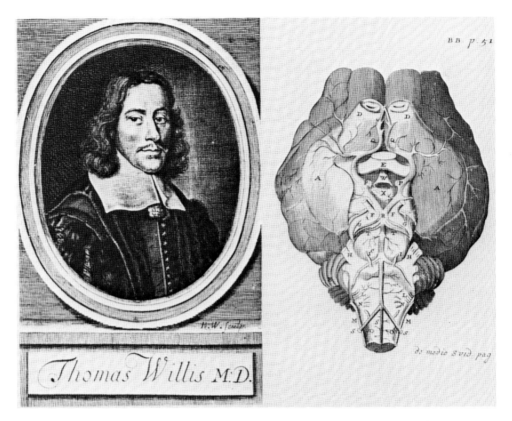

FIG. 35. Thomas Willis at the age of 45 with his dissection of a sheep's brain drawn by Christopher Wren, a strong contrast to Descartes' sketch made in the slaughterhouse.

"being moved about the middle of the brain, and from thence outwardly towards the nervous system."[19]

The corporeal soul was closely linked in Willis' thinking to animal spirits: "For the Animal Spirits, which being within the Brain, there constitute the chief Faculties of the Soul, and from thence flow into the Nervous stock, for the performing of the Spontaneous Acts of Sense and Motion."[20] These spirits, according to Willis, get "worn out and tyred" and need to be refreshed by sleep, although they are "not granted a Vacation." He made a discrimination among categories of animal spirits, some "as it were of a Superior Order, at those times keep Holy-day; but others, whose task is more assiduously required, for the Preservation of Life, are wholly inhibited." (Only those may sleep.)

Willis carried his belief in the ancient concept of animal spirits into his clinical work, especially in his explanation of convulsions. In a treatise published in 1667, *Pathologiae Cerebri*, summarized in an anonymous review in the *Philosophical Transactions* (December 9, 1667), the following appeared:

> The knowledge of the Diseases which use to affect these parts, is esteemed very difficult and intricate, and particularly the true Causes of *Convulsions* are of a very deep research. For the clearing of them up, this Author Philosophiseth after this manner. He teacheth, that

[19]*Dr. Willis' Practice of Physick*. Pordage translation, London, 1684.
[20]*De Anima Brutorum*. 1672.

there are indeed *Animal* Spirits; that they constitute the *Being* of the *Corporeal* Soul, and are also the *next* and *immediate* Instruments of all Animal motions, producing them by a kind of Explosion or Shooting, upon which *Elastick*, or *Explosive* power he establish's his whole *Doctrine* of *Convulsions*.

Writing 10 years after the posthumous publication of Descartes' *De Homine*, Willis also assigned to man alone an immaterial "Rational Soul" in command of the material corporeal soul he shares with brutes.[21] The "superior" soul "inhabits the Body, and is the Supream and principal form of the whole Man: But after Death, the Corporeal Soul being extinct, this survives and is immortal." To Willis the soul was a vital flame, reminiscent of the "feu sans lumière" of Descartes. In Willis' words, "... the soul of the Brute is Corporeal and Fiery." He had some trouble explaining away the lack of palpable heat in what he calls "the less perfect or frigid Animals." These, too, he believed to have a corporeal soul, which "seems to be as it were the specter, or the shadowy hag of the body." He gave several paragraphs of description to what he termed the "Pineal Glandula or Kernel" and commented that "we can scarce believe this to be the seat of the Soul."

In 1667, after the Great Fire of London, Willis moved to the City and there became engrossed in a thriving clinical practice until his death in 1675. His long-time assistant, Richard Lower, inherited the practice.

Willis had returned to a London devastated by the Great Fire, which had raged for four days, destroying more than three-fifths of the city. Almost immediately plans for rebuilding began under the leadership of Charles II. Several of the scientists associated with Gresham College (which escaped the fire) and from the Royal Society were involved in the plans and, although not trained architects, they produced individual charts for reconstruction of the city. Even John Evelyn, the diarist, and a lecturer at Gresham College,[22] submitted a plan. Another was Robert Hooke,[23] the microscopist and Curator of Experiments to the Royal Society, whose plan for the whole city was presented first to the Royal Society. He was appointed by the City to the main planning group, as was Christopher Wren, the experimenter on venous feeding and illustrator for Willis' anatomy. Wren was appointed by the King as one of "His Majesty's commissioners for Rebuilding," and later "Surveyor-General to the Royal Works." Coming from the anatomical dissecting room and a professorship in astronomy, he nevertheless had more architectural experience than Hooke, having designed the Sheldonian Theatre in Oxford. He, too, had a plan for city-wide rebuilding.[24] In the end, neither plan of these two scientists was adopted, although Wren left his mark on London with his designs for parish churches and for St. Paul's Cathedral, and Hooke left his on the hospital nicknamed Bedlam. In the 1940s London suffered far more widespread and more disastrous destruction from the German bombs, and much of the 17th-century planning was wiped out.

Richard Lower (1631–1691)

Richard Lower, born of puritan stock, entered Oxford (then a stronghold of Cromwell's party) in 1649, the year Charles I was beheaded. He proceeded through the usual premedical degrees to qualify as a doctor of physic in 1665. Then began a close association with Thomas Willis, the Sedleian Professor of Natural Philosophy, an association lasting beyond their

[21]*De Anima Brutorum.* 1672.

[22]*The Diary of John Evelyn*, edited by E. S. de Beer, 6 vols. Oxford, 1955.

[23]*The Diary of Robert Hooke 1672–1680*, edited by H. W. Robinson and W. Adams. London, 1935.

[24]Wren's plan is in the British Museum (Add. MS 6193). There is a print in the Library of the Society of Antiquaries.

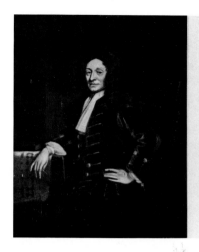 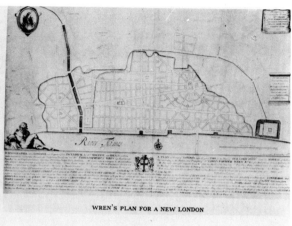

WREN'S PLAN FOR A NEW LONDON

FIG. 36. **Left**: Sir Christopher Wren, illustrator of Willis' *Cerebri Anatome*, architect of St. Paul's Cathedral, and Professor of Astronomy at Oxford. (Portrait by Kneller in the National Portrait Gallery, London.) **Right**: Wren's plan for the rebuilding of London was one of those invited by the King but not adopted. (Courtesy of the British Museum.)

Oxford days and into their years of clinical practice in London. They appear to have complemented each other well: Willis the anatomist and Lower a pioneer of experimentation. Willis acknowledged this help in the preface to *Cerebri Anatome*. A year after moving to London, Lower was elected to membership in the Royal Society.

The interests of the group of outstanding experimenters at Oxford at this time were primarily focused on the blood—perhaps because of Harvey's spectacular demonstration. Less attention was given to the functions of the nervous system in spite of Willis' fine contribution to anatomy of the brain. It was the role of the blood that captured attention: the part it played in respiration, in nutrition, and in life. In an age when intravenous feeding was unknown, there was growing interest at Oxford in the possibility not only of introducing nutrients and drugs into the blood stream as had been achieved by Christopher Wren,[25] but also of transfusing blood from one animal to another; it is with this early endeavor that Lower's name is often associated. In view of Harvey's discovery it seems strange that Lower should first attempt transfusion from vein to vein. Claude Perrault, working in Paris, had succeeded well, illustrating the technique in a drawing still preserved in the Archives of the Academie des Sciences. Lower was testing his hypothesis, as a scientist should, a hypothesis he spelled out in letters to his patron, Robert Boyle,[26] published after his death. His experiment was "to try how long a dog may live without meat, by syringing into a vein a due quantity of good broth." With the encouragement and cooperation of Boyle, he moved from this experiment to one in which he successfully transfused blood from one dog to another, as others had succeeded before him. There is also a detailed record[27] of a successful transfusion from a sheep to a man. Since the patient survived, one can only presume that his life was saved by a blood clot; however, Lower claims that he repeated the transfusion many times in the same patient.

In the context of contribution to our understanding of the nervous system, Lower's interest came through his overwhelming preoccupation with the blood, an interest shared with his

[25]A way to convey liquors immediately into the mass of the blood. *Phil. Trans. roy. Soc.*, 1:128–130 (1665).
[26]*The Works of the Honorable Robert Boyle*, edited by T. Birch. Millar, London, 1744.
[27]*Phil. Trans. roy. Soc.*, 2:1577 (1667).

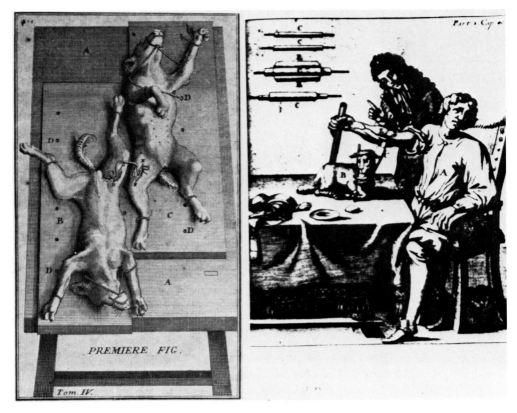

FIG. 37.   Left: Transfusion experiment of Claude Perrault. Within a tube, which he called a "siphon," he led the blood from the crural artery of one dog into the crural vein of the other. (Perrault, C. *Essais de Physique*, Vol. 4. Coegnard, Paris, 1688.)   **Right**: A sketch made at the time to illustrate the attempt by Richard Lower and Edward King to transfuse from sheep to man.

teacher, Willis. The colors of venous and arterial blood were still a puzzle and it was Lower who, by experimentation, detected that the change of color took place in the lungs by virtue of some property of the air. This problem is expanded in Lower's best known work, *Tractatus de Corde*,[28] an exhaustive description of his many experiments, published in 1669. In this book, he maintained that the heartbeat was controlled by the brain although he still believed in animal spirits collected in the "brain and cerebellum." He held that these spirits flowed by gravity from the head to the heart through the 8th pair of nerves (Willis' numbering for the vagus). Again we find Lower testing his hypothesis: He ligatured these nerves in the neck of a dog and noticed the profound change in the heartbeat.[29] More than a century and a half were to pass before the inhibitory action of the vagus on the heart was clarified by the Webers. Lower made a most intensive study of the structure of heart muscle. He boiled it, as had Baglivi, in order to study the fibers, and he was impressed by the extent of the nerve supply that he found. Another experiment on the nervous system demonstrated the effect on respiratory movements of sectioning the phrenic nerves.

Lower became involved in a controversy, aired in the meetings of the Royal Society[30] over a period of five months, concerning Steno's report (in *Musculi Description Geometrica*)

---

[28]*Tractatus de Corde*, p. 86.

[29]John Ward. *Diary*, 16 vols.

[30]T. Birch. *The History of the Royal Society*, Vol. 2. 1756.

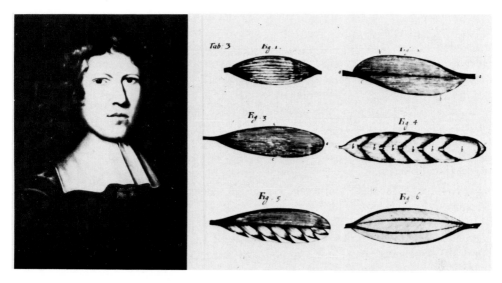

FIG. 38. **Left**: Portrait of Lower from a private collection. (Courtesy of the Wellcome Institute.) **Right**: Lower's figures to illustrate his view of limb muscles with their fibers (*b*) inserted into tendons (*a*). His *Fig. 4* shows multiple muscles, the tendons of each attached to separate vertebrae. *Fig. 6*, from the leg of a sheep, is reminiscent of Steno's diagrams. (From *Tractatus de Corde*, 1669.)

that "tying up the artery descending from the head deprived the animal immediately of all motions." This was an experiment made by Steno during his stay with Thévenot in Paris. As reported by the Dane Ole Borch:[31]

> A dog's back was pierced with a curved needle and the descending aorta bound up; the dog's back legs became completely numb and lifeless because of this, and its pulse stopped. When the binding was loosened after a few moments the legs and tail began to move again and the aorta began to pulse in the abdomen.

Some members were so sceptical that Lower was asked to repeat the experiment. On the first try he did not ligature the aorta but merely pressed with his finger. This did not stop the dog's struggles. Croone therefore requested him to repeat more exactly Steno's experiment and this he did. The animal, being freed of restraints but with the ligature still in place, bounded to its feet; to Willis and all others convinced of the primary role of the blood in muscular contraction this seemed unbelievable. Experiments were therefore repeated until finally another member, Edmund King, succeeded in confirming the original observation by Steno. The blood was vindicated.

Although Lower accepted an influence of "animal spirits" or "succus nervosus," he was unwilling, without testing by experiment, to accept a current theory that these were the origin of sperm. He searched unsuccessfully for the presence of nerves in the testicles of a boar[32] and remained sceptical.

Lower, by experiment, was able to rule out a long-standing theory about the brain, namely, that the fluids of catarrh originated in the ventricles of the brain and flowed down into the nostrils via the cribriform plate and into the mouth via the pituitary gland. Experiments on the brain of a calf convinced him that these assertions were ridiculous. He applied the same technique of injecting ink that he had used when testing Willis' claims for the "circle" at the base of the brain. It was his experimental ligaturing of the carotid and vertebral arteries that proved that Willis had indeed found an anastomosis.

[31]Ole Borch. Diary preserved in manuscript in Copenhagen. (Translation by G. Scherz).
[32]John Ward. *Diary*, 16 vols.

After many experiments, Lower became convinced that the fluids of catarrh and tears came from the serum of the blood and in no way involved the brain, "the ruling site of body and soul" (*regiam illam corporis et animae sedem*). He divined the roles of the lachrymal and maxillary glands and quoted Steno's work as support.[32a] In a definite statement of disbelief, he declared that animal spirits were contained in the ventricles as believed by the ancients and by many of his contemporaries.[33] In 1672 Lower published his work on catarrh in a small tract,[34] now rare, although reissued more than once in the following year. It carried a small section describing safe procedure for venipuncture, for he carried his views on the role of the serum to treatment of his patients whose secretions in catarrhs and phthisis stemmed, he felt, from excess of serum in the blood. Throughout his work, one perceives a clinical goal.

Lower, the puritan, had succeeded well in the quietly Catholic London of Charles II, eventually becoming Court Physician, and his book, *Tractatus de Corde* was well received. But times changed after the death of King Charles and the incoming reign of the openly Catholic James II. Lower lost his appointment to the Court and left London for his native Cornwall. He returned with the accession of William and Mary, but died shortly afterward, in 1691.

John Mayow (1641–1679)

The works of Steno had become well known in England, and we have in Oldenburg's letters the note that he received in December 1667 "Stenosis Musculi Description Geometrica." The English anatomists were still greatly influenced by Willis and found the novel mathematical approach of Steno disturbing. One of the Oxford group, resistant to Steno's contention that the change of shape of the muscle in contraction did not involve the addition of any fluid, was John Mayow.

Mayow, a Cornishman, born in 1641, became, in the brief 38 years of his life, the outstanding experimenter on respiration. Having been engaged for some years in studies of its chemistry, he was a convinced believer in the "nitro-aërial" constituents of the air we breathe (oxygen as yet undiscovered). When he wrote the five sections of his *Tractatus*, the first of these was on *Sal-nitro et Spiritu Nitro-aëreo*, but the fourth was *De Motu Musculari et Spiritibus Animalibus* (published 12 years after Steno's treatise).

Mayow's work on muscular motion was printed by a press that had recently been established in the basement of the Sheldonian Theatre in Oxford,[35] an event of great importance for the scholarly world because at the time there existed no general free press. Printers had to be licensed by the Stationers' Company, an edict from Henry VIII, who suspected the power of the printed word that had developed since Gutenberg's invention of movable type. The immense expansion of literacy that followed this achievement had earlier also frightened the Pope who, recognizing the force of Martin Luther's use of the printed word to spread his Protestant revolution, had issued a Papal Bull in 1501 restricting printed books and subjecting them to inspection. In Protestant England, the Star Chamber, to quell sedition, shut down all printing presses except those of the City of London and the two universities,

---

[32a]N. Steno. *De Musculis et Glandulis Observationum Specimen*. 1664.

[33]"Non quod credem species ipsas per eorum cavitates in ventriculos cerebri deferri, aut spiritus animales in ventriculis cerebri hospitari, prout veteres sentiebant."

[34]*De catarrhis*. 1672.

[35]One of the rare existing copies of Mayow's Treatise, printed at the Sheldonian, can be seen at the Wellcome Historical Library in London and a copy presented by Mayow himself is in the library of All Souls, Oxford.

Oxford and Cambridge. A famous voice was raised against this form of censorship and suppression: In 1644 John Milton privately printed his protest ("hee who destroyes a good Booke, kills reason it selfe . . ."),[36] the famous *Areopagitica* that remains to this day a clarion call for freedom and distribution of ideas, although relief did not come until the Star Chamber was destroyed.

Mayow was a young contemporary of John Milton who, though not himself a scientist, championed the search for new science. Milton traveled to see Galileo in his old age[37] and there is a poignancy about a visit to the old blind astronomer from the poet about to become blind.

Students of the nervous system, all had their works printed by university presses or across the Channel during the period of the ban, and, when writing on such sensitive subjects as man's brain and soul, were understandably cautious in wording their ideas—especially about the soul. Willis's *De Anima Brutorum* was printed first in Leyden, Harvey's *De Motu Cordis* in Frankfurt, and the first appearance of John Locke's famous *Essay Concerning Humane Understanding* appeared in France two years before the English printing in London.[38]

Mayow opened his discussion of muscular motion by declaring his stand on the importance of the "nitro-aërial spirit" for "aëration" of the blood, and went on to insist on its part in muscular contraction:[39]

> That Nitro-aerial Spirit is, by means of respiration, transmitted into the mass of the blood, and that the fermentation and heating of the blood are produced by it, has been elsewhere shown by us. But I shall now further add concerning the use of that inspired spirit, that it takes the chief part in the origination of animal motions, an opinion which I published now a good while ago, and still firmly hold; not that I have set myself to stick to it, as fixed to a pre-conceived hypothesis, but because I consider it most agreeable to reason.

Mayow's belief in an "explosion" of the "nitro-aërial" spirits within the fibers of the muscles made him protest Steno's concept of parallelograms of muscle fibers together with his statement that:[40]

> If a muscle should change from an oblique-angled parallelogram into a parallelogram the angles of which are less acute, as is supposed to happen in the contraction of the muscle, then it will be contracted in length, and will also swell up, without the addition of any new matter.

Mayow would not accept this concept of Steno's for he held that the muscular contraction was chiefly caused, not by the conspicuous "fleshy fibres" (which he agreed with Steno are inserted obliquely into the tendons), but by finer fibrils inserted transversely into the muscle fibers.

In order to demonstrate what he felt to be the error of Steno's model, he illustrated it in one of the plates for his own treatise.

> . . . let a, b, c, d, be the muscle, c, d, a, f, the same contracted, and although it be of the same magnitude as before, and has had no new matter added to it, has yet undergone contraction as to length, and besides, rises at f into a tumour. But, indeed, it is hardly to

[36]John Milton (1608–1674). *Areopagitica*. A speech for the Liberty of Unlicensed Printing to the Parliament of England. 1644.

[37]"There it was, in Italy," he wrote, "that I found and visited the famous Galileo, grown old a prisoner in the Inquisition, for thinking in astronomy otherwise than the Franciscan and Dominican licensers thought." *The Poetical Works of John Milton*. Nelson, London, 1851.

[38]John Locke (1632–1702). *Extrait d'un Livre Anglais que n'est pas encore publié, intitulé ESSAIE PHILO-SOPHIQUE concernant l'ENTENDEMENT ou l'on montre quelle est l'entendue de nos connoissances certaines et la manière dont nous y pervenons*. Bibliothèque Naturelle et Historique, Paris, 1688.

[39]John Mayow (1641–1679). *Tractatus Quinque Medico-physicae*. Sheldonian, Oxford, 1674.

[40]John Mayow, *Tractatus Quinque*.

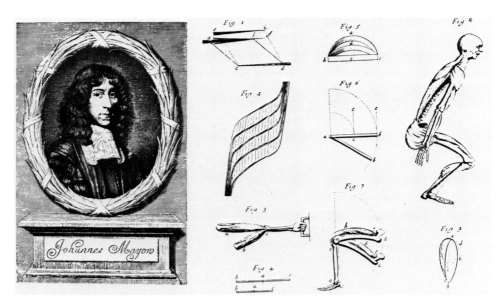

FIG. 39. Left: Portrait of John Mayow (All Souls, Oxford). **Right:** Mayow's illustration for his *Tractatus Quinque*. At the upper left is a representation of Steno's proposal of a muscle parallelogram, which Mayow criticises adversely in his text. Below this is sketched Mayow's concept of transverse fibrils responsible for the contraction of muscle. (*Tractatus Quinque.* Sheldonian, Oxford, 1674.)

> be believed that muscular fibres should be ready to start this sort of motion unless some new matter were added for that end.

Below the parallelogram of Steno's model he drew his own concept of the transverse fibrils (marked in his plate: Fig. 2) to show "the series of fibres and of fibrils, as they are seen in muscles that have been boiled for a sufficiently long time." This startling treatment of the tissue seems drastic to today's anatomist but was common procedure in the days before hardening and staining and was the technique used by many, including his contemporary, Malpighi.

In discussing his drawing, Mayow emphasized that "...in our opinion (which I should wish to express with all respect) not the fibres but the fibrils inserted transversely into them, take the chief part in muscular contraction...."

It was for the contraction of these fibrils that he needed his "nitro-aërial" spirit which he equated with the animal spirits of Willis, his powerful Oxford contemporary. Engrossed as he was with his work on respiration he proposed that the inspired "nitro-aërial" spirit was the precursor of these animal spirits, that they were carried in blood from the lungs to the dura mater, which, he was convinced, pulsated. These pulsations pressed the "nitro-aërial" spirits into the brain, where they became the animal spirits distributed through nerves to the muscles. There, they encountered "sulphureous particles" exuded from the blood, the result being an "effervescence" that inflated the muscle.[41]

> ...that for the contraction of the muscles there is as we have indicated above, absolute need, not only of animal spirits, brought by the nerves from the brain, but in addition, of other particles supplied by the blood.

Mayow was aware of some difficulties in view of commonly held beliefs and the recent demonstrations that the nerves had no cavities to carry the animal spirits to the muscles.

---

[41]A similar proposal was made for heart muscle by Pierre Chirac of Montpellier. (*De motu cordis adversaria analytica.* Montpellier, 1698.)

Nevertheless, he held that "they pass in a moment through filaments of the nerve, although these have no visible cavity," and describes them as "so slender that they are at once dissipated and leave no vestige of themselves."

More disturbing to him was the general belief that identified the animal spirits with the soul.

> I may note here, by the way, that while I hold that nitro-aërial particles are the animal spirits, I do not wish to be so understood as if I thought nitro-aërial spirit to be the sensitive soul itself: for we must suppose that the sensitive soul is something quite different from animal spirits and that it consists of a special subtle and ethereal matter but that the nitro-aërial particles, i.e. the animal spirits, are its chief instrument. For, indeed, as to the sensitive soul, I can form no other notion about it than that it is some more divine aura, endowed with sense from the first creation and co-existensive with the whole world, and that a little portion of it, contained in a properly disposed subject, exercises functions of the kind which we observe and admire in the bodies of animals; but that that spiritual material, existing out of the bodies of living things, is not to be supposed either to perceive or to do anything but to lie quite dormant and inert, being much as is the case with the sensitive soul when the animal is buried in sleep.

Mayow's concept, outlined in 1668 and developed more fully in 1674, clearly owed a great deal to the views of Thomas Willis on muscular contraction, although he did not accept them entirely. He quoted the following paragraph from *De Anima Brutorum* to indicate his opinion of the author's theories:[42]

> That an impulse transmitted by the nerves, as it were a token, is required, and that this is done by other spirits sent from the brain, while, namely these inflowing spirits, by their varying approach to the muscles, regulate the innate spirits in their various movements, whether of expansions or of retreats.

Mayow remarked that "This theory of the learned author is certainly very ingenious, but I am not sure that it is in the same degree in accordance with truth." Mayow thought it essential that of the two agents needed for "effervescence," one had to be delivered by the blood. Another famous Oxonian (Richard Lower) had, from his own experiments, concluded that "the blood in its passage through the lungs absorbs air."[43] Mayow's interest lay in its passage from the blood to the tissues and, most importantly, to the muscles.

Mayow was elected to the Royal Society in 1678, a year before his early death. This recognition came to him essentially because of his contributions to unraveling the puzzle of respiration. In his first treatise, *Tractatus de Respiratione*, written at the age of 25, he had declared the air we breathe to contain some combustible element essential to life. As worded in a contemporary review of his *Tractatus*, he held that "there is something in the Air absolutely necessary to life, which is conveyed into the Blood, which, whatever it may be, being exhausted, the rest of the Air is made useless and no more fit for Respiration."[44] This was 100 years before Lavoisier's recognition of the role of oxygen in animal life.[45]

In this period there was a common link among men of science—an ardent search for some clue to the power of man's brain. Their work introduced problems that had previously lain in the realm of philosophy. The questions they raised were fundamental, for they began to lead away from the long reign of Aristotelianism; philosophers were thus inevitably drawn into discussions of the actual neural findings of the experimenters. The growing recognition of the importance of the brain was beginning to challenge the concepts of free will and, for

[42]Thomas Willis (1621–1674). *De Anima Brutorum quae hominis vitalis ac sensitiva est, exertationes duae.* Oxford, 1672.

[43]Richard Lower (1631–1691). *Tractatus de Corde; item de Motu et Colore Sanguinis.* 1669.

[44]*Phil. Trans. roy. Soc.* (1668), p. 833.

[45]Antoine-Laurent Lavoisier (1743–1794). *Mémoire sur les changements que le sang éprouve dans les poumons et sur le méchanisme de la respiration.* Procès-verbaux de l'Académie des Sciences, 1777.

the theologians, the supremacy of the soul. The 17th century is the first in which we meet this shared interest and actual interplay between the experimental scientist and the concept-seeking philosopher.

BIBLIOGRAPHY

Walter Charleton (1619–1707)

Selected Writings

The Darkness of Atheism Dispelled by the Light of Nature. A Physico-theological treatise. London, 1652.

Physiologia Epicuro-Gassendo-Charltoniana: or a Fabrick of Science Natural, upon the Hypothesis of Atoms. Newcomb, London 1654. (Available in facsimile in: *Sources of Science*, No. 31, edited by Hugh Kargon, 1966.)

The Immortality of the Human Soul, Demonstrated by the Light of Nature. William Wilfem, London, 1657.

Exercitiones Physico-anatomicae sive Oeconomia Animalis in Medicina Hypothesibus Superstructurae. Ravesteynium, Amsterdam, 1659.

Natural History of Nutrition, Life and Voluntary Motion. Herringman, London, 1659.

The Harmony of Natural and Positive Divine Laws. London, 1682.

Secondary Sources

Pagel, W. The reaction to Aristotle in Seventeenth-Century Biological Thought. In *History, Philosophy and Sociology of Science*, Vol. 1, edited by E. A. Underwood, pp. 489–509. Oxford University Press, London, 1953.

Pierre Gassendi (1592–1655)

Selected Writings

Exercitationem paradoxicarum adversus Aristoteleos, libre septem. Grenoble, 1624.

De Vita et Moribus Epicuri, libri octo. Lyons, 1647.

Animadversiones in decimum librum Diogenis Laertii, qui est de vita, moribus placitisque Epicuri, 3 vols. Lyons, 1649.

Philosophiae Epicuri Syntagma, cum refutationibus dogmatum quae contra fidem christianam ab eo asserta sunt, oppositis per Petrum Gassendum. The Hague, 1649.

Syntagma Philosophicum (logica, physica, ethica) (posthumous), 1658.

Secondary Sources

Bloch, O. R. *La Philosophie de Gassendi: Nominalism, Matérialism et Métaphysique.* Paris, 1971.

Sortais, G. *La Philosophie Moderne*, Vol. 2. Lethielleux, Paris, 1920.

Spink, J. S. *Free Thought from Gassendi to Voltaire.* Athlone Press, London, 1960.

Francis Glisson (1597–1677)

Selected Writings

De rachitide, sive morbo puerili, qui vulgo the rickets dicitur. London, 1650. (English translation, *A Treatise of the Rickets*, by P. Armin. London, 1651.)

Tractatus de Anatomia Hepatis. Pullein, London, 1654.

Tractatus de Natura Substantiae Energetica. Brome and Hooke, London, 1672.

Tractatus de Ventriculo et Intestinis. Brome, London, 1677.

Secondary Sources

Bastholm, E. The history of muscle physiology. *Act. Hist. Sci. Nat. Med.* 7:1–253 (1950).

Grmek, M. D. La motion de fibre vivante chez les médecins de l'école iatrophysique. *Clio. Med.*, 5:297–318 (1970).

William Croone (1633–1684)

Selected Writings

De Ratione Motus Musculorum. (Published anonymously, bound with Thomas Willis' *Cerebri Anatome.*) Hayes, London, 1665. Amsterdam, 1667.

An hypothesis of the structure of a muscle, and the reason of its contraction; read in the Surgeons Theatre, Anno 1674. *Philosophical Collections*, No. 2:22–25 (1681).

Secondary Sources

Ward, John. *The Lives of the Professors of Gresham College.* London, 1740.

Wilson, L. G. William Croone's theory of muscular contraction. *Royal Society Notes and Records*, 16:158–178 (1960).

Thomas Willis (1621–1675)

Selected Writings

Diatribae duae Medico-philosophicae, quarum prior agit de fermentatione sive de motu intestino particularum in quovis corpore. Martyn and Allestry, London, 1659. [In: *Dr. Willis' Practice of Physick, Being the Whole Works* (translated by S. Pordage). London, 1664.]

Cerebri Anatome cui accessit nervorum descriptio et usus. Martyn and Allestry, London, 1664.

Pathologiae Cerebri, et Nervosi Generis Specimen. In *Quo agitur de morbis convulsivus, et de scorbuto.* Allestry, Oxford, 1667.

De Anima Brutorum quae hominis vitalis ac sensitiva est. Davis, Sheldonian, Oxford, 1672. (Translation by S. Pordage: *Two Discourses concerning the Soul of Brutes which is that of the Vital and Sensitive of Man.* Stationers' Hall, London, 1683.)

The London Practice of Physick, being the Practical Part of Physick containing the works of the famous Dr. Willis (translated by S. Pordage). London, 1684.

The Anatomy of the Brain and the Description and Use of the Nerves. [Facsimile of Samuel Pordage's translation (1681) of *Cerebri Anatome*, entitled *The Remaining Medical Works of that Famous and Renowned Physician Dr. Thomas Willis*, edited by W. Feindel.] McGill University Press, Montreal, 1965.

Secondary Sources

Dewhurst, K. *Thomas Willis's Oxford Lectures*. Sandford, Oxford, 1980.

Feindel, W. (Ed.). Tercentenary edition of Pordage's translation of *Cerebri Anatome*. McGill University Press, Montreal, 1965.

Foster, M. *Lectures on the History of Physiology during the 16th, 17th and 18th centuries*. Cambridge University Press, London, 1901. (Reprinted: Dover, New York, 1970.)

Frank, R. *Harvey and the Oxford Physiologists*. University of California Press, Berkeley, 1980.

Isler, H. *Thomas Willis 1621–1675. Doctor and Scientist*. Hafner, New York, 1968.

Meyer, A., and Hierons, R. A note on Thomas Willis' views on the corpus striatum and the internal capsule. *J. Neurol. Sci.*, 1:547–554 (1964).

Richard Lower (1631–1691)

Selected Writings

Diatribae Thomae Willisii MD et Prof. Oxon. De febribus vindicatio, adversus Edm. de Meara Ormondiensem Hibern, MD. Martyn and Allestry, London, 1665.

Tractatus de Corde item de motu et colore sanguinis et chyli in eum transitu. Allestry, London, 1669. Elzevir, Amsterdam, 1669. (English translation by K. J. Franklin and facsimile in: *Early Science in Oxford*, Vol. 9, edited by R. T. Gunther, 1923.)

De Catarrhis. London, 1672. (English translation by R. Hunter and I. Macalpine. Dawsons, London, 1963.)

Secondary Sources

Hoff, E. C., and Hoff, P. M. The life and times of Richard Lower, physiologist and physician. *Bull. Inst. Hist. Med.*, 4:517–535 (1936).

Frank, R. *Harvey and the Oxford Physiologists*. University of California Press, Berkeley, 1981.

John Mayow (1641–1679)

Selected Writings

Tractatus duo Quorum prior agit de Respiratione: Alter de Rhachitide. Oxford, 1668.

Tractatus Quinque Medico-Physici. Quorum primus agit de Sal-Nitro, et Spiritu Nitro-aëreo. Secundus de Respiratione. Tertius de Respiratione foetus in utero, et ovo. Quartus de Motu Musculari, et Spiritibus animalibus. Ultimus de Rhachitide. Oxonii, e. Theatro Sheldoniano, Oxford, 1674.

Secondary Sources

Gotch, Francis. *Two Oxford Physiologists*. Clarendon Press, Oxford, 1908.

Partington, J. R. The life and work of John Mayow (1643–1679). *ISIS*, 47:217–230, 405–417 (1956).

The Medical-Physical Works of John Mayow LLD, MD, 1674. Published by the Alemic Club. Livingston, London, 1957.

CHAPTER V

Emphasis on Structure

(In a period when experiment was beginning to invade the peripheral nervous system very few had attempted to test the ancient concepts of the brain other than by anatomical studies such as those of Willis. Only in the living animal could function of the brain be studied, and the pioneers of ablation technique were few compared with their successors in the next century. Surgical techniques were so primitive, and understanding of cerebral circulation so scant, that the animals frequently succumbed to the procedures, and the early attempts at surgery were so drastic that results were rarely specific./ For example, the experimental results that led Willis to believe the cerebellum to be a vital center were probably due to his animals having succumbed to injuries near the fourth ventricle. Another experimenter with ablation techniques, facing the same difficulties, was Perrault.

Claude Perrault (1613–1688)

Claude Perrault wanted to test whether the brain alone was the seat of the soul, since he could not accept that its control over the whole body was effected by effusion of animal spirits from the brain. Although he did accept the flow of spirits in nerves, total control by such a process seemed mechanically impossible; moreover, in many zoological studies he had seen snakes wriggle away after being partially dissected. Perrault was not satisfied with such a localized control center, and, to test if the soul permeated the whole organism, he set about some experiments on dogs to examine their faculties after surgical interference with their brains. One wishes he had had more success: His dogs did not live long enough to be really useful for study. He was an indefatigable dissector of all kinds of animals, a pioneer in comparative anatomy. A picture in the Museum d'Histoire Naturelle (now in the Jardin des Plantes) depicts Perrault overseeing the dissection of a fox taking place in the "cabinet d'Histoire naturelle du Jardin du

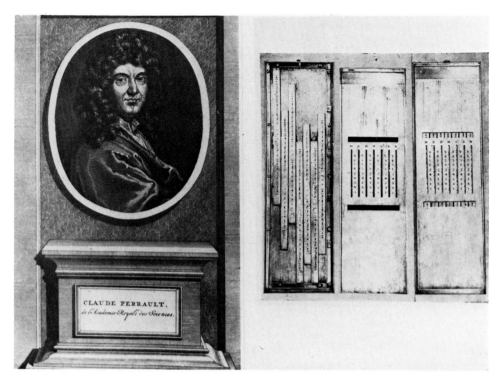

FIG. 40. **Left:** Claude Perrault (1613–1688), explorer of the nervous system, designer of the co-lonnade of the East wing of the Louvre, and a founding member of the Académie des Sciences. (Copy of portrait by Philippe de Champaigne in the Archives of the Académie des Sci-ences.) **Right:** Perrault's "Abaque Rhabdologique" for addition and subtraction. (Courtesy of the Conservatoire des Arts et Métiers.)

Roi," with Duverney behind him being shown an illustration from Perrault's book, which includes extensive studies of animals—of touch, taste, smell, and the questioned role played by the soul. Perrault's concept of muscle contraction was in sharp contrast to that of his contemporaries. He held that spirits "which come from the brain" act to relax the antagonist, contraction of the opposing muscle being a passive and secondary reaction.

Perrault was a brilliant man, eminent as a scientist, zoologist, physician, and architect. One sees his talent in the design of the whole east wing of the Louvre, with its pillared façade, and also in the Observatory. This many-faceted genius also designed a calculating machine (machine à l'addition), which he called the "Abaque rhabdologique," a design entirely independent of Pascal's, working on a system of sliding rulers. He died before he could construct more than one machine, but a detailed description of its operation was published in the large tome entitled *Oeuvres Diverses de Physique et de Mécanique*, and the instrument is preserved in the Conservatoire des Arts et Métiers in Paris. These mechanically driven sliding rulers are reminiscent of "Napier's Bones," which were operated manually and were the precursors of logarithms.[1]

Giovanni Alphonso Borelli (1608–1679)

At a time when, in England, Willis was proposing fermentation as a force blowing up the muscle during contraction, the same general principle was being tested by Giovanni Alphonso

[1]J. Napier (1550–1617). *Rabdologiae, seu numerationis per virgulas.* Edinburgh, 1617.

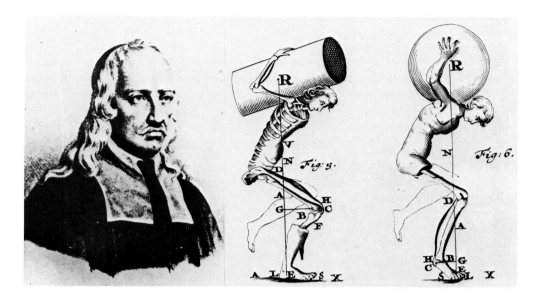

FIG. 41. Giovanni Alphonso Borelli and one of his sketches showing the center of gravity when carrying a load. (From *De motu animalium*. Bernado, Rome, 1680–1.)

Borelli in Pisa. Borelli, an heir to the Renaissance and destined to experience its decline, was born in 1608 in Naples in the Kingdom of the Two Sicilies. A talented mathematician, who trained in Rome, he taught mathematics at the University of Messina for 13 years until in 1656 he was appointed to the professorship of mathematics at Pisa. In a still fragmented Italy, both Naples and Messina were under Spanish domination. The move to Pisa was to Tuscany and the patronage of the Medici brothers.

It was at Pisa that Borelli formed a lasting friendship with Malpighi, a friendship that was to yield an intense correspondence that has become a classic.[2] It was also at Pisa that Borelli focused his mathematical mind on muscles, establishing an anatomical laboratory in his house to study their structure.

Although a prolific writer, Borelli did not live to see the publication of his major work in biological science *(De motu animalium)*, although some of the studies had been heralded by earlier publications. In *De vi percussionis* (1667) he examined mathematically the impact on bodies of accelerating forces, and in *De motionibus naturalibus a gravitate pendentibus* (1670) he wrote of his studies on floating bodies.

In the great posthumous book, *De motu animalium*, which is profusely illustrated, his studies are of the mechanics of men and animals when standing or walking under burdens of different weights, when running, and of the flight of birds.[3] He was fascinated by the swim bladders of fish, and argued from them to the design for a scuba diver. His arguments

[2]H. B. Adelmann (Ed.). *The Correspondence of Marcello Malpighi*, 5 vols. Cornell University Press, Ithaca and London, 1975.

[3]Translation in *Aeronautical Classics #6*. London, 1911.

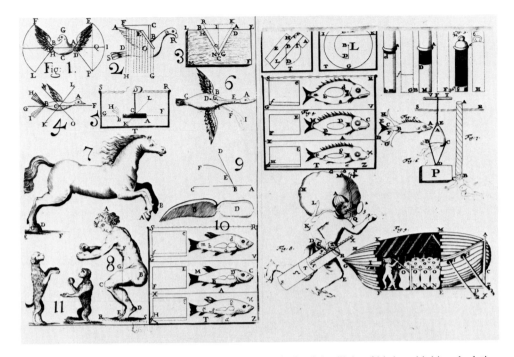

FIG. 42.   Left: Among other diagrams, Borelli's analysis of the flight of birds, with his calculation of the quantity of air acted upon by the wing span *(fig. 1)*; the motion of the wings for level flight *(fig. 2)*; the movement of the tail for upward or downward flight *(fig. 4)*; and the turning of the neck to move right or left *(fig. 6)*. **Right:** Analysis of the swim bladder of fishes changing at different depths *(fig. 4)* and the argument from this for an underwater boat *(fig. 9)*. Several sketches to show how a man underwater could continue to breathe air *(figs. 7 and 8)*. (From *De motu animalium*, Vol. I, 1680.)

were all clearly influenced by the mechanical teachings of Galileo, who had also questioned the mechanics by which fish achieve hydrostatic equilibrium.[4]

What is clearest in Borelli's writing on the flight of birds is the mathematical relation of the strength of the muscles in the movement of the wings, the velocity of wingbeat, and the weight of the bird. (The hollow structure of the bird's wing bones was not yet known.) He calculated that, in order to achieve flight, the weight of the pectoral muscles needs to be large in proportion to body weight, and he declared that man's failure to fly, even with enormous wings attached to his arms, was due to the low proportion of the pectoral muscles in the total weight of the body. Consequently he doubted the possibility of the mythical flight of Icarus.

In Borelli's second volume of *De motu animalium* he questioned the inner "chemistry" of the contracting muscle and laid to rest the concept of an action by gaseous spirits. Peripheral muscles were still regarded to be rather like balloons, inflated by nervous fluid or gaseous spirits reaching them through hollow nerves. Borelli conceived and performed an ingenious experiment in which he submerged a struggling animal in water and then slit its muscles, demonstrating that the spirits could not be gaseous since no bubbles appeared in spite of the violent contractions. Therefore, he concluded, muscle inflation and contraction could not be due to gaseous spirits ("Igitur non a spiritibus corporeis inflantur & moventur"). This

---

[4]Galileo. *Discorsi e dimostrazioni matematiche intorno a due nuove scienze attenenti alla mecanica e i movimenti locali*, 1638.

experiment led him to the suggestion of a liquid medium (a "succus nerveus") coming from the nerve and mixing in the muscle to cause a contraction by explosive fermentation ("ebullitio et displosio"). Borelli wrote that, upon cutting a nerve, "spiritous droplets" were squeezed out. One feels he would not have been surprised by the 20th century discovery of axoplasmic transport.

Borelli's letters reveal that he was familiar with Descartes' mathematics in *Discours de la Méthode*, but we find no reference to the *Traité de l'Homme*. The concept of a chemical interaction being involved in muscle contraction has some similarity to the short treatise by Croone although, as this was published anonymously, there is no mention of his name in Borelli's writings. Unlike Croone, however, Borelli recognized that the muscle does not increase in volume during contraction (presumably, he heard of Swammerdam's unpublished experiment from Steno when he came to live in Tuscany). In other letters he writes about Glisson's *Anatomia Hepatis*, but there is no mention of his reading the treatise on the stomach and intestines[5] in which Glisson reports Goddard's experiment to test whether a man's arm contracting under water causes the water level to rise.

Borelli concerned himself also with the actual structure of muscle in which he recognized two sorts of contraction: an elasticity, or tonus, and the active limb movement. From his correspondence we know that he was using the new technical aid that Malpighi had introduced at Pisa—the microscope. He was also familiar with Steno's concept that the fleshy part of the muscle was attached in the form of a parallelepiped to noncontractile tendons at each end. Borelli accepted that the tendons did not contract and could not be stretched but he developed a different concept of the geometrical arrangement of the muscle fibers, favoring rhomboids, which became shortened and hardened on inflation by fermentation. For fermentation, he argued, two agents are needed: one coming from the nerve (which it does not inflate) and another derived from the blood but already in the muscle, with which it reacts with "ebullition." The initiation of this movement of the liquid in the nerve was held to be a physical disturbance or agitation arising in the brain.

Contraction was a continuing puzzle, not only in respect to limb muscles; at that time, attention was drawn to the heart by the publication of William Harvey's magnificent treatise *De Motu Cordis*.[6] This small book (72 pages) disproved the long-held doctrine that the motion of the blood in the arterial and venous systems was a tidal ebb and flow, independent except for some leakage through Galen's (hypothetical) "pores" in the interventricular septum.[7] By experimental sequential ligaturing of arteries and veins, Harvey proved his own hypothesis "that the blood in the animal body is impelled in a circle, and is in a state of ceaseless motion."

Historians have found that Harvey's statement that "the beat of the heart produces a perpetual circular motion of the blood" was made several years before publication of his book. In the previous century, in order to provide for the study of anatomy, Henry VIII (whose encouragement of anatomy was acknowledged by the dedication to him of Vesalius' *Epitome*) granted a charter in 1540 to the Barber-Surgeons giving permission to use the bodies of felons for experiments. A quarter of a century later, his daughter Elizabeth extended the charter to the College of Physicians, and it was in their halls, in his position as Lumleian Lecturer, that Harvey made his first announcement of the circulation of the blood in 1616.

---

[5]Francis Glisson (1597–1677). *Tractatus de ventriculo et intestinis.* Henry Brome, London, 1677.

[6]William Harvey (1578–1657). *Exercitatio anatomica de motu cordis et sanguinis in animalibus.* Fitzeri, Frankfurt, 1628.

[7]Although depicted by Leonardo da Vinci, no pores exist in the interventricular wall.

The handwritten notes (in Latin) in which Harvey made this momentous statement can be seen in the Sloane collection in the British Museum.[8] But even this triumph of the empirical method did not unseat Harvey's belief in a soul located in the blood ("anima ipsa esse sanguis"). Harvey was Galenist enough to accept the *rete mirabile* as the destination of the blood within the cranium, although doubt as to the existence of a rete in man had already been raised by Berengario da Carpi,[9] the great surgeon-anatomist of Bologna, 100 years earlier.

Harvey had his own views on nervous function. "I believe," he wrote, "that in the nerves there is no progression of spirits, but irradiation; and that the actions from which sensation and motion result are brought about as light is in air, perhaps as the flux and reflux of the sea." He came to the defense of Aristotle on the primacy of the heart, stating in his final chapter: "We must not disagree with Aristotle concerning the principality of the heart by asking whether it receives motion and sensation from the brain...." His contemporary, Willis, granted that the brain was the organ of sense (Aristotle's "sensorium commune"), but held it to have only a controlling, not an initiating, action on the muscles. He also believed that the muscular walls of the heart thickened on contraction. For the mathematician Borelli, such a view left open the role of the nerves in the working of the heart as a mechanical pump.

Whether or not the blood was involved in muscular contraction was of such importance to Borelli's concept that he necessarily became concerned with its circulation, credit for the clarification of which he gave to both Cesalpino and Harvey.[10] Cesalpino,[11] who had been Professor of Medicine at Pisa in the previous century, had indeed reached a concept, somewhat similar to Harvey's: a systole sending blood not only throughout the system via the aorta, but also by a different route to the lungs, where it was cooled and then returned to the heart. But, unlike Harvey, he did not recognize the function of the venous valves and made no experimental proof of his concept beyond the dissection of the blood vessels.

That the contraction of the heart must be the energy source to drive the blood throughout the body intrigued the mathematical mind of Borelli who wrote several propositions on the subject with calculations and illustrations.

While in Pisa, Borelli became one of the group drawn together by the Medici brothers, admirers of science, in the famous, but short-lived, Accademia del Cimento. Founded in 1657, this was a gathering of nine savants, all greatly influenced by Torricelli and by the views of Galileo (who had died in the previous decade). Borelli took an active part in planning and in experimental demonstrations, traveling to Florence for the rather sporadic meetings in the Pitti Palace. Essentially mathematicians, physicists, and philosophers, the group's one publication (in which their contributions were anonymous) contains no biological observations except that small animals fail to survive in a vacuum (and to report that toads are not generated from rain as had been reported by Della Porta[12]). Entitled *Saggi di naturali esperienze*,[13] this now famous book followed Galileo's custom of writing in the vernacular

[8]William Harvey. *Praelectiones anatomicae universalis*, edited by Royal College of Physicians (edited notes of Harvey's Lumleian Lectures, 1616–1656). Churchill, London, 1886. English translation by C. D. O'Malley, F. N. L. Poynter, and K. F. Russel.

[9]G. Berengario da Carpi (1460–1550). *Isagogae breves, perlucidae*. In: *Anatomiam humani corporis, ad suorum scholasticorum preces in lucam edisae*. Bologna, 1522. (English translation by H. Jackson. *A Description of the Body of Man, Being a Practical Anatomy*. London, 1664.)

[10]*De motu animalium*, Vol. 2, p. 44.

[11]Andrea Cesalpino (1524–1603). *Questionum Peripateticarum Libri*. Venice, 1571.

[12]Giambattista Della Porta (1535–1615). *Magia naturalis*. Naples, 1558.

[13]*Saggi di naturali esperienze fatte nell'Accademia del Cimento*. Cocchini, Firenze, 1666–1667.

and was published in Italian in 1666–7, attracting little attention until translated, in 1731, into Latin, the language of scholars, by the Dutchman Pietrus van Musschenbroek, Professor of Mathematics at Leyden.

The Accademia closed in 1667, some members having moved away, including Borelli who left Tuscany to return to Messina. The city of Florence has preserved many scientific instruments of the Accademians (including some of Borelli's) in its Museum of the History of Science[14] and many manuscripts in the Collezione Galileiana at the Biblioteca Nazionale Centrale.

Of the Medicis, those great patrons of science, Ferdinand, the Grand Duke, died in 1670; Leopold, his younger brother, was elected a Cardinal and died in 1675. Their deaths brought to an end the Renaissance.

When Borelli returned to the University at Messina, he began systematically to write out his work. Already a prolific writer on mathematical and physical subjects, including astronomy, his last work was concerned with biological science and he combined his knowledge of mathematics with the results of his anatomical studies in Pisa. These were not published until after his death. The anatomical studies were found to consist of two parts: the external movements of the skeletal system and the internal movements of the viscera—in particular, the heart. The two sections were combined under the title *De motu animalium*. (Borelli's book did not please all mathematicians. One critic was Sir Christopher Wren, then president of the Royal Society.) When the second edition was published in 1743, bound with it was a dissertation filled with calculations inspired by Borelli's proposals: *De motu musculorum*, by Johann Bernoulli, a scion of the famous mathematical family of Basel. The calculations on effervescence and fermentation were republished separately in 1690.[15] Bernoulli's comments highlight the arguments between the iatrochemists, represented by Mayow and Willis, and the iatromechanists.

During the last decade of his life Borelli left Messina because of the uprising against Spanish domination, in which his life was threatened. He went to Rome, gained the patronage of Queen Christina, and joined the "Accademia Reale," which she had founded in 1674. It is to her patronage that we owe the publication of the two-volume *De motu animalium*, following his death in 1679.

Marcello Malpighi (1628–1694)

Malpighi, friend of Borelli and one of the outstanding microscopists of the 17th century, made his major contributions in areas other than the nervous system. His most famous treatise is *De pulmonibus*, in which the intimate structure of lung tissue was revealed for the first time. This work did not appear first as a formal treatise but as two letters written to Borelli in 1661. And it is in other letters that we find Malpighi's first writings on the brain. In a letter dated 1664 to Carlo Fracassati, Professor of Medicine at Pisa, Malpighi wrote his short account *De cerebro*. This evoked a longer dissertation *(Dissertatio epistolica responsoria de cerebro)* from Fracassati.[16] Published later (1669) in Amsterdam, Malpighi's letter was illustrated by insert drawings: one of the optic lobes and one said to depict the intimate structure of the optic nerve. Both stemmed from his dissections of fish, studies of whose brains led him to conclude that the ventricles served no useful purpose, and to speculate

[14]Maria Luisa Righini Bonelli. In: *Celebrazione della Accademia del Cimento nel Tricentenario della Fondazione*. Pisa, 1958.

[15]Johann Bernoulli (1667–1748). *De effervescentia et fermentatione*. Basel, 1690.

[16]Fracassati. *Epistolica de Lingua ad D. To. Alphronsum Borellium Casparum Commelinsum*. Amsterdam, 1669.

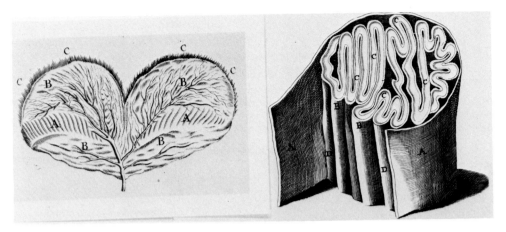

FIG. 43. Drawings pasted into the 1669 edition of Malpighi's letter to Fracassati. **Left:** Optic lobes of a fish opened to show: **A,** white fibers coursing out of the ventricles; **B,** outer section of the cortex through which pass blood vessels; **C,** white fibers of the brain running subcortically. **Right:** Drawing of the white matter of the optic lobes of the fish. **A,** outer membrane; **B,** thin membrane enclosing bundles of nerves and their blood supply; **C,** transverse cut through nerve substance.

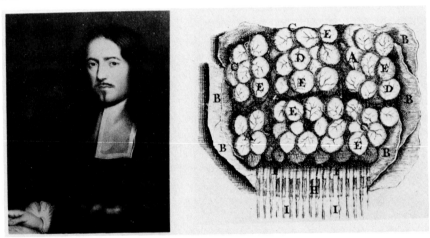

FIG. 44. **Left:** Marcello Malpighi. (Portrait in the Galleria Borghese in Rome.) **Right:** Malpighi's illustration of "minute glands" which he saw through his primitive microscope when he examined brain tissue. They were artifacts contributed by his having boiled the tissue in aqueous solution. (From Malpighi, *De cerebri cortice*, as published by Bidloo in *Anatomia humani corporis*, Amsterdam, 1685.)

that they were formed by an accident of nature.[17] In discussing the optic system he comments that Descartes' *Dioptrics* was plausible and an "inventium famigeratissimi."

Where Malpighi's interpretations of what he saw through the microscope misled him was in his studies of the cortex, published in 1666 in *De viscerum structura exercitatio anatomica*. He described a mass of very small glands with fibrils extending from the cortex down into the white matter of the brain. He provided no drawing but when Bidloo[18] included this short

[17]"Cerebri ventriculos nullius usus gratia, sed per accidens a Natura suisse efformatos."

[18]G. Bidloo. *Anatomia humani corporis*. Someren, Amsterdam, 1685.

essay in his major work he employed an artist to illustrate it. Unfortunately, Malpighi was misled by formations in the preparation of his specimens (which he boiled) and, although earlier claimed by some as nerve cells, these objects are now certainly recognized as artifacts. Believing them to be nerve cells, Malpighi himself held to old concepts that they received material from the blood transformed into a nervous fluid in the gland from whence it flowed down hollow nerves.

Another study in the nervous system was Malpighi's detection of sensory receptors in the papillae of the tongue, described first in a letter to Borelli in 1664 (*Exercitatio epistolica de lingua*), an important discovery that led him to look for, and find, sensory receptors in the skin.

Malpighi is claimed as a distinguished son by the Bolognese, having spent the first half of his life there and gaining his first professorship in medicine at its University in 1656. He moved to Tuscany when he received an appointment at the University of Pisa, and there he met and was influenced by Borelli. He was to return shortly to Bologna and then move to the University of Messina where Borelli himself spent his final productive years. Malpighi returned to teach in Bologna for 25 years, in the Teatro Anatomico built for him in the beautiful 16th-century Archiginnasio. Massively damaged in World War II, this fine lecture theatre has been meticulously restored, leaving no trace of the disaster.

In his work on plant and animal tissues, Malpighi came close to major discoveries such as the capillaries in the lungs (also seen and sketched by Leeuwenhoek), although the universal role of capillary networks in the circulation escaped him (as they had also escaped Harvey). He thought that the movement of the lungs in respiration pumped the blood through these capillaries. He also described what we know to be blood corpuscles; he thought they were globules of fat. Although his contribution to knowledge of the nervous system was meager, his work on the viscera (liver, kidneys, spleen) was outstanding for his time, as was his work in embryology. He became renowned in Europe, receiving invitations to send his reports to the Royal Society, which also undertook the publication of some of his books.[19]

The correspondence with Malpighi originated with Oldenburg, Secretary to the Royal Society. This was a time when the king (James I) was pressing for an increase in the silk industry and cultivation of the silkworm (the natural history of which was one of Malpighi's interests). The favorite food of the silkworm is the leaf of the mulberry tree, introduced in England for that reason in 1609; many Londoners today owe the presence in their gardens of these long-lived, lavishly fruit-bearing trees to the royal initiative (and perhaps indirectly to Malpighi).

Malpighi, who had been honored with membership by the Royal Society, died in Rome where he had been acting as physician to Pope Innocent XII. As was the custom one of his pupils, Georgio Baglivi, performed the autopsy. Originally written in Italian and circulated, as was also the custom, to all of Malpighi's friends, the manuscript can be seen in the Archives of the University of Bologna. (The diagnosis was apoplexy.) Later, Baglivi published it in Latin in his *De Proxi Medica* (1696).

Giorgio Baglivi (1668–1706)

Toward the end of the 17th century a new voice was heard. As the century had progressed and the use of the microscope had turned men's minds toward the structural elements composing the organs, an all-embracing theory was promulgated by Giorgio Baglivi, namely,

[19]*Phil. Trans. roy Soc.*, 14:601–608, 630–646 (1684).

that the functional element in all tissues was the fiber. (Two centuries later physiologists were to insist it was the cell.) Leaving the iatrochemists to their fluids and their spirits, he proceeded to give all his attention to the mechanics of fiber structure.

Giorgio Baglivi was born in 1668 at Ragusa, on the Adriatic, then a city-state in fee to the Ottoman empire and today, after the period of Austrian Dalmatia, a Yugoslavian city named Dubrovnik. After his early education there by Jesuits he moved to Italy where he trained as a physician (and remained for the rest of his life). After a period in Bologna, where he had the good fortune to be a pupil of Malpighi, he followed him later to Rome. The influence of his great teacher is found throughout all of Baglivi's work, and with Malpighi's encouragement he pursued the surgical and microscopical techniques that led to the experiments that lay behind his hypotheses.[20]

Armed with a compound microscope (with four lenses), he used the tissues of animals and human cadavers dissected in the anatomical theater in Rome. He prepared his specimens by soaking them first in ordinary water, then in spirits of wine, and finally in a mild acid solution;[21] as had Malpighi, his teacher, he boiled his specimens. When it came to the question of muscle, he was able to differentiate the contractile fibers (*fibrae motrices seu masculares*) from those of tendons and meninges (*fibrae membranaceae*).[22]

Baglivi was delighted with the visible detail of the many fibrils constituting the fascicles of the muscle substance, which could not be seen without the microscope. He held that they originated from solidification of blood (which accounted for their color), whereas the membranous fibers (the only ones that could also carry sensation) were formed from solidified nervous juice secreted in the membranes surrounding the brain. These he (mistakenly) thought pulsated continuously, yielding a periodic oscillation; borrowing Descartes' image, Baglivi likened it to a clock.

Under the microscope he could see two arrangements of fibers in muscle itself: one running parallel to the length of the muscle and the other transversely. This observation has been interpreted by some as a differentiation between striped and smooth muscle. To see these different fibers more distinctly, Baglivi boiled the tissues in almond oil and looked at them through his microscope lit by strong sunlight.

He concluded that the initiation of the actual fibrillary contraction did not come directly from the brain for he had observed the beating of the excised heart and had found that even the isolated muscle fiber, seen under the microscope, contracted when touched. So important to Baglivi was the flow of the blood between the fibers that he thought the corpuscles excited the fibrils by contact as they flowed between them. In other words, the force necessary for contraction came from the blood and hence originated in the heart, the corpuscles working on the innate elasticity (*tonus fibrarum*) of the muscle. The influence of the brain, under direction from the soul, operated through the continually oscillating membranes surrounding it (the *dura mater*), but could affect only the membranous fibers (*fibrae membranaceae*) of which all membranes were constructed—those enclosing the nerves, the muscles, the blood vessels, and even the bones. This influence could alter the pressure of the blood corpuscles against the motor fibers (*fibrae carneae*) by changing their shape and thus modify the contraction.

A strong point in Baglivi's theory was that, as this efferent action was a pulsation of the meninges, the speed of conduction from brain to periphery would be much faster than that of any juice flowing inside a nerve canal. The motor fiber, being in a continuous oscillation

[20]Letter from Malpighi to Baglivi, 5 January 1692 (in the Osler collection at McGill University).

[21]"Ideò, ut fibram carneam humanam diligentius examinarem, infudi primò eam in aqua communi mox in spiritu vini, demum in aqua aceto temperata."

[22]*De Fibra Motrice et Morbosa.* Letter to Pascoli. Published: Perugia, 1700.

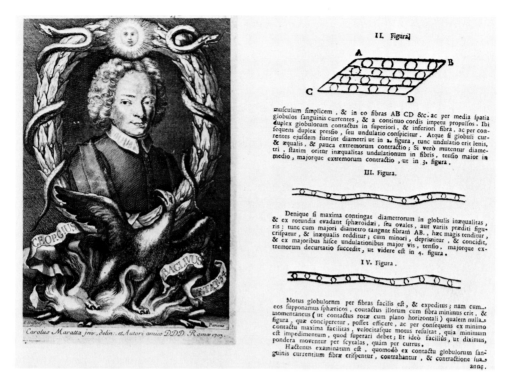

FIG. 45. Giorgio Baglivi (1668–1707) rising like a phoenix from the flames and his own sketch of blood corpuscles stimulating muscle fibers by contact, causing different reactions as they change in shape or flow. (From *De fibra motrice et morbosa*, 1700.)

(a kind of tonus), was ready for the message when it came. Gone, therefore, was the age-old concept of juice making a time-consuming flow down the nerve; it merely needed a push to convey a change in its oscillating pulsations. He likened these to systole and diastole. Baglivi agreed with Steno that the tendons did not contract—they were his fibrae membranaceae, and he accepted Borelli's tenet that nervous spirits did not enter into the muscle to expand its volume. Although essentially a mechanist, he still retained a role for this fluid through its action on the flow of the corpuscles.

After Malpighi's death, Baglivi gave more and more time to his work as a physician. A successful clinician, among his patients was the Pope, who was influential in his appointment as Professor of Anatomy at the College of Sapienza in Rome and, later, Professor of Theoretical Medicine (an apt title for this philosopher). His reputation spread throughout Europe and brought him membership in the Royal Society before he was thirty. He died in 1706.

BIBLIOGRAPHY

Claude Perrault (1613–1688)

Selected Writings

Mémoires pour servir à l'histoire des animaux. Académie des Sciences, Paris, 1671–1676.

Essais de Physique, ou Receuil de Plusieurs Traités Touchant les Choses Naturelles, 4 vols. Paris, 1680–1688.

Receuil de Plusieurs Machines de Nouvelle Invention. Coignard, Paris, 1700.

Oeuvres Diverses de Physique et de Mécanique, 2 vols. Vander, Leyden, 1721.

Abaque Rhabdologique inventé par M. Perrault. *Machines et Inventions approuvées par l'Académie Royale des Sciences (1666–1701)*, 1:55–58 (1734).

Giovanni Alphonso Borelli (1608–1679)

Selected Writings

De Vi Percussionis. Bologna, 1667.

De Motionibus Naturalibus a Gravitate Pendentibus. Reggio di Calabria, Bologna, 1670.

De Motu Animalium. 2 vols. (posthumous). Bernado, Rome, 1680–1681.

Secondary Sources

Bastholm, E. The history of muscle physiology. *Acta Hist. Sci. Nat. Med.*, 7:178–189 (1950).

Foster, M. *Lectures in the History of Physiology.* Cambridge University Press, London, 1924.

Fulton, J. F. *Selected Readings in the History of Physiology.* Baillière, Tindall and Cox, London, 1930.

Nordenskiöld, E. *The History of Biology.* Tudor Publ. Co., New York, 1928.

Wolf, A. *A History of Science, Technology, and Philosophy in the 16th and 17th Centuries.* Allen and Unwin, London, 1935.

Marcello Malpighi (1628–1694)

Selected Writings

De pulmonibus Observationes Anatomicae. Ferronius, Bologna, 1661.

Epistolae Anatomicae de Cerebro, ac Lingua. Bologna, 1665.

De cerebri cortice. In *De Viscerium Structura Exercitatio Anatomica.* Montius, Bologna, 1666.

Dissertatio Epistolica de Formatione Pulli in Ovo. London, 1673.

Secondary Sources

Adelmann, H. B. *Marcello Malpighi and the Evolution of Embryology.* Cornell University Press, Ithaca, NY, 1966.

Belloni, L. La neuroanatomia di Marcello Malpighi. *Physis*, 8:253–266 (1966).

Meyer, A. *Historical Aspects of Cerebral Anatomy.* Oxford University Press, London, 1971.

Giorgio Baglivi (1668–1706)

Selected Writings

De Praxi Medica ad Priscam Observandi Rationem Revocanda, libro duo. Caesaretti, Rome, 1696. (French translation by J. Boucher. Labé, Paris, 1851.) (English translation *The Practice of Physick.* London, 1704.)

De Fibra Motrice et Morbosa. Epistola ad Alexandrum Pascoli. Constantinum, Perugia, 1700.

De Anatome Fibrarum, de Motu Musculorum. 1700.

Specimen Quatuor Librorum de Fibra Motrice et Morbosa. Buagni, Rome, 1702. Leigh and Midwinter, London, 1703.

Opera Omina Medico-practica Anatomica. Anisson and Posuel, Lyons, 1704.

Secondary Sources

Bastholm, E. The history of muscle physiology. *Acta Hist. Sci. Nat. Med.*, 7:178–189 (1950).

Grmek, M. D. La notion de fibre vivante chez les médecins de l'école iatrophysique. *Clio. Med.*, 5:297–318 (1970).

CHAPTER VI

The Impact on Philosophers and Mathematicians

The growing recognition of the importance of the brain was beginning to challenge the concepts of free will and, for theologians, the supremacy of the soul. The 17th century was the first in which one meets this shared interest and actual interplay between the experimental scientist and the concept-seeking philosopher.

John Locke (1632–1704)

Outstanding among the philosophers was a friend of Richard Lower's, John Locke. Not a scientist himself, although later a practicing physician, he was a student of Willis and one of the few who met for discussions in the home of Robert Boyle. Born in Somerset and educated at the famous Westminster School in London, Locke had a multifaceted career: as an experimentalist in Oxford, a diplomat in Europe during the war with the Dutch, Secretary to the Lords Proprietors of Carolina in the New World (for which he wrote a constitution), and an exile in Holland (where he met Leeuwenhoek) and in Montpellier (a thriving center of physiological thought). During his exile in Holland he wrote his masterpiece, *Essay Concerning Humane Understanding*.[1]

While Locke was still a schoolboy, Descartes died. Revolutionary as he had been in drawing "perception" into the nervous system, Descartes nevertheless believed some ideas to be innate and that certainty of truth could be reached by reasoning. This reasoning stemmed

---

[1]First published in the Bibliothèque Naturelle et Historique in French translation, *Extrait d'un Livre Anglois qui n'est pas encore publié, intitulé "ESSAI PHILOSOPHIQUE CONCERNANT L'ENTENDEMENT,"* 1688, and two years later in English under the title *Essay Concerning Humane Understanding*, 4 vols. London, 1690.

from the rational soul, which he gave uniquely to man. It was essentially on these issues that Locke's concepts diverged from those of Descartes and, in doing so, ushered in a new age in the theories of brain science to tease the experimentalists. Locke insisted that all knowledge comes from sensory observations and from reflection on them, and that the mind is incapable of formulating ideas from any source other then the senses, to the exclusion of all *a priori* knowledge, "without the help of any innate impressions." Extracts from Locke's famous *Essay* appeared in French in Pierre Coste's translation two years before its printing in London. In England, the *Essay* received immediate recognition and monetary reward, earning for its author more than was paid to John Milton for *Paradise Lost*. The following century was to write harshly of Locke but, in his own time, he received acclaim and support from his friend and correspondent, Isaac Newton.

Compressed into a single quotation from the draft of his famous *Essay Concerning Humane Understanding*, Locke's argument is that "all knowledge is founded on and ultimately derives itself from sense, or something analogous to it, which may be called sensation." Locke's model also contained a storage mechanism, for it was necessary to have a repository serving those ideas

> . . . which the senses provided when the understanding is once stored with these simple ideas, it has the power to repeat, compare, and unite them, even to an infinite variety, and so can make at pleasure new complex ideas. But it is not in the power of the most exalted wit, or enlarged understanding, by any quickness or variety of thought, to invent or frame one new simple idea in the mind not taken in by the ways aforementioned.

Perhaps the most difficult task that Locke's model presents is explained by the fact that Locke was not purely an empiricist: He felt impelled to bring his religious beliefs into his overall theory. Unprepared to accept theological dogma that was open to disproof by the empirical method, he was nevertheless willing to admit on "faith" (as contrasted with "reason") religious tenets that were immune to proof or disproof. One example Locke gave is that the dead shall rise again—a proposition he accepted not only because it is stated in the gospels, but because its truth or untruth is impossible to test. He did not attempt a neural explanation of faith, although he considered the existence of God to be proven.[2] Locke died in 1704.

Isaac Newton (1642–1727)

Locke was a personal friend of the giant of his century, Isaac Newton, and they corresponded on the movements of the planets, politics, and religious tenets.[3] Newton, born in the year Galileo died, was ten years younger than Locke, but his genius flowered early. It is not an exaggeration to say that he transformed the mathematics of Galileo and Descartes. His only assay into problems of the nervous system came later—in the set of thirty-one queries in the second edition of *Opticks*. To his *Principia* he had added the theory of an all-pervading "aether," and being impatient with lingering concepts of animal spirits in nerves, he wrote:[4]

> Is not Animal Motion perform'd by the Vibrations of this Medium, excited in the Brain by the Power of the Will, and propagated from thence through the solid, perlucid, and uniform Capillamenta of the Nerves and the Muscles, for contracting and dilating them?

[2] *Essay*, Book. IV, Chapter X.

[3] *The Correspondence of John Locke*, 4 vols., edited by E. S. De Beer. Oxford University Press, Oxford, 1977–1978.

[4] Isaac Newton. *Opticks: or a Treatise of the Reflections, Refractions, Inflections and Colours of Light*, 2nd edn, Query 22. London, 1730.

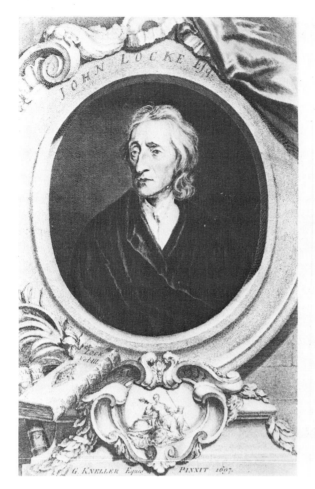

& Hiftorique de l'Année 1688. 49

<hr>

II.

Extrait d'un Livre. Anglois qui n'eft pas encore publié, intitulé ESSAI PHI-LOSOPHIQUE *concernant* L'EN-TENDEMENT, *où l'on montre quel-le eft l'étenduë de nos connoiffances certaines, & la maniere dont nous y par-venons.* Communiqué par Monfieur LOCKE.

Livre Premier.

D ANS les penfées que j'ai euës, concernant nôtre Entende-ment, j'ai tâché d'abord de prouver que nôtre Efprit eft au com-mencement ce qu'on appelle *tabu-la rafa;* c'eft à dire, fans idées & fans connoiffance. Mais comme ce n'a été que pour détruire les préjugez de quel-ques Philofophes, j'ai cru que dans ce petit Abregé de mes principes, je de-vois paffer toutes les Difputes Préli-minaires, qui compofent le premier Li-vre. Je prétends de montrer, dans les fuivans, la fource de laquelle nous ti-rons toutes les idées, qui entrent dans nos raifonnemens, & la maniere dont elles nous viennent.
Tome VIII.   C   *Livre*

FIG. 46.   Left: The well-known portrait by Kneller of John Locke in his later years.   **Right:** the opening section of Locke's *Essay Concerning Humane Understanding*, published first in the Biblio-thèque Naturelle et Historique in 1688.

Newton died half a century before the revelations of the role of electricity in nerves startled the world of science.

The suggestion that "aether" might be the agent for nerve conduction was immediately embraced by many contemporary writers. One of them, Bryan Robinson,[5] was so enthusiastic that he claimed "Sir Isaac Newton discovered the Causes of Muscular Motion and Secretion," and went on to argue that "the agent by which the nerves propagate to the muscles the power of the will is no less than Newton's aether." In this way, he could account for the invisible nature of the nervous force and the speed of its action. Another writer, William Smith,[6] granted that this "aether" was so fine as to be invisible to man, but suggested that cats and owls might be able to see it.

Newton's concern with nerves was related to his work on optics. He was interested in a contemporary book, *Theory of Vision*, written in 1687 by an ophthalmologist named William

[5]Bryan Robinson. *A Treatise of the Animal Economy*, 3rd edn, 2 vols. Innys, London, 1738.
[6]William Smith. *Dissertation Upon the Nerves*. W. Owen, London 1768.

Briggs. The question that puzzled Newton was that of binocular vision and how the fibers of the optic nerve would need to be at different degrees of stretch ("nervos opticos ex capillamentis varie tensis constare supponis") in order for the two images to superimpose.[7] His theory was discussed at a meeting of the Royal Society and met with some objections.[8]

Newton's eminence as a mathematician and his work on gravitation brought him not only membership in the Royal Society (which published *Principia*[9]) but also its presidency—a role he filled for nearly a quarter of a century, and in 1705 it brought him a knighthood. In no way a recluse, he served as member of parliament for the University of Cambridge in the short-lived Convention Parliament set up in 1689 on the accession of William and Mary to the throne. Any account of the Newtonian era that is restricted, as is this, to its impact on neural sciences, of necessity does little justice to his mathematical achievements although, 200 years later, mathematics invaded the study of the nervous system. Calculus, the discovery by those two giants, Newton and Leibniz, who quarreled so bitterly over priority, became a common tool for neurophysiologists and biophysicists interested in calculating rate of change. And Newton's analysis of the nature of light, set out in *Opticks*, is relevant to all studies of the visual system. Like Descartes before him, Newton strove to analyze the way in which the eye receives light rays; he thought light was corpuscular in nature (and wave theory still lay in the future).

For the last 30 years of his life Newton was Warden of the Mint, at first retaining his appointment at Trinity College, Cambridge. During his tenure, the old hand-struck coins were withdrawn from circulation and Christopher Wren's plea for a decimal coinage was rejected—postponed for another 260 years.

Newton died in 1727. In papers found after his death, a great number of theological manuscripts were found, revealing how deep were his studies of theology, an interest he shared in his correspondence with John Locke. Newton was not the only mathematician concerned with the propositions in Locke's *Essay* or with the mathematics of Descartes. Gottfried Wilhelm Leibniz was critical of both.

Gottfried Wilhelm Leibniz (1646–1716)

Leibniz was born in Leipzig in 1646 and was schooled in Aristotelianism at its university. He soon became known as an outstanding mathematician and an ingenious designer. As Pascal had before him, he designed a mechanical calculator, and commented that "It is unworthy of excellent men to lose hours like slaves in the labour of calculation which could safely be relegated to anyone else if machines were used."

In 1672 Leibniz was invited to demonstrate his calculator (which he claimed could also multiply) to the Royal Society, but it did not work well.[10] The Society's Curator of Experiments, Robert Hooke, challenged Leibniz saying he would design "an arithmetical machine much more simply that that of Mons. Leibniz produced before the Society on the 22nd of January." On February 26, Hooke did produce a machine and was challenged to show how it differed from that of Leibniz (who was not present). Leibniz did not return, but his designs

---

[7]Letter to William Briggs, April 25, 1685. In: *The Correspondence of Isaac Newton*, Vol. II, edited by H. W. Turnbull. Cambridge University Press, London, 1960.

[8]Thomas Birch. *The History of the Royal Society*, Vol. 4, p. 136. London, 1757.

[9]Isaac Newton. *Philosophiae Naturalis Principia Mathematica*. London, 1687.

[10]T. Birch. *History of the Royal Society*, Vol. III.

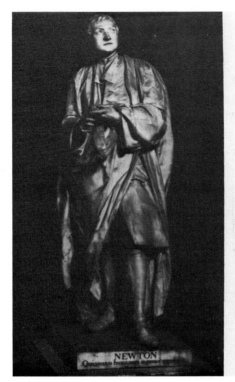 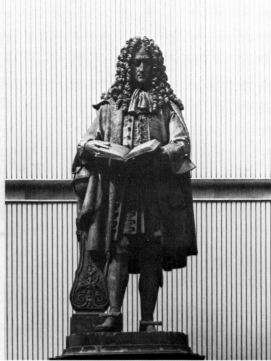

FIG. 47.   Two famous mathematicians drawn into the growing concepts of brain function, and rival inventors of differential calculus.   **Left:** Isaac Newton. Statue in the Ante-Chapel of Trinity College, Cambridge.   **Right:** Gottfried Wilhelm Leibniz. Statue outside the Karl-Marx University in Leipzig. This statue originally stood outside the St. Thomas Church in Leipzig where, from 1723, to his death in 1750, Johann Sebastion Bach was the organist. (Courtesy of Dr. A. Nicolai.)

can be seen in the Niedersächsische Landesbibliothek in Hannover;[11] a model made from them in modern times can be seen in the Deutsches Museum in Munich.

Much traveled and well-read, Leibniz had met Leeuwenhoek in Holland and Malpighi in Rome. In England he met with the men of the Royal Society, but apparently not with Locke. With his own interest in how the mind worked (about which he had written in 1684[12]) he seized on Locke's *Essay* and wrote an almost chapter-by-chapter criticism of it. (He could not read English, and had to wait for the French translation by Pierre Coste in 1688).[13] Leibniz's view of mental activity contrasted vitally with Locke's: he thought that the mind contained the essence of ideas, which the senses could then call forth. Leibniz's criticism of Locke, *Nouveaux Essais sur l'Entendement Humain*, was an extremely long treatise that was never published in full because, as Leibniz wrote to a friend, "the death of Locke has taken away my desire to publish my remarks upon his works." The complete work was published 50 years after his own death.[14]

[11]Letter from Oldenburg to Leibniz, 26 July 1676. In: Gerhardt. *Leibnitzens Mathematische Schriften*, Vol. 1, p. 100, 1850.

[12]G. W. Leibniz. *Meditationes de Cognitione, Veritate et Ideis*, 1684.

[13]P. Coste. *Essai philosophique concernant l'entendement humain par M. Locke*, 5 vols. Amsterdam, 1688.

[14]G. W. Leibniz. *Nouveaux Essais sur l'Entendement Humain*, 1765. English translation by A. G. Langley. *New Essays Concerning Human Understanding*. Open Court Publ., La Salle, 1896.

Leibniz's opinions about Descartes' works appear in his letters: "I do not hesitate to say that I approve more things in the books of Aristotle than in the Meditations of Descartes."[15] He scolds the Cartesians for not distinguishing space from matter and for their allegiance to the pineal gland. Of his view of nerve action on the soul he wrote:

> The nerves and the membranes are the parts that receive sensation for us, more than other parts, and it is perhaps only through them that we perceive the others, which happens apparently, because the movements of the nerves or of the fluids belonging to them imitate more closely sensations and confuse them less, so the more distinct expressions of the soul correspond to the more distinct impressions of the body. It is not that the nerves act upon the soul, to speak metaphysically, but that the one represents the state of the other by reason of a spontaneous relation.

Throughout Leibniz's writings he refers to Descartes—sometimes agreeing with him, but more often criticizing. He shared the Cartesian tenet that a single science could explain all phenomena. He also agreed that a vacuum could not exist and corresponded about this with Guericke. At first he embraced a corpuscular theory, preferring this Cartesian concept to the atomism of Gassendi, but later the Cartesian Method led to his own theory of monads: centers of energy that direct our conscious lives. Like Newton, Leibniz believed in an "aether" responsible for motion, although, unlike Newton, he did not suggest that it was the agent that moved the impulse down the nerve.

It was from his intense studies of force and motion (in which he disagreed fundamentally with Descartes) that he developed his method of differential calculus, over which a bitter quarrel for priority was to develop with Newton. Both were concerned with the necessity for a mathematical method of calculating rates of change of a quantity (or "fluxions," as Newton called them). Both solved the problem and both had to design a method of notation. Subsequent scientists found Leibniz's symbols, dx and dy,[16] more useful than Newton's "dot."

Leibniz moved in diplomatic circles throughout the centers of European nobility. A man of many interests, he was appointed librarian to the Court of Hannover, and was elected a member in the Royal Society in 1673. He was a founding member of the Berlin Academy of Sciences in 1700 and became its president for life. Leibniz died in 1716. A fine statue of him stands outside his old university in Leipzig.

These philosophers and mathematicians, Locke, Newton, Leibniz, so critical of Descartes, were themselves to meet a more powerful critic: Voltaire. He chides Newton for being a follower of Democritus and Epicurus and especially of Gassendi.[17] He criticizes Locke for his denial of innate ideas, which leads to the absence of any notion of good and evil. Descartes is scolded for his speculations, for inventing so much. ("Descartes aurait été le plus grand Philosophe de la Terre, s'il eût moins inventé.") Voltaire attacks Leibniz for his scheme of monads, one of which is said to be the soul. But one feels that, of these men, Descartes was the one who most interested Voltaire.

On his death, Voltaire's library was sold by his niece to Catherine the Great, and it can be seen now in the Public Library in Leningrad. All of Descartes' books are in the collection, but it is not their number that is so interesting. It is that Voltaire, a great man for marginalia, has annotated them so plentifully.

[15]Leibniz's letter to Jacob Thomasius, April 20, 1669. Latin manuscript in the Library in Hannover. Niedersächsische Landesbibliothek.

[16]*Nova methodus pro meximis et minimis.* Acta Eruditorum, 1684.

[17]Voltaire. *Eleméns de Philosophie de Newton*, 1745. En trois parties.

BIBLIOGRAPHY

Selected Writings of Locke, Newton, and Leibniz

Locke, John. *Essay Concerning Humane Understanding*, 4 vols., London, 1690. Translated into French by P. Coste. *Essai Philosophique Concernant l'Entendement Humain par M. Locke*, 5 vols. Amsterdam, 1688.

————.*The Correspondence of John Locke*, 4 vols, edited by E. S. De Beer. Oxford University Press, 1977–1978.

————.*Oxford Lectures of Dr. Thomas Willis*. Translated into English by K. Dewhurst. *Willis's Oxford Lectures*. Sandford, Oxford, 1980.

Newton, Isaac. *Opticks: or a Treatise of the Reflections, Refractions, Inflections and Colours of Light*, 2nd edn (with queries). London, 1703.

Leibniz, Gottfried Wilhelm. *Meditationes de Cognitione, Veritate et Ideis*, 1684.

————.*Miscellanea Berolinensia*, Vol. 1. 1710.

————.*Nouveaux Essais sur l'Entendement Humain*, 1765.

   English translation by A. G. Langley. La Salle: Open Court, 1896.

Secondary Sources

Andrade, E. N. Da C. *Isaac Newton*. London, 1950.

Anthony, H. D. *Sir Isaac Newton*, Abelard-Schuman, London, 1960.

Balavel, Y. *Leibniz Critique de Descartes*. Paris, 1960.

Cranston, M. *John Locke: a Biography*. London, 1957.

Gibson, J. *Locke's Theory of Knowledge*. Cambridge, 1917.

Guitton, J. *Pascal et Leibniz*. Paris, 1951.

Meyer, R. W. *Leibniz and the 17th Century Revolution*. Glasgow, 1956.

CHAPTER VII

Academies and Societies of Science

By the close of the 17th century three great advances had been made that benefited all scientists: the formation of powerful scientific societies supplanting the group meetings in private homes, the founding of scientific journals, and the establishment of publishing houses as outlets for their books.

Small scientific groups of a few dedicated scientists had appeared in every European country, some to flourish for a short time, usually the active period of their few members, and some to go on to become academies of renown. In all cases they were generated by the enthusiasm of small groups gathered around a central figure. In Naples, in the Kingdom of the Two Sicilies, a group met in the house of Giambattista della Porta and called themselves the Accademia Secretorum Naturae. As the name suggests, they were devoted to alchemy and magic, although they encouraged experiment. An extraordinary book came from della Porta in 1558: *Magia naturalis*, revised and expanded in 1589 and translated into many languages. Among the great number of observations, magical and otherwise, there are a few which border on the sciences that were to develop in the 17th century: observations on lenses used in telescopes and some experiments on the lodestone. In his old age, della Porta accused Gilbert of having plagiarized his work and ridiculed him for believing that the earth revolved.[1] Gilbert, in turn, wrote that della Porta's book was "full of most erroneous experiments,"[2] although he credits him with describing how to prepare iron for a magnet. Della Porta's field was alchemy and he made many attempts to transform metals. References to della Porta are found throughout Gilbert's *De Magnete*, mostly critical in nature.

Della Porta's small "academy" existed for only a few years—in part, because it was suspected by the Church of trafficking with the occult. A later edition of his book contains

[1]Giambattista della Porta (1535–1615). *Magia naturalis*, Italian edition. Naples, 1611.
[2]William Gilbert. *De Magnete*. Mottelay translation, 1893.

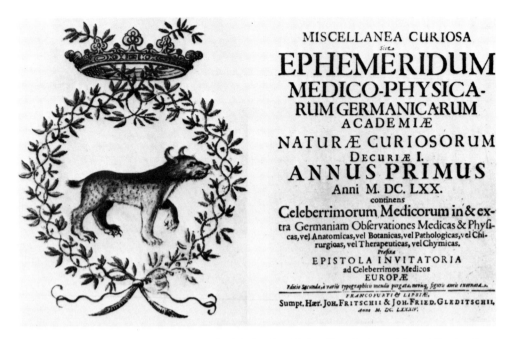

MISCELLANEA CURIOSA
Sive
EPHEMERIDUM
MEDICO-PHYSICA-
RUM GERMANICARUM
ACADEMIÆ
NATURÆ CURIOSORUM
DECURIÆ I.
ANNUS PRIMUS
Anni M. DC. LXX.
continens
Celeberrimorum Medicorum in & ex-
tra Germaniam Obſervationes Medicas & Phyſi-
cas, vel Anatomicas, vel Botanicas, vel Pathologicas, vel Chi-
rurgicas, vel Therapeuticas, vel Chymicas.
Præfixa
EPISTOLA INVITATORIA
ad Celeberrimos Medicos
EUROPÆ
Editio Secunda, à variis typographicis mendis purgata, novis, figuris aucta exornata.
FRANCOFURTI & LIPSIÆ,
Sumpt. Hær. JOH. FRITSCHII & JOH. FRIED. GLEDITSCHII,
Anno M. DC. LXXXIV.

FIG. 48. **Left:** The seal of the Accademia dei Lincei. **Right:** Frontispiece of the publication from the German Academy in Halle, claimed to be the first journal in natural history.

noticeably less magic. His most important contribution was his help in promoting a truly scientific society: the famous Accademia dei Lincei, an academy that flourished in Rome from 1603 to 1630 and was revived several times. Named for the clear-eyed lynx, the society grew under the patronage of Duke Federico Cesi, himself a naturalist. This small academy gave its members the opportunity to publish their work, and two publications carry Galileo's name; one on sunspots,[3] the other his famous polemic *Saggiatore*.[4] The Academy contributed little to the neural sciences, although there were some published descriptions of the use of the microscope in biology.[5] With the death of Cesi in 1630, the Academy closed. Several efforts to revive it failed: one favored by Napoleon in 1801, one in 1847 by a statute of the Pope, dubbing it a pontifical academy, and, finally, when, after the struggles of the Risorgimento and Rome became the capital of a united Italy, the Academy used the name "Reale," competing with the Accademia d'Italia that had been founded by Descartes' friend, Queen Christina.

Another bleak period followed during the Fascist regime and the occupation by the German armies, but on the liberation of Rome in 1944 this persistent organization was reborn, largely by the efforts of Benedetto Croce; it occupies the magnificent Corsini Palace, with its splendid libraries, and great treasure troves of science and the arts. Among its elected members are some of the world's distinguished scholars, including two whom neurophysiology can claim as its own. In free Italy the lynxes call themselves the Accademia Nazionale dei Lincei.

The next short-lived (but perhaps more famous) academy was the Accademia del Cimento, founded in 1657 in Tuscany and closing in 1667. Again, survival was dependent largely on

[3]Galileo. *Istoria e dimonstrazione intorno alle machie solari*. Lyncaei, 1613.

[4]*Il saggiatore*. Lyncaei, 1623.

[5]Francesco Stelluti (1577–1652). *Apiarium*. Lyncaei, 1623.

patronage; in this case, the Medici brothers. Unlike the Lincei, the members of the Cimento met to collaborate on experimental problems. It was the realization of what Bacon was urging in England. In *New Atlantis*,[6] he had insisted that the secrets of nature were so great and so complex that organization and cooperative effort were necessary to seek the solutions. Bacon described an imaginary society in which a college existed to bring experimenters together, providing them with laboratory instruments. The work of the group was then "interpreted" in order to "raise the former discoveries by experiments into great observations, axioms and aphorisms." The value of this fantasy is that it illustrates what in fact influenced those who, after his death, met in such groups; in his own country, there was the founding of the Royal Society.

So strong was the collaborative feeling of the members of the Cimento that, in the sole report that they published *(Saggi di naturali esperienze)*, no individual names are given. We are fortunate that the Academy kept a diary in manuscript, now lost but not before the Florentine Targione Tozzetti had made a copy that is well preserved in the Biblioteca Nazionale in Florence, together with some other manuscript notes. From these two sources, scholars have gained more information about the experiments carried out at the Academy than from the *Saggi* itself. Few experiments were concerned with neural science, since the group of eight men and a secretary who formed the nucleus were overwhelmingly influenced by the philosophy and works of Galileo and Torricelli, both of whom had died within a few years of each other in the previous decade. There are many experiments on air pressure and on the lingering problem of the vacuum—experiments which would no doubt have pleased Pascal and Descartes. The question as to whether or not small animals could survive in a vacuum was explored, a subject later explained by John Mayow in England.

One who made a stir at that time was Gassendi with his atomistic explanation of our nervous systems; although alluded to in the *Saggi*, it was only his views on the speed of sound that interested the group. Many experiments were made on magnets (without reference to Gilbert, although surviving manuscripts from the Academy mention him); other experiments in the *Saggi* report the effect of friction on amber and the properties of gems as "electric power" (virtu elettrica and potenza elettrica). The Academy closed in 1667, and its members dispersed.

It was also in the first half of the 17th century that an academy that became famous for the journal it founded began in Halle, in the Duchy of Hannover; known today as the Deutschen Akademie der Naturforscher, it was famous for three centuries as the "Leopoldina," named for Kaiser Leopold II, who founded it in 1652. (Its full name was "Sacri Romani Imperii Academia Caesareo-Leopoldina Naturae Curiosurum.")

The initial idea of forming a group to pursue the curiosities of nature came from Johann Lorenz Bausch, a physician from Schweinfurt. Greatly influenced by Bacon's *Novum Organum* and *New Atlantis*, his goal was to replace "credo" with "ratio." When this bold movement toward the encouragement of science was launched, there was not yet a university in Halle, although one was to open at the end of the century. The most outstanding contribution of this academy was the establishment of a publication, *Ephemeridum medico-physicarium* (claimed to be the first natural history journal), which later became the famous *Nova Acta Leopoldina*. Surviving through the 20th century, this was the journal chosen to carry a long review by the first man to demonstrate the electrical activity of the human brain,[7] a phenomenon already known in the lower animals.

[6]Francis Bacon (1561–1626). *New Atlantis* (posthumous). 1627.

[7]H. Berger. Das Elektrenkephalogram des Menschen. *Acta Nova Leopoldina*, 6:173–309 (1938).

There were growing movements in England and France to found truly lasting academies from the scattered groups of scientists who, like Bacon, believed in the value of collaborative effort and free exchange of ideas. The English and French academies came into full existence within a few years of each other, the Royal Society in 1662 and the Académie Royale des Sciences in 1666. Both owed their establishment to men in high places who enlisted patronage from the respective monarch.

In England groups of scientists had been meeting in private houses since the opening of the century. In Oxford the famous group dubbed "the invisible college" met in the house of Robert Boyle, and later in 1660 in the rooms of Gresham College in London. When the end of the civil war came and with it restoration of the monarchy, Charles II, declaring himself the Founder, gave the group a charter. With the charter, Charles presented his portrait by Sir Peter Lely (which hangs in the Royal Society's rooms to this day), the mace, and the Charter Book in which all Fellows still sign.

Many histories of the Royal Society have been written; one of the first (and rather unreliable) was that of Bishop Sprat. However, his account is valuable for its picture of the contemporary scene in the founding years of the Society. In 1756 a classic history was published, in four volumes, by Thomas Birch[8] (also a man of the church and biographer of Robert Boyle), from which we can follow its development into one of the leading centers of knowledge in Europe; Birch copied the items from the register kept at every meeting.

Membership was not limited to scientists; in fact, in the 17th century they comprised, together with physicians and surgeons, approximately one-third of those elected. The Fellows who contributed to the development of neurophysiology in the earliest years of the Society were Christopher Wren, Robert Boyle, Walter Charleton, William Croone, Francis Glisson, Jonathan Goddard, Robert Hooke, John Locke, Robert Lower, John Mayow, Isaac Newton, and Thomas Willis. (Locke and Lower were later forced to resign for nonpayment of dues.) They were joined by such famous men from other fields as John Aubrey, John Evelyn, and Samuel Pepys. Their manuscripts give us the most vivid pictures of the distinguished men of their times.[9]

Among the proceedings that Birch copied from the Register are some that concern this science, for example, Charleton's observations on comparative anatomy of the brain,[10] opinions conflicting with those of Willis. The Society ordered that this disagreement be settled in private. Stranger experiments on the brain were reported by Croone,[11] including putting wine into the ventricles of a fresh cadaver and tracing it through the gut. And Goddard's experiment on the lack of volume increase in muscle contraction is faithfully reported by Birch.[12] Letters from the foreign members give a vivid picture of activities across the channel. Most were written in Latin and translated into English by the secretary, Henry Oldenburg.

Bacon died before England achieved its Royal Society, but his influence was not forgotten by Sprat when he wrote his history. The frontispiece (only in the first edition) shows a bust of the King, with Bacon on his left and Viscount Brounckner, a Society president, on his right. Perhaps the most concise declaration of goals of the Royal Society is found in Hooke's

[8]Thomas Birch, *The History of the Royal Society of London*, 4 vols. Millar, London, 1756.

[9]John Aubrey. *Brief Lives*, edited by O. L. Dick. Secker and Warburg, London, 1949. John Evelyn. *The Diary of John Evelyn*, 6 vols, edited by E. S. de Beer. Oxford, 1955 (first published in 1818). Samuel Pepys. *Diary 1660–1669*.

[10]Thomas Birch. *The History of the Royal Society of London*, vol. I, p. 436.

[11]Thomas Birch. *The History of the Royal Society of London*, vol. II, p. 232.

[12]Thomas Birch. *The History of the Royal Society of London*, vol. II, p. 356.

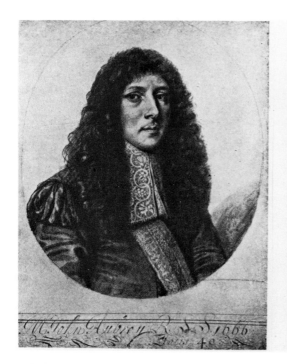
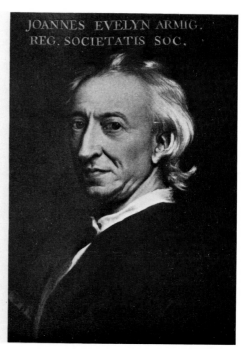

FIG. 49. **Left:** John Aubrey F.R.S. (1626–1697), whose rich descriptions of the men of his times give us the most intimate light on the 17th century. The manuscripts in four folios are preserved in the Bodleian Library. (From the drawing by Faithorne in 1666.) **Right:** John Evelyn F.R.S. (1620–1706), the diarist. Unsuccessful competitor with his design for the rebuilding of London after the Great Fire. (From the portrait by Kneller. Courtesy of the Royal Society.)

papers written in 1663:[13] "To improve the knowledge of natural things, and all useful Arts, Manufactures, Mechanic practices, Engynes and Inventions by Experiments—(not meddling with Divinity, Metaphysics, Moralls, Politicks, Grammar, Rhetorick, or Logick)."

By rule of the Society members could have copies of all papers read but were forbidden to distribute any except their own. However, in 1665 the famous journal *Philosophical Transactions of the Royal Society* was established. It has continued to this day with only one hiatus at the death of Henry Oldenburg. Robert Hooke filled the gap with *Philosophical Collections* until, in 1783, the journal resumed its original name. Unfortunately, unlike the French Academy, which devoted a room in the Louvre for the purpose, the Royal Society did not preserve the scientific apparatus of its famous experimenters. No instruments of Harvey, Boyle, or Lower remain.

The Académie des Sciences followed the Royal Society in 1666, but in France its prehistory was very different. The ministers of King Louis XIV, in particular, Richelieu and Colbert, had influenced the founding of several academies. Many small groups calling themselves academies had grown up on their own, but when the powerful Cardinal Richelieu persuaded Louis XIV to give regal support, the Académie Française was established.

Earlier academies of, for example, poetry and music became overshadowed, but for science the precursors were found (as described in earlier chapters) in the house of Thévenot, in the cell of Mersenne in the convent of the Minimes, and in the establishment of Montmor. From

[13]C. R. Weld. *History of the Royal Society.* London, 1848.

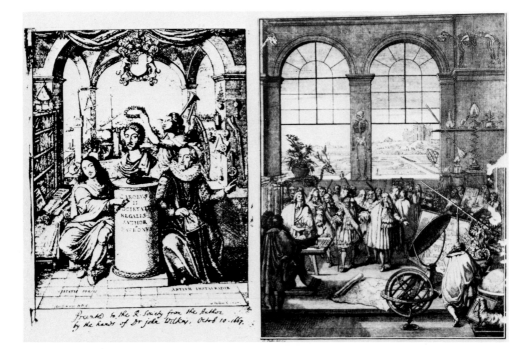

FIG. 50. Left: The frontispiece of a few (only) copies of the first edition of Thomas Sprat's *History of the Royal Society*. Charles II, according to the inscription, is founder and patron of the Royal Society. At his left sits Bacon who, having died in 1626, did not see the opening of the Society for whose founding his views were so influential. **Right:** Visit of Louis XIV accompanied by Colbert and his court to the Cabinet de Physique du Jardin du Roi. Through the window is seen the Observatory under construction. (Engraving by Sebastian Leclerc in Claude Perrault's book: *Memoires pour Servir a l'Histoire des Animaux*, 1671.)

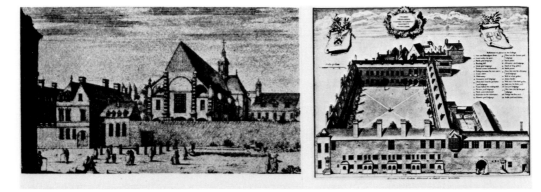

FIG. 51. Two centers for the gathering of scientists that proved to be precursors of, in one case, the Académie Française and, in the other, the Royal Society. **Left:** Convent of the Minimes where the group around Mersenne met. Closed in the Revolution, only vestiges of the chapel remain and a beautiful staircase. **Right:** Gresham College, built by a London merchant, and first home of the Royal Society. Miraculously escaping the Great Fire, which destroyed almost all its neighbors, the College was taken over to house the Royal Exchange and the Society had to move to Arundel House.

1620 to his death, the cell of Mersenne, himself an experimental scientist and a musician, and advocate of an international academy, was the meeting place of European intellectuals and, for those who could not make the journey, the center for an exchange of knowledge by voluminous correspondence. On his death the scientists met in the houses of François de Pailleur and Habert de Montmor, the latter becoming in its turn a little academy. Although an ardent supporter of Cartesian philosophy, Montmor, an aristocrat, was also a friend of Descartes' opponent Gassendi, and gave him lodging, which then drew to his house the group that had previously surrounded Mersenne. There they met for discussion and to perform experiments and correspond with the Royal Society in London. In spite of the membership of Gassendi, there is little record of discussion of the nervous system, interest focusing instead on physics, mathematics, and astronomy. Such biological discussions as there were in the Académie Montmor tended to be on spontaneous generation. There is a report that they discussed the brain—but what they said we are not told. They questioned whether "toutes les connoissances sont dépendantes des sens" (but did not mention Locke). The house where they met still stands, in the street now called Rue du Temple. Inner dissension, led by the secretary, Sorbière, led to the disintegration of this small academy in 1664.

When it was founded in 1635, the Académie Française was essentially limited to a group of literary men entrusted with the preservation of the French language and the preparation of a dictionary. In 1663 Colbert, minister to Louis XIV, added two more academies—Académie royale des Inscriptions et Belles Lettres in 1663 and the Académie royale des Sciences founded by royal charter in 1666. They were followed in 1669 by the Académie royale de Musique and, in 1671, the Académie royale d'Architecture. One of the most influential supporters was Charles, the brother of Claude Perrault. The structure of the Académie des Sciences (one of its principal goals being to build an observatory) was, therefore, totally different from that of the Royal Society, which embraced more than science, and was independent of the state, because its members were unsalaried. Not only did the French Academicians receive a pension from the king, but also financial assistance for their researches. Thévenot, de Montmor, and Perrault were among the first members, and the first meetings took place in the Bibliothèque du Roi, where Thévenot was librarian; they later moved to rooms in the Louvre in 1669. The Académie des Sciences contributed little at first to the science of physiology; the meetings were essentially devoted to technology: the invention of instruments and machines.

When first formed, the Académie had two sections: mathematics and physics; the latter included anatomy, i.e., structure, but not function of our bodies. Some anatomists were members: Perrault himself, DuVerney, his friend, Duhamel, and Pequet, discoverer of the thoracic duct. Their researches consisted essentially of the dissection of enormous numbers of species of animals that can still be studied in the Musée de l'Histoire Naturelle, in what is now called the Jardin des Plantes. At the entrance is a monument honoring the evolution of man: a statue of Lamarck. The distinguished Dutch mathematician and astronomer, Christiaan Huygens, already a member of the Royal Society, was invited to join the Académie and remained there until the revocation of the Edict of Nantes in 1685 offended his Protestant beliefs. He wrote his famous *Traité de la Lumière* while there, but it was published later, on his return to the Hague.

In the following century, all royal academies were dissolved by the Revolution in 1793; and in 1795 came the inauguration of the Institut National, encouraged by Napoleon, and bringing under its aegis the previously independent academies. Now housed on the banks of the Seine where Mazarin's Collège de Quatre Nations once flourished, the magestic dome of the Institut surveys three courtyards—in one of which Voltaire was honored by his nude statue. (The statue has been moved to the Louvre in exchange for a portrait of Mazarin to hang in his own building.) Unlike the Royal Society, which required no formal attire, since 1806 the Académie Française has had a mandatory "habit vert" for the select few who receive the honor of membership.

Two more great academies appeared in the next century: Leibniz's Berlin Academy of Science (in 1700) and Peter the Great's Academy of Sciences (in 1725). It is of some interest that for many years (until 1804) the Berlin Academy published its proceedings in Latin (*Miscellanea Berolinensia*, starting in 1710). The Russian Academy used both French and Latin until 1918.

In the 17th century, museums, sources for scientific inquiry, were still essentially "cabinets of the curiosities" and only one heralded what was to come. It was the Ashmolean Museum at Oxford, which opened in 1683 as a university museum of art and archeology. Beginning with the gifts of Tradescant, a botanist, and of Ashmole, a collector of "rarities," it was strengthened by its collection of books, although these were later transferred to the Bodleian Library. The Ashmolean remains essentially a museum of art and natural history, not truly of science. But it was a pioneer (the British Museum did not open until 1759). The French Académie's treasury of books and manuscripts was the Bibliothèque du Roi and the British Museum's was the incorporation of the Royal Libraries, collections dating back to Edward IV in the 15th century.

BIBLIOGRAPHY

References for the Scientific Academies

Italian Academies of the 17th Century

Celebrazione della Accademia del Cimento nel Tricentenario della fondazione. Domus Galileiana, Pisa, 1958.

Della Porta, Giambattista (1535–1615). *Magiae naturalis.* Naples, 1558. Second enlarged edition, 5. (English translation by Wright. London, 1658. Reissued by the Smithsonian Institution, edited by D. J. Price. Basic Books, New York, 1957.)

Middleton, W. E. K. *The Experimenters. A Study of the Accademia del Cimento.* Johns Hopkins University Press, Baltimore, 1971.

Saggi di naturali esperienze fatte nell'Accademia del Cimento sotto la protezione del Serenissimo Principe Leopoldo di Toscana e descritte dal segretario di essa Accademia. Cocchini, Florence, 1667. (English translation by R. Waller, Alsop, London, 1684.)

Targioni-Tozzetti, G. *Atti e memorie inedite dell'Accademia del Cimento.* 3 vols. Ranieri, Florence, 1780.

——*Notizie degli aggrandimenti delle scienze fisiche accaduti in Toscana nel corso di anni LX del secolo XVII.* Ranieri, Florence, 1780.

French Academies of the 17th Century

Brown, H. *Scientific Organisations in Seventeenth Century France (1620–1680).* Williams & Wilkins, Baltimore, 1934.

Daumas, M. *Les Instruments Scientifiques aux XVIIè et XVIIIè Siècles.* Presses Universitaires de France, Paris, 1953.

Hahn, R. *The Anatomy of a Scientific Institution. The Paris Academy of Sciences (1666–1803).* University of California Press, Berkeley, 1971.

Histoire et Prestige de l'Académie des Sciences (1666–1966). Musée du Conservatoire National des Arts et Métiers, Paris, 1966.

Lenoble, R. *Mersenne, ou la Naissance du Mécanisme*. Vrin, Paris, 1943.

Mémoires de l'Académie Royale des Sciences depuis 1666 jusqu'à 1699, 9 vols. Paris, 1729–1732.

Mémoires de l'Institut National des Sciences et arts. Sciences, Mathématiques et Physiques, 6 vols. Paris, 1798–1806.

Ornstein, M. *The Role of Scientific Societies in the Seventeenth Century*. University of Chicago Press, Chicago, 1928 and 1938.

Pelisson, F. P. *Histoire de l'Académie Française jusqu'en 1652*. Paris, 1653.

Taton, R. *Les Origines de l'Académie Royale des Sciences*. Presses Universitaires de France, Paris, 1966.

German Academies of the 17th Century

Buchner, A. E. *Sacrae Caesareae Majestatis Mandato et Privilegio Leges*. Halle, 1756.

Deutsche Akademie der Naturforscher "Leopoldina." Halle, 1952.

Malpertius, P-L. de. *Histoire de l'Académie Royale des Sciences et Belles Lettres de Berlin depuis son Origine jusqu'au Présent (1750)*. Berlin, 1752.

English Academies in the 17th Century

Birch, T. *The History of the Royal Society of London*, 4 vols. Millar, London, 1756.

Hall, M. B. Sources for the history of the Royal Society in the 17th Century. *History of Science*, 5:62–76 (1966).

Record of the Royal Society. London, 1897.

Sprat, T. *The History of the Royal Society of London, for the Improving of Natural Knowledge*. Martyn and Allestry, London, 1667.

Weld, C. R. *History of the Royal Society*. Parker, London, 1848.

Envoi

The 17th century ended with a glorious record of all that contributes to man's progress, not only in the growth of understanding of the nervous system (which is the core of this study) but also in the activities occurring simultaneously in all fields. In architecture, Wren transformed London with the domineering dome of St. Paul's and his eloquent, spired churches (55 in all, 21 of which were destroyed in the bombings). Mansart, in France, architect to the King, was responsible for the famous Gallerie des Glaces at Versailles (centuries later the site of a momentous treaty) and the solidity of the Hôtel des Invalides, built not as a tomb but as a hospital; and Bernini in Rome had his great colonnade. In drama, the first half of the century witnessed the eruption of the Shakespeare plays; in the second half the theaters of Paris saw for the first time Racine's *Phèdre* and *Le Cid*. Molière, no longer a medical student of Gassendi's, intrigued Paris with his series of plays, giving *La Malade Imaginaire* just before he died. In music, this was the great century of the baroque in which London saw the birth of Purcell, Leipzig the birth of Bach, Venice the birth of Vivaldi, and Darmstadt that of Telemann, a promise of delight for the next century and for all time.

And what had the students of nervous activity achieved as a heritage for the next generation? They had begun to unseat Aristotle and Galen as explainers of the nervous system; they had begun the microscopic examination of its parts; they had undermined the age-old view of the nerve impulse as the passage of animal spirits; they had recognized (but not assigned to nerve) electricity, the invisible power that the next generation would begin to elucidate; they had drawn to them the great mathematicians and philosophers of the age; they had introduced mensuration into experiment and seen the precursors of the computer. Their comrade in another field had proven that blood moves, not as an ebb and flow, but as a circulation through our bodies. But unlike him, those concerned with the nervous system had moved away from vitalism and, by introducing experiment to test their concepts, had launched the mechanistic explanation that receives recognition today. Essentially the 17th is the century of attack on tradition and the expansion of intellectual freedom.

PART II
The Rise of Electrophysiology
in the 18th Century

Prologue

The 18th century had inherited from the 17th the urge to replace conjecture by demonstration and proof. This goal was sought for the nervous system by groups of workers in the older centers of learning in the Italies, the Netherlands, England, and France with the encouragement of the kings and princes of the great empires and of the duchys and principalities of what would two centuries later become Germany. Influential in this drive to replace unsupported concept by demonstrated fact was the most famous and controversial philosopher of that period: Descartes. Though not himself an experimenter, his statement expressed their goal, namely, that he must have no doubts before he can believe.[1] Progress was remarkable for an age when mighty forces were ranged against any departure from the 1500-year-old Galenic views of nervous action, when the teaching of Aristoteleanism was still mandatory at the ancient universities of Oxford and the Sorbonne, and when acceptance of the heliocentric universe still invoked papal displeasure.

The end of the 17th century had seen a breakaway from some of these earlier restraints for in its closing years two great scientists, Newton and Leibniz, rose into prominence, to be followed by the widely read promoter, Voltaire. But for the nervous system the part having the greatest difficulty for release from vitalism was the brain, so inevitably identified with the soul. And still persisting throughout the 18th century was the concept that some form of animal spirits was responsible for nervous transmission, although in its last decade the crucial experiments on animal electricity were to shake the world. A role for electricity, tentatively suggested in the past by Boyle, and queried by Newton, became in the 1800s the power that was to replace animal spirits. The century closed nine years after the seminal disclosure of Galvani's *Commentary*, but it would be the following one that would offer proof.

---

[1] "... quelquechoses en ma créance qui fust entièrement indubitable."

CHAPTER VIII

The Great Teachers

By the beginning of the 18th century the patient searching and growing understanding by individual explorers of the nervous system began to invade teaching in the medical schools. In the north, at the outstanding center of medicine, which was to send its scholars throughout Europe, Boerhaave was teaching at the University of Leyden. Once again leadership was coming from the Dutch.

Herman Boerhaave (1669–1738)

Boerhaave was descended from a family in Flanders, a country with a past in the Holy Roman Empire but subsequently torn between the French, the Austrian Hapsburgs, Spain, and in the 19th century by the creation of Belgium. During Boerhaave's lifetime, one portion was annexed by Louis XIV, remaining a part of France as the Departement du Nord, an industrial section centering on Lille. To the north was the country of the United Netherlands, with a lively history of standing against all domination, free and independent since the Treaty of Westphalia in 1648 at the end of the Thirty Years' War. Boerhaave was born there, near Leyden, in 1669. Schooled in philosophy, divinity, and mathematics, in 1701 Boerhaave received his first appointment at the University of Leyden, founded in 1575. It was to be his intellectual home for the rest of his life, to which his brilliant career brought fame.

Boerhaave's prominence lies in his teaching. Not himself an essentially investigative scientist, he nevertheless familiarized himself with current knowledge of botany, chemistry, embryology, and anatomy so that he could teach these subjects within the context of medicine. In botany he inspired his pupil, Linnaeus, to produce the famous classification of plant life *(Index plantarium)*, and in chemistry he produced his own classic, *Elementa Chemiae*. As a student of philosophy before graduating in medicine, Boerhaave had written theses on the human mind[1] in which the influence of Descartes' dualism emerges; he wrote of "the soul, the organ of thought being intimately united to the body" and that "animals can feel but they do not think." After his teaching appointment at Leyden he gave a speech on "Mechanistic Reasoning in Medicine."[2] In this early public lecture, Boerhaave revealed his strong belief in the use of mechanistic explanations in medicine, a position he was to hold all his life.

Boerhaave's most famous writings are his *Institutiones Medicae*, published first in 1708, beginning a series of new editions running until 1735. In terms of our present search for the history of the nervous system, the contents are meager. But it is to his devotion to collecting the writings and drawings of Swammerdam that students in this field owe him a debt, not only for their publication (in the *Bible of Nature*), but also for an intimate biographical account of this fine experimenter. Willed by Swammerdam to his friend Thévenot, these manuscripts were sold by him to the painter Joubert and later to Duverney. Boerhaave relentlessly followed the trail of the manuscripts and bought them for a large sum. They were of course in Dutch, and he was then faced with the task of translation to Latin. There were 52 copper plates of Swammerdam's drawings (they can now be seen in the Museum Boerhaave in Leyden). The two volumes occupied much of Boerhaave's later years, the second published just before his death in 1738.

We are told that Boerhaave did not take courses in medicine at the University but molded his work as a physician on the clinical medicine practiced by Thomas Sydenham, whom he greatly admired for his emphasis on bedside teaching.[3] Boerhaave's scientific training was in botany, important for making medications, and in chemistry, leading him to align himself against the iatrochemists. At Leyden there was a botanical garden, created in 1587; Boerhaave, as Professor of Medicine and Botany, was influential in its development, using its herbs to teach their use in medicine. He encouraged botanists there to attempt to grow, in the cold Dutch climate, some of the exotic fruits brought back from the Dutch East Indies. Their techniques included spraying the plants each day with warm water, and it is recorded that they succeeded with the banana plant.

Boerhaave was closer to experiment in chemistry as well as anatomy, where, it is known, he studied dissections. He was a great admirer of Vesalius. Boerhaave's very important contribution was his great influence as a teacher when he became Professor of Medicine and Chemistry. Strongly averse to the iatrochemists' view that the chemistry of the body mimicked the reactions of substances in laboratory reports, he definitely aligned himself with the iatrophysicists.

In describing his general view of the nervous system and the working of the body in his famous *Aphorisms*, Boerhaave emphasized the dichotomy of solids and fluids. Solids were constituted by the vessels (nerves and blood vessels), within which fluids passed. He described the two as though they were parts of a building: In the body the solid components formed the support, the pillars, the girders, the bastions, and the coverings, which, in order to produce movement, acted like a wine press to propel, by levers and pulleys, the movements of the nonsolid elements, as if by bellows, sieves, canals, troughs, and reservoirs. Fluids were contained within this system and moved solely by solids, which, by their actions, could mix them, separate them, change them. There was no metaphysical influence involved— their mechanical movements followed the laws of hydrostatics and hydraulics.[4]

---

[1]*De mente humana* 1687–1688. In: G. A. Lindeboom (Ed.). *Bibliographia Boerhaaviana*, 1–4, 1959.

[2]*De usu ratiocinii Mechanici in Medicina*. Verbessel, Leyden, 1703.

[3]G. A. Lindeboom. *Herman Boerhaave*. Methuen, London, 1968.

[4]*Aphorisms*, Nos. 40 and 41.

Boerhaave's system covered all secretions: blood, chyle, lymph, tears, and nervous fluid, preserving the old concept of humors.[5] He was a firm believer in a succus nervosa furnished by the brain and the spinal cord, and he supported Malpighi's idea that the cortex had a glandular structure for secreting the nervous fluid essential for muscular movement.

To locate Boerhaave's ideas about the nervous system we have to look at a series of lectures on nervous diseases,[6] begun late in life, eight years before he died, and published after his death.[7] Again, we find no discoveries but we do encounter the doctrines with which this great teacher aligned himself. Largely anatomical in context, his description of the sensory nerves being soft and the motor nerves hard reminds one of Galen. He numbered the cranial nerves as 10, and counted the spinal nerves as 30 pairs. He taught circulation by discussion of the cerebral arteries. Considering the capillaries of the lungs, Boerhaave held that here the blood cells were crushed and broken and that this explained the red color found there. (The same error had been made by Leeuwenhoek who, ignorant of haemolysis, studied the blood corpuscles he had discovered in blood diluted with water.) Without mention of Baglivi, Boerhaave rejected pulsations of the dura mater as a nervous phenomenon, assigning them to distant action from the heart: a purely physical interpretation. According to Boerhaave, sensory and motor nerves met in a sensorium commune in the brain and spinal cord, but how they traveled and what mechanism carried the message resembled Descartes' minute particles, commonly accepted by such 17th-century writers as Gassendi and Charleton.

In his lectures on the nervous system, Boerhaave taught that "The Ventricles of the Brain have also many Uses or Advantages in Life, such as the perpetual Exhalation of a thin Vapour or Dew." Although himself a chemist, he made no experiments to test his theories. He was content to teach that:[8]

> Tho' the nervous Juice or Spirits separated in the Brain are the most subtile and moveable of any Humour throughout the whole Body, yet are they formed like the rest from the same thicker Fluid the Blood, passing thro' many Degrees of Attenuation, till its Parts become small enough to pervade the last Series of Vessels in the Cortex, and there it becomes the subtile Fluid of the Brain and Nerves.

These pronouncements are difficult to reconcile with the exhortation expressed in his *Aphorisms*, that attention to facts and observations is the best means of promoting medical knowledge. It is also disappointing to find Boerhaave teaching so many outdated concepts of nervous structure, for example, that the nervous system was glandular and that subtle juices flowed down tubular nerves. He passed over the work of so many from the previous century on this subject. Little change was made in these lectures from Descartes' description, although according to Boerhaave the juices bearing minute particles brought to the brain by the blood were there transformed, not by the pineal, but by the sensorium commune in the cortex. They then passed into the medulla and down the nerves without awareness or control by the will. Some, he said, passed from afferent to efferent in a sensorium commune in the spinal marrow: an essentially mechanistic procedure. Strangely, Boerhaave considered the

[5]*Aphorisms*, No. 403.

[6]J. Van Eems. *Hermanni Boerhaave. Praelectiones Academicae de morbis nervorum.* Leyden, 1761. Berne, 1762.

[7]*Dr. Boerhaave's Academical Lectures on the Theory of Physics, Being a Genuine Translation of his Institutes and Explanatory Comment*, 6 vols. London, 1747.

[8]From the anonymous translation of Boerhaave's *Institutiones Medicae*, entitled *Academical Lectures on the Theory of Physic, being a genuine translation of his Institutes, and Explanatory Comment*, 5 vols. Innys, London 1743.

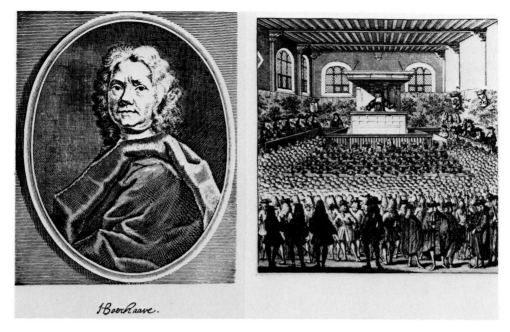

FIG. 52. **Left:** Herman Boerhaave (1669–1738) the great teacher of the early 18th century. (Portrait after Jan Wandelaar.) **Right:** Boerhaave giving a lecture in the Auditorium of the University of Leyden. (Title page to Boerhaave's oration: *De comparando certo in physicis.* 1715.)

nerves to be continuous at their peripheral endings with the finest fibers of the muscles they served.[9]

Boerhaave differentiated between voluntary muscles, which he stated were derived from the cerebrum, and involuntary muscles, on which the mind had no influence. These, he stated, must therefore derive their power of movement from the cerebellum and be concerned with vital functions, such as those of the heart, the stomach, and the lungs.

Carrying his views of the brain into his experiences in clinical situations, Boerhaave taught that conditions of delirium and frenzy ("phrenitis") were due to inflammation of the brain and that the apoplexy caused by head trauma was caused by compression of the brain. These teachings were spread throughout Europe by his admiring students; he was a man of great popularity. In 1730 he was elected to membership in the Royal Society, and in 1731 to the French Académie des Sciences.

There is a contemporary description of his habits and also his looks: "He had a large head, short neck, florid complexion, light brown hair (for he did not wear a wig), and open countenance, and resembled Socrates in the flatness of his nose. . . ."[10]

Boerhaave's chief relaxation was music and he played several instruments, of which his favorite was the lute. He discarded his wig as a gesture symbolic of the Netherlands' rupture from France and Spain. He died of gout in 1738.

Boerhaave's influence on the teaching of medicine should not be underestimated. His pupils came from many countries and left to found schools of medicine with teaching methods based on his own, including the medical school of Edinburgh where the famous Monro

[9]G. van Swieten. trans. *Commentaries upon Boerhaave's Aphorisms concerning the knowledge and Cure of Diseases*, 18 vols. Edinburgh, 1776.

[10]William Burton. *An account of the Life and Writings of Herman Boerhaave.* Lintot, London, 1743.

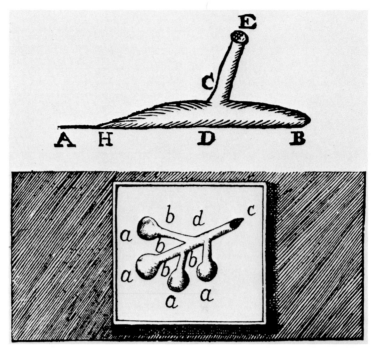

FIG. 53. **Above:** Boerhaave's concept of the neuromuscular junction. He believed that the nerve (EC) flowed directly into the substance of the muscle (HB). (From his *Institutiones medicae*, page 91. Leyden, 1734.) **Below:** Boerhaave's concept of a gland which, in opposition to the views of Ruysch, he maintained was a separate structure and not merely a distorted vessel. (From: Frederick Ruysch. In: *Opusculum anatomicum de fabrica glandularum in corpore humano*. Leyden, 1722.)

family was active; his most influential pupils were van Swieten and Albrecht Haller. Boerhaave's reputation was not limited to physicians: Samuel Johnson, the lexicographer, wrote "Life of Dr. Herman Boerhaave."[11] In a history restricted to the nervous system, Boerhaave's chief legacy was not his own work but Swammerdam's, in the magnificent *Bible of Nature*, and his championship of a mechanistic approach to physiology. He is memorialized by a statue outside the Academisch Ziekenhuis, Leyden's University Hospital.

Among his pupils, Boerhaave numbered all the prominent students of the nervous system, men who followed his precept that the goal of the learning taught in the classroom was its application to clinical medicine at the bedside: Monro, Pringle, Cullen, De Haen, Haller, and van Swieten are the well-known names among his pupils. The last two were responsible for spreading the teaching of Boerhaave by reproducing their lecture notes for circulation.

G. L. B. van Swieten (1700–1772)

Gerhard van Swieten was a Dutch Catholic, which gave him little chance of success in the protestant universities of the Netherlands. He obtained his degree in medicine and spent some time in clinical practice. Although clearly a competent teacher, his appointment to succeed Boerhaave was denied by the Senate. In 1745, at the invitation of Maria Theresia,

---

[11]Samuel Johnson. Life of Dr. Herman Boerhaave, late professor of physic in the University of Leyden in Holland. *Gentleman's Magazine*, 9:37–172 (1739). Life of Dr. Herman Boerhaave. *Universal Magazine*, 10:48–97 (1752).

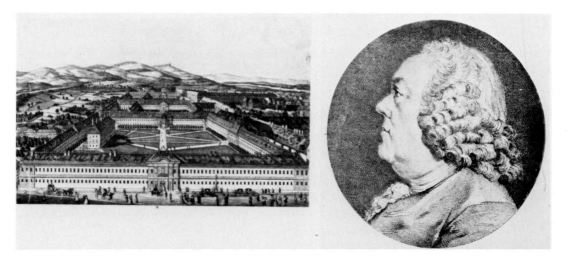

FIG. 54. Left: The famous Allgemeines Krankenhaus in Vienna, founded through the efforts of van Swieten to provide a general hospital for the sick. (From an early colored copper plate by Joseph and Peter Schaffer, 1784.) **Right:** Gerhard van Swieten, pupil of Boerhaave and publisher of his lectures.

the young Empress of Austria-Hungary, van Swieten moved to Vienna as Professor of Medicine, where an earlier student of Boerhaave's, Joannes Baptista Bassand, was physician at the Imperial Court. Bassand, a Frenchman, had come from Burgundy to learn from Boerhaave, but he, too, could not expect success in the protestant Netherlands.

In Austria there was a heritage of Jesuit teaching in the universities. In reaction to the rapid spread of Martin Luther's Reformation, Ferdinand I had appealed to Ignatius Loyola in 1550 to send him priests. The result was the founding of many Jesuit colleges, first in Vienna and later throughout Austria, with an increase in scholasticism but little advance in medicine. In 1625 the Jesuits had moved from their monastery in the Am Hof to the Universitätsplatz to take over the old University of Vienna, founded in 1365. By the 18th century, physics, astronomy, and chemistry were taught in Jesuit colleges throughout the provinces. However, the tide was turning and in 1773 the Society of Jesus was banned in Austria, and the Jesuit Order left the country, while the Catholic Counter Reformation movement prospered.

Empress Maria Theresia was eager to develop a school of medicine for Vienna's University and van Swieten was given the task. As a true follower of Boerhaave, he set up a procedure based on his experience in Leyden. His conviction was that hospitals were not only for treatment of the sick but also for teaching. His beliefs influenced Maria Theresia's son Joseph to found, in 1784, the Allgemeines Krankenhaus, a great general hospital, and the Academy of Medicine and Surgery in Vienna. Largely through the work of van Swieten, teaching in the University was reorganized, especially in the area of medicine and the natural sciences. Innovations in technique were also welcomed, including the use of percussion as a diagnostic tool, introduced by Joseph Leopold Auenbrugger, a pupil of van Swieten.[12] The clinical thermometer, whose use was advanced by Anton de Haen, was brought to Vienna by van Swieten.

---

[12]J. L. Auenbrugger (1722–1809), *Inventum novum ex percussione thoracis humani ut signo abstrusas interni pectoris morbos detegendi*. Vienna, 1761.

Van Swieten did not live to see the development of the great general hospital from his early teaching wards at the Bürgerspital in Vienna. That city hospital had only twelve beds, six for men and six for women. One must note van Swieten's organizational success, in his determination to upgrade the care of the sick and to make the hospitals centers for learning. To this end, he wrote commentaries of Boerhaave's teaching from the shorthand notes he had taken as a student in Leyden.[13] His method was to reproduce the actual words of Boerhaave as he had taken them down during the lecture and then add, in a different handwriting, his own commentary. It is from these commentaries that we learn so much of Boerhaave's medicine. Some of van Swieten's own views appear, including his conviction that epilepsy is congenital and caused by a fright to the mother during pregnancy.

Van Swieten's mostly uncritical commentaries on Boerhaave's views were preserved without change until the early 19th century. Some of Boerhaave's own notes were taken to Russia by his nephews as conditions for receiving appointments from the Car and, though never published, are now preserved in Leningrad. Microfilms of these manuscripts can be studied in the library of the University of Leyden and positive prints of them in the Boerhaave Museum.

Van Swieten had been honored by membership in the French Academy of Sciences and on his death in 1772 his place went to Benjamin Franklin as "associé étranger," the first American to receive this honor.

Johannes de Gorter (1689–1762)

Another of Boerhaave's students revived an idea from the previous century—the concept of the irritability of all tissues, not only muscle and nerve. This had been proposed by Francis Glisson[14] in a theory suggesting a kind of "tonus," or readiness to react. The hypothesis lay fallow for many years until a somewhat similar idea was revived briefly by Boerhaave's pupil, the surgeon Johannes de Gorter.

In 1734 de Gorter published the volume which brought out of obscurity the concept of the intrinsic irritability of tissues.[15] It is not clear whether de Gorter owed any of his ideas to Glisson. He presented a dynamic scheme, in which movements of muscles and nerves acted mechanically on each other with a vital oscillatory motion without which, he claimed, the heart would be unable to maintain the circulation.[16] Incorporated in his plan was a vitalistic component, a "motus vitalis," present in all living matter including plants (and therefore not identified with the soul). In this respect his view differed greatly from Glisson's, although he retained the idea of the "will" initiating muscular contractions.

De Gorter's view of muscle contraction was indeed novel. He held that the nerve made no contribution whatsoever to the "motus vitalis." He pictured the individual muscle fibers as longitudinal hollow strings criss-crossed by transverse nerve fibrils containing animal spirits. These nerve fibrils sectioned the muscle fibers into chains of vesicles which, when the "will" initiated a contraction, shortened in length and swelled in width. His concept of blood corpuscles and their travel through the circulatory system was that they became smaller

---

[13]G. L. B. van Swieten (1700–1772). *Commentaria in Hermanni Boerhaave, aphorismos, de cognoscendis et curandis morbis*, 6 vols. Verbeek, Leyden, 1742–1776.

[14]F. Glisson. *Anatomia hepatis.* Pullein, London, 1654.

[15]Johannes de Gorter (1689–1762). *Exercitationes medicae, I. De Motu vitale.* Amsterdam, 1734.

[16]*Exercitationes medicae, V. De actione viventium particulari.* Amsterdam, 1748.

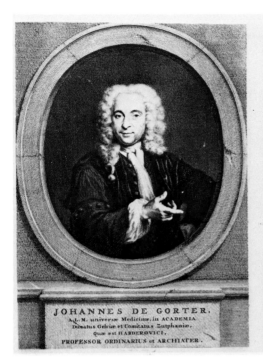 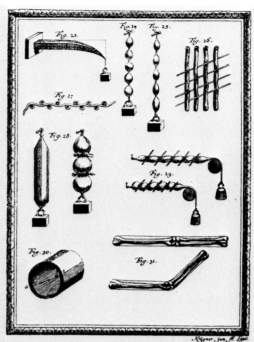

FIG. 55. **Left:** Johannes de Gorter (1689–1762). Engraving in the Boerhaave Museum in Leyden (after the portrait by J. M. Quinkhard). **Right:** Gorter's schema for muscle contraction. His drawing shows a single muscle fiber in contraction *(Fig. 24)* and when relaxed *(Fig. 25)* and the network of hollow longitudinal fibrils and transverse nerve fibers *(Fig. 26)* which constrict the long fibers into vesicles. On contraction to lift weights these vesicles swell *(Fig. 29)*. This results in shortening of the muscle and increase in width (From: de Gorter. *Medicinae Compendium*. Leipzig, 1749.)

and smaller as the blood vessels narrowed, thus maintaining their irritating effect. He gave a striking illustration of this in *Opuscula varia medico-theoretica*.[17]

At the end of the previous century Peter the Great, himself a physician, had visited Holland and (as we are told by Voltaire,[18] his first biographer) had sought to persuade Dutch scientists and medical men to come to Russia to strengthen his move to found an Academy of Science. Several went, including Boerhaave's two nephews, the anatomist Ruysch, and eventually de Gorter. Peter's success in bringing these scientists to Russia accounts for the fact that his capital, St. Petersburg, was the home of Ruysch's anatomical collections and several manuscripts of Boerhaave. De Gorter's attempt to explain the nervous system in terms of intrinsic irritability of tissues went practically unnoticed. It was in a different form that this view was revived yet again by Boerhaave's student, Haller.

Albrecht Haller (1708–1777)

Of Boerhaave's many famous pupils, one who was to have a great impact on concepts of the nervous system was Albrecht Haller, born in 1708 in Berne, the future capital of

[17]J. de Gorter. *Opuscula varia medico-theoretica*. Manfre, Leyden, 1751.

[18]François Marie Arouet Voltaire (1694–1778). *L'histoire de l'Empire de Russie sous Pierre le Grand*. Paris, 1759–1763.

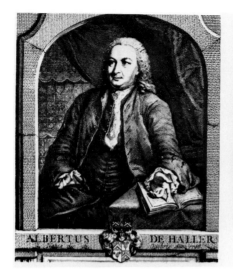
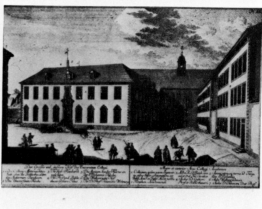

FIG. 56. **Left:** Albrecht von Haller (1708–1777), the influential teacher of physiology in the eighteenth century. (The portrait is from the frontispiece of his *Elementa Physiologiae* and is an engraving by Tardieu.) **Right:** The University of Göttingen, founded in 1737 by George II of England, Elector of Hannover. Haller spent his most scientifically productive years here as Professor of Anatomy, Botany and Surgery.

Switzerland. After beginning his medical training at Tübingen in its ancient university built in 1477, he was drawn by Boerhaave's fame to Leyden where he graduated in 1727 as a doctor of medicine. In 1736 he was appointed by George II, King of England and Elector of Hannover, to be Professor of Anatomy, Botany, and Surgery in Göttingen. This town in the Electorate of Hannover had just founded its university. Haller spent eleven years there, the experimental part of his career, until his love for the Alps and Switzerland drew him home again to pursue his interests in anatomy, botany, and poetry. While in Göttingen Haller's experiments were many and diverse; those directed toward investigation of the nervous system relied on vivisection.

His views became generally known after two lectures he gave before the Societatis Regiae scientiarum (George II's "Royal Society") in Göttingen in 1752. They were published the following year as *De partibus corporis humani sensibilibus et irritabilibus*.[19] This dissertation discussed the role of irritability as the property of muscle and sensibility as the property of nerve. Haller's notion of irritability, although scarcely differentiated from contractility, was the forerunner of the modern physiologic concept of excitability. His theory also differed fundamentally from that of Glisson,[20] for it lacked the intermediate element of psychic perception between the irritation and the contraction. Glisson had introduced the action of the soul to explain our voluntary movements. Haller defined the dual properties of irritability as follows:

> I call that part of the human body irritable, which becomes shorter on being touched; very irritable if it contracts upon slight touch, and the contrary if by a violent touch it contracts but little. I call that a sensible part of the human body, which on being touched transmits the impression of it to the soul; and in brutes, in which the existence of a soul is not so

[19]De partibus corporis humani sensibilibus et irritabilibus. *Comm. Soc. reg. Sci. Göttingen*, 2:114–158 (1753). Translated into English, anonymously (from Tissot's French translation). Nourse, London, 1755.

[20]Francis Glisson (1597–1677). *Tractatus de ventriculo et intestinis*. Brome, London, 1677.

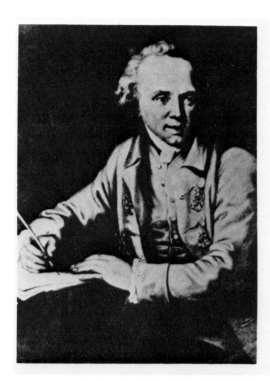 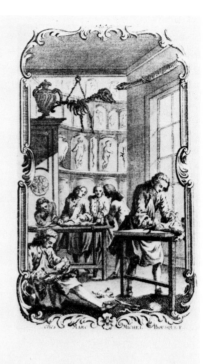

FIG. 57. **Left:** Samuel August David Tissot, physician in Lausanne, friend of Haller and translator and conserver of his correspondence. **Right:** Illustration depicting experiments with intravascular injection. (From: Haller. *Deux mémoires sur le mouvement du Sang et sur les effets de la Saignée, fondées sur les Expériences faites sur les Animaux.* Translation by A. Tissot. Bousquet, Lausanne, 1756.)

> clear, I call those parts sensible, the Irritation of which occasions evident signs of pain and disquiet in the animal.

This distinction between the action of sensation on man and on lower animals is reminiscent of Descartes. No doubt the "absence" of the soul in his experimental animals lessened Haller's misgivings about vivisection.[21]

> I took living animals of different kind, and different ages, and after laying bare that part which I wanted to examine, I waited till the animal ceased to struggle and complain, after which I irritated the part, by blowing, heat, spirit of wine, the scalpel, lapis infinalis, oil of vinegar, and bitter antimony. I examined attentively, whether upon touching, cutting, burning, or lacerating the part, the animal seemed disquieted, made a noise, struggled, or pulled back the wounded limb, if the part was convulsed, or if nothing of all this happened.

As one reads through his vast series of experiments (he discusses 190), many done in collaboration with Zimmermann,[22] one cannot escape some feeling of revulsion at their cruelty, and Haller himself felt some apology was due. He writes of it as "a species of cruelty for which I felt such reluctance, as could only be overcome by the desire of contributing to the benefit of mankind."

[21]Quotations are from the anonymous translation published by Nourse, London, 1755.
[22]Johann Georg Zimmermann (1728–1795).

Haller recognized that nerves are "the source of all sensibility," but applied his dichotomy between irritability and sensibility to various types of nerves, noting that all nerves are not irritable according to his definition, and insisting on resultant contraction. He thus came close to differentiating motor and sensory nerves. Yet he still included in his hypothesis the 1600-year-old concept of nervous fluid within the nerves—in spite of his being aware (as he tells us)[23] of the work of Swammerdam. The only competing hypothesis, tentatively suggested and little supported, was that the nerves were cords that communicated sensation to the brain by their vibrations. This proposal was rejected by Haller's teacher Boerhaave, who declared it to be "repugnant to the Nature of the soft, pulpy and flaccid nerves," and was also rejected by Haller.

In considering how a fluid could possibly flow as swiftly as nerves can be observed to act, Haller proposed that it must indeed be a very subtle fluid imperceptible to the eye yet more substantial than heat, vapor, electricity, or magnetism. The velocity with which a nervous fluid would need to travel to cause an observable reaction was an intrinsic difficulty for all who still believed in a fluid. Haller calculated that the fluid would have to travel as fast as 9,000 feet per second. De Sauvages, at the University of Montpellier, calculated that no less than 32,000 feet per second would be necessary.

Haller defined nervous fluid as "an element of its own kind unlike everything else. An element too subtle to be grasped by any of the senses, but more gross than fire, or aether or electrical or magnetic matter, since it can be contained in channels and restrained by bonds, and moreover is clearly produced out of and is nourished by the food." It is of interest that Haller had noted (and rejected) Newton's suggestion that the invisible power might be aether.[24]

He did allow that electricity was a most powerful stimulus to nerves but he thought it improbable that the body's internal stimulus was itself electrical in nature. Thinking in terms of electricity flowing down a wire, Haller, like so many physiologists after him, felt that the lack of insulation around the nerve was a critical argument against nervous influence being electrical. But during his lifetime, the suggestion was to come up again and again and was brought into prominence within twenty years of his death.

Haller held that the heart was independent of the nervous system, and the most irritable organ of the body whose muscle fibers were stimulated to contract in systole by the incoming blood. In his treatise on the movement of the blood, he reports that he could find no action on the heart by the nerves. Stimulation of the phrenic nerve caused no effect on the heartbeat and even when he irritated the spinal marrow until the animal had a convulsion, he found no change in the heartbeat. "Tous les muscles," he noted, "entrent en convulsion mais le coeur est excepté de cette loi et il conserve la regularité de ses bâtimens."[25] He was not surprised when it was shown that the heart of the frog continues to beat after destruction of its brain and spinal cord. Haller, in fact, opposed many of the views of the famous scientists of the 17th century: he denied the vibration theory of nerves proposed by Baglivi and scorned Steno's geometric structure of muscle and Willis' regard for the corpus callosum as the seat of the soul.

Haller was not only a great experimenter, he was also an indefatigable scholar. He compiled vast bibliographies of anatomy, botany, surgery, and medicine that contain thousands of

[23]*De Partibus corporis sensibilibus et irritabilibus*, Section II, 1753.

[24]Isaac Newton. *Opticks*, 2nd ed., 24th query. London, 1717.

[25]*Deux mémoires sur le mouvement du sang et sur les effets de la saignée*, translation by A. Tissot, p. 147. Bousquet, Paris, 1756.

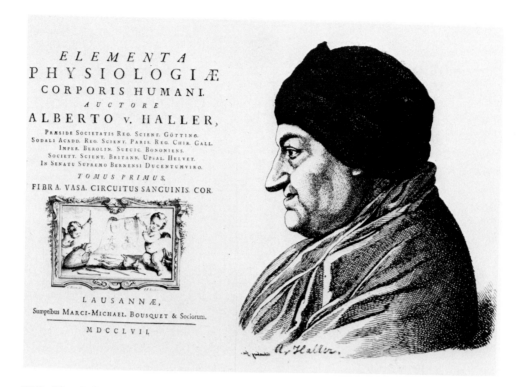

FIG. 58. **Left:** The title page to Haller's famous book on physiology. One of the putti holds a measuring rod and the other some anatomical drawings. Below is an excised heart and a comparatively miniscule dog. **Right:** Haller in his old age when he had retired to Berne where he pursued his love of botany and wrote poetry.

references. These were published in the many volumed *Elementa Physiologiae Corporis Humani*.[26] He died in 1777, a much revered figure, commemorated in many portraits, medallions, and statues, many of which have been collected in a book of iconography.[27] His views outlasted him, and Hallerian physiology remained influential until the end of the 18th century.

In the 17th century a mechanistic view of the animal and human body was evolving, an approach that received some backing from experimentation in the nervous system. In the 18th century, this disturbing view inevitably began to filter into the medical schools and, in fact, we find the great leaders there giving more time to polemics than to the laboratory. Descartes' views and writings still received more consideration than those of any contemporary. We find them discussed by Boerhaave, Gorter, van Swieten, and Haller. The nucleus of concern to all of these men was the question of the degree to which they would acknowledge a mechanistic explanation of the nervous system. Their concern was highlighted by another pupil of Boerhaave: Julien Offray de la Mettrie.

Julien Offray de la Mettrie (1709–1751)

La Mettrie, although in Leyden only briefly after obtaining his baccalaureate in medicine at Rheims, left a continuing contribution in that he too spread the teachings of the master

[26]*Elementa Physiologiae Corporis Humani.* Lausanne, 1762. (Translation by M. Foster. *Lectures on the History of Physiology.* Cambridge, 1901.)

[27]A. Weese. *Die Bildnisse Albrecht von Hallers.* Francke, Bern, 1909.

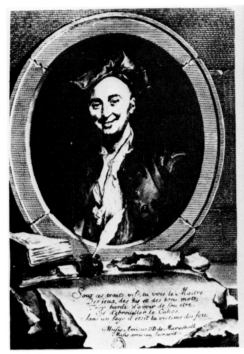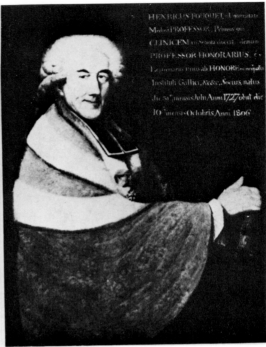

FIG. 59. Two distinguished men who offended Haller: **Left:** Julien Offray de la Mettrie (1709–1751) who dedicated his materialistic treatise, *L'homme machine*, to Haller. The portrait is an engraving by Tardieu (reproduced here by permission of the Bibliothèque Nationale), the original pastel being by Maurice Quentin de la Tour.   **Right:**   Henri Fouquet (1727–1806) prominent physician at Montpellier who wrote a long attack on Haller's theory of irritability and sensibility in Diderot's *Encyclopédie* (Vol. 15, pp. 38–52). (Oil painting in the Faculté de Médecine at Montpellier. Reproduced by permission from the University of Montpellier.)

by translating them into French. In fact, la Mettrie's rendering of Boerhaave's teachings are the clearest we have. La Mettrie was a Breton, born at St. Malo in 1709. He worked as an army doctor and then as a medical officer in Paris until some of his writings brought him trouble—in particular, *Histoire naturelle de l'âme* (1745), which was condemned by the Parliament of Paris the following year. A much traveled man, he visited China as a ship's doctor and, on returning to Paris, wrote a satire about his fellow physicians pretending it was a translation from the Chinese of "Dr. Fum Ho Ham."[28] The doors of Paris were then closed to him and he moved to Leyden and wrote *L'Homme Machine*, which forced him into exile once again. The book (it is really not much longer than a pamphlet) was published anonymously with a notice to this effect by the printer and with a quotation from Voltaire on the title page. He dedicated it to Haller whom he had never met.

In the text, la Mettrie began with an attack on the dualism of Descartes and proceeded to argue that what is called the "soul" is in fact a reflection of the body itself, varying with the food eaten, the body temperature, and sleep ("l'âme et le corps s'endorment ensemble"). He also discussed the effect of inflammation. Food, he maintained was all important, for the brain and nerves depended on the firmness of solids ingested and reflected their influence.

[28]*La politique du médecin de Lachiavel ou le chemin de la fortune ouvert aux médecins.* Bernard, Amsterdam, 1746.

Raw meat, for example, made animals savage (the English, he said, were fierce because they did not cook their meat enough). Heavy food made a dull and lazy mind. All of these arguments were used to demonstrate the oneness of body and soul.

La Mettrie studied brain size and cortical convolutions, both superior in man, noting that Lancisi put the site of the soul in the corpus callosum, a structure that was nonexistent in the fish which he put lowest on the ladder of the animal kingdom. He spurned the proposal that the soul was in the cerebellum, citing Haller's observations.[29]

Unlike Descartes, la Mettrie was no dualist. He believed that all of the body's operations, in man as in animals, were driven by a mechanical force. He made no distinction between man and lower animals and emphasized this by his title "Man the Machine." In fact, because of the provocative way in which it was written, his book appeared to be much more disruptive to the thought of his time than the writings of others. The book, which caused so much stir, presented a totally materialistic view of mental activity, describing it in terms of physiological states without any reliance on direction from a soul. Although he retained the presence of animal spirits, he relied heavily on the concept of irritability for explaining spontaneous motion. This probably explains his satirical dedication to Haller, the prophet of irritability, with whom he had quarreled and who was not pleased with the dedication for he considered la Mettrie's system "impious."[30]

La Mettrie relied on classic experiments that demonstrated the reaction to stimulation of isolated muscles. He also cited Steno in declaring that the isolated muscle fiber can move and needs no directive from a nerve, brain, or soul. The negative reaction to his work in Holland hastened la Mettrie's acceptance of an invitation to the court of Frederick the Great in Potsdam where a free-thinking group which included Voltaire lived and worked. He spent the rest of his life there, honored by an appointment to the Prussian Academy of Science, and when he died in 1751, Frederick wrote his eulogy.

La Mettrie's irreverent approach to what we now call the mind–body problem was disturbing to another of Boerhaave's pupils, Jerome David Gaub.

Jerome David Gaub (1705–1780)

Scientists owe a debt to Gaub, a professor of chemistry at Leyden, for it was he who translated Swammerdam's classic works from Dutch into Latin so that all scholars could read the *Biblia Naturae* that Boerhaave had collected for publication.

Gaub was a clinician as well as a professor, and it was his experience with patients that generated his interest in the role of the mind in the actions of the body. He believed the role of the mind was exaggerated and that many so-called "mental states" were curable by treatment of the body. Later he was to give somewhat more emphasis to the role of the mind in disease as had Galen before him. In 1747 Gaub published a lecture on this subject.[31] He was distressed when, in the same year, the provocative *Man the Machine* was published by la Mettrie who had attended the lecture. Gaub did not wish to be associated with such an extreme view and was careful to state this in his next publication.

In the context of the nervous system, Gaub declared that the mind was intimately involved with sensation and muscular motion which operated through an agent, which he named "enormon," flowing in the nerves—an old concept, with a new name. He believed this agent

---

[29]Albrecht von Haller. Observatio de Schirro Cerebelli. *Phil. Trans. roy. Soc.*, 43:100–101 (1744).

[30]Albrecht von Haller. *Mémoires sur la nature sensible et irritable des parties du corps animal*, Vol. 1, p. 90. Lausanne, 1756.

[31]*De regimine mentis*, Leyden 1747. (Translated into English by J. Trapell under the title: *On the Passions*.)

of the mind acted on the muscles by irritation which triggered the release of their innate vital power (vis vitalis). But in his *Institutiones* he provides the unexpected suggestion that this vital power could be electrical in nature, a vis electrica. He was searching for a force that could trigger movement of the muscles for, as the translator of Swammerdam, he knew that no agent, even his own "enormon" flowed into the muscle and expanded it. These concepts were elaborated in his textbook, *Institutiones Pathologiae Medicinalis*.[32]

Gaub, born in Heidelberg, was not Dutch but, after initial schooling in Halle, he was drawn to Leyden by the magnetic Boerhaave. He studied medicine there and achieved his degree at the age of 20; and it was to Leyden that he returned six years later when appointed by Boerhaave as a lecturer in chemistry. His appointment as professor of medicine in 1734 brought him into the clinical world where he gained prominence and membership in foreign societies, including the Académie des Sciences in Paris and the Royal Society in London. But offers from other centers, including St. Peterburg, could not persuade him to leave Leyden where he also served as Rector no less than three times. He died there in 1780 at the age of 75.

BIBLIOGRAPHY

Herman Boerhaave (1669–1738)

Selected Writings

De Usu Ratiocinii Mechanici in Medicina. Leyden, 1703.

Institutiones Medicae, in Usus Annuae Exertationis Domesticos Digestae ab Hermanno Boerhaave. Leyden, 1708, 1713, 1720, 1727, 1735.

Aphorismi de Cognoscendis et Curandis Morbis in Usum Doctrinae Domesticae. Leyden, 1709.

Elementa Chemiae, quae Anniversario Labore Docuit, in Publicis, Privatisque, Scholis, Hermannus Boerhaave, 2 vols. Severinus, Leyden, 1732.

Bijbel der Natuure, door Jan Swammerdam, 2 vols. In Dutch and Latin. Leyden, 1737–1738. (English translation by T. Flloyd. London, 1758.) Facsimile edition, edited by G. A. Lindeboom. Leyden, 1982.

[Van Eems, J.] *Hermanni Boerhaave Praelectiones Academicae de Morbis Nervorum*. Leyden, 1761.

[van Swieten, G.] *Commentaries upon Boerhaave's "Aphorisms Concerning the Knowledge and Cure of Diseases."* Translated from the Latin, 18 vols. London, 1759. Edinburgh, 1776.

Secondary Sources

Burton, W. *An Account of the Life and Writings of Herman Boerhaave*. London, 1743.

Daremberg, C. *Histoire de Sciences Médicales*, Vol. 2. Ballière, Paris, 1870.

Haller, A. *Hermanni Boerhaave*. Praelectiones academicae in propriis. Amsterdam, 1742.

King, L. *The Medical World of the Eighteenth Century*. University of Chicago Press, 1958.

La Mettrie, J. O. de. *Institutions de Medecine de M. Herman Boerhaave*, 2 vols. Paris.

Lindeboom, G. A. *Boerhaave's Correspondence*, 2 vols. Leyden, 1962 and 1964.

Lindeboom, G. A. *Herman Boerhaave*. Methuen, London, 1968.

Lindeboom, G. A. Boerhaave's concept of the basic structure of the body. *Clio Medica*, 5:203–208 (1970).

---

[32]*Institutiones pathologiae medicinalis*. Leyden, 1758. (Translated into English by C. Erskine. Edinburgh, 1778.)

G. L. B. van Swieten (1700–1772)

Selected Writings

Commentaria in Hermanni Boerhaave, Aphorismos, de Cognoscendis et Curandis Morbis, 6 vols. Verbeek, Leyden, 1742–1776. (English translation: *Commentaries upon Boerhaave's "Aphorisms Concerning the Knowledge and Cure of Diseases,"* 18 vols. Edinburgh, 1776.)

Secondary Sources

Lindeboom, G. A. *Herman Boerhaave*. Methuen, London, 1968.

King, L. S. *The Medical World of the Eighteenth Century*. University of Chicago Press, 1958.

Lesky, E. *The Vienna Medical School of the 19th Century*. The Johns Hopkins University Press, Baltimore, 1976.

Johannes de Gorter (1689–1762)

Selected Writings

De perspiratione insensibili. Vander, Leyden, 1736.

Exercitationes Medicae, 5 vols. I, *De motu vitale*, 1734. II, *Sommo et vigilia*, 1736. III, *De fame*, 1736. IV, *De siti*, 1737. V, *De actione viventium particulari*, 1748. Amsterdam.

Medicinae Compendium. Frankfurt and Leipzig, 1749.

Opuscula varia medico-theoretica. Manfre, Leyden, 1751.

Albrecht Haller (1708–1777)

Selected Writings

Primae Lineae Physiologiae in Usum Praelectionium Academicarium. Vanderhoeck, Göttingen, 1747. (English translation by W. Cullen. Edinburgh, 1779.)

De Partibus Corporis Humani Sensibilibus et Irritabilibus. In: *Commentarii Societatis Regiae Scientium Gottingensis*, Vol. 2, pp. 114–158. 1753. (Translated into French by A. Tissot, 1754, and into English anonymously. Nourse, London, 1755.)

Icones Anatomicae. Vandenhoeck, Göttingen, 1743–1756.

Elementa Physiologiae Corporis Humani, Hemmerde Vols. 1–5. Bousquet, Lausanne, 1757–1763. Vols. 6–8, Bern, 1764–1766. 8 vols., 1757–1765.

Mémoires sur les Parties Sensibles et Irritables du Corps Animal, 3 vols. Lausanne, 1760.

Bibliotheca Botanica. Orell, Zurich, 1771–1772.

Bibliotheca Chirurgica. Schweighauser, Basle, 1774.

Bibliotheca Medicinae Practicae. Schweighauser, Basle, 1776.

Bibliotheca Anatomica. Orell, Zurich, 1774–1777.

[Hermann Boerhaave] *Praelectiones Academicae in Propries Institutiones Rei Medicae Edidit*, 7 vols. Vandenhoeck, Göttingen 1739–1744.

[Hintzsche, E.] *Albrecht von Haller's Briefe an August Tissot*. 1754–1777. Huber, Bern, 1977.

Secondary Sources

Foster, M. *Lectures on the History of Physiology During the Sixteenth, Seventeenth and Eighteenth Centuries*. Cambridge University Press, Cambridge 1924.

Hintzsche, E. *Albrecht von Haller–Marcantonio Caldani. Briefwechsel 1756–1768.* Bern, 1964.

Rudolph, G. Haller's Lehre von Irritabilität und Sensibilität. In: *Von Boerhaave bis Berger*, edited by K. E. Rothschuh pp. 14–34. Stuttgart, 1964.

Temkin, O. Dissertation on the sensible and irritable parts of animals by Albrecht von Haller. (English translation) *Bull. Hist. Med.*, 4:651–699 (1936).

Julien Offray de la Mettrie (1709–1751)

Selected Writings

Systeme de M. Boerhaave sur les Maladies Veneriennes. 1735.

Aphorismes sur la Connaissance. 1738.

Aphorismes de Mr Herman Boerhaave sur la Connaissance et cure des Maladies. Huart et Brisson, Paris 1739.

Traité de la Matière Medicale. 1739.

Les Institutions de Medicine. 1740.

Abrège de la Théorie Chimique. 1741.

Traité de l'Histoire Naturelle de l'Ame. The Hague, 1745.

La Politique du Médecine de Machiavel ou le Chemin de la Fortune ouvert aux Médecins. Bernard, Amsterdam, 1746.

L'Homme Machine (anonymous). Luzac, Leyden, 1748. (English translation by E. Luzac. G. Smith, London, 1750; and by G. C. Bussey, Chicago, 1912.)

Secondary Sources

Lemee, P. *Julien Offray de la Mettrie.* Mortain, 1954.

Rosenfield, L. C. *From Beast-Machine to Man-Machine.* Oxford University Press, 1940.

de Saussure, R. Haller and la Mettrie. *J. Hist. Med.*, 4:431–449 (1949).

CHAPTER IX

The Vitalists

Georg Ernst Stahl (1659–1734)

In the German states the most powerful figure to emerge after the Thirty Years' War was Georg Ernst Stahl. He was born in 1659 in Ansbach, a strongly Lutheran city in what is now Bavaria but was then a Hohenzollern principality. After study at the University of Jena (founded in 1558), where he received a medical degree, he began to give lectures in chemistry. In these he promoted his theory of phlogiston as a crucial element in combustion, a theory accepted by Priestley but eventually disproved by Lavoisier. In 1687 he was appointed court physician to the Duke of Saxe-Weimar, then a leading center of the arts. The court organist was Johann Sebastian Bach and a culture was developing that would attract Goethe and Schiller and, in the following century, Franz Liszt. It was at Jena that Schiller wrote his Wallenstein trilogy. In 1693 the University of Halle was founded,[1] and when it opened a year later Stahl was appointed as second professor of medicine. He stayed until 1716 when he was called to Berlin as personal physician to Frederick William, King of Prussia.

He was destined to create the strongest (and last) center of vitalism outside of the Church. In attack of the mechanistic view of the animal body that was gaining popularity in the rest of Europe, he wrote a dissertation on the difference between organs and machines.[2] No machine, he held, could create on its own such wonderful esthetic experiences as the "anima," which he believed regulated all bodily activity.

In opposition to both the chemical and mathematical schools of thought that had been gaining ground, he reintroduced an immaterial anima which he believed was the sole activating principle of the body parts. Since the search for an immaterial agent lies outside the

---

[1] Now named the Martin-Luther-Universität Halle-Wittenberg.

[2] *Dissertatio inauguralis medica de medicina medicinae curiosae.* Halle, 1714.

scope of science, Stahl's doctrines, promulgated with arrogance and dogmatism, virtually extinguished experimental inquiry among his followers. Even writers sympathetic to his viewpoint found that in attempting to follow his arguments they became "involved in a labyrinth of metaphysical subtlety."[3] The metaphysical approach of Stahl came under criticism from Vicq d'Azyr, the great anatomist, who suggested that the use of an imaginary soul to resolve those phenomena that could not yet be explained by the laws of physics and chemistry was merely a cloak for ignorance.

The chief impact of Stahl's teaching was on the concepts of the brain. His adverse influence on the growth of experimental neurophysiology had a very negative impact on the development of knowledge about the nervous system, for he dethroned the brain from the ruling seat. For Stahl the "anima" in living creatures was totally separate from the matter of bodily organs and ruled them through operations that might indeed be mechanistic in detail. This in a nonmaterial anima placed not only the nervous system but all bodily functions outside the realm of scientific exploration. According to this concept, at death the anima left the body and the activities it once controlled, circulation, respiration, etc., all ceased. Thus, Stahl maintained, the living body was under this immaterial control. It was the anima that caused movement of the muscles hence there was no need to postulate animal spirits as the agent. This strongly vitalistic philosophy contained no element of deism and was not connected to the teachings of the Church. Stahl was a member of the Pietists, a group derived from Martin Luther's Reformation. An able clinician, he worked these beliefs into his concepts of disease and treatment. Such a position, coming from so prominent a man, was bound to slow the growing recognition of materialist explanations of the human body.

One of the readers of Stahl's *Theoria medica vera*, who was most perturbed by his vitalistic theory, was the aging Leibniz. For Leibniz the soul was so distinct that it had no influence whatsoever on the physical properties of the body. He emphatically denied Stahl's teachings. The interchange of argument between Stahl in Halle and Leibniz in Leipzig was pursued not in German but in Latin and continued for eight years until Leibniz died in 1716. Four years later Stahl published the entire debate under the title *Negotium otiosum*.[4]

In 17th century Holland, Italy, France, and England, there was a strong movement from concept to experiment. In Germany however, this development was overpowered by Stahl's doctrine of vitalism.

Friedrich Hoffmann (1660–1742)

Friedrich Hoffmann, born in Halle in 1660, went first to the ancient university of Erfurt (where Martin Luther had also studied) and then to Jena where he received his medical degree. He was appointed Professor of Medicine at Halle by the Elector of Brandenburg when a university was founded there in 1693. In contrast to Stahl, who followed him to Halle the following year, Hoffmann was receptive to many of the tenets of the mechanistic interpreters of the nervous system. He accepted animal spirits but declared them to be composed of material particles circulated in a "nerve juice."[5] He derived this nerve fluid from an aether, as did Newton, and believed it to be present in the blood. Others, for example, Baglivi,[6] had postulated a pulsation of the brain as the force which circulated nerve

[3]John Bostock (1773–1846). *Sketch of the History of Medicine from Its Origins to the Commencement of the Nineteenth Century.* Sherwood, Gilbert, and Pipa, London, 1835.

[4]English translation by L. J. Rather and J. B. Frerichs. *Clio Medica*, 3:21–40 (1968) and 5:53–67 (1970).

[5]*Fundamenta medicinae.* Huebner, Halle, 1695.

[6]G. Baglivi. *De fibra motrice et morbosa.* Perugia, 1700.

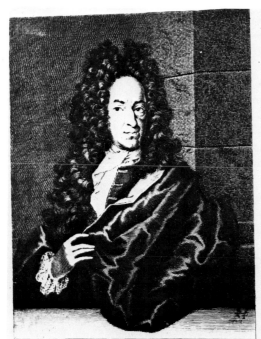

GEORGII ERNESTI STAHL,

THEORIA
MEDICAVERA.
PHYSIOLOGIAM
&
PATHOLOGIAM,
TANQVAM
DOCTRINAE MEDICAE PARTES
VERE CONTEMPLATIVAS,
e NATVRAE & ARTIS
VERIS FVNDAMENTIS,
Intaminata ratione, & inconcuffa Ex-
perientia fiftens.

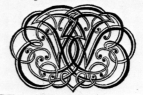

HALAE, *LITERIS ORPHANOTROPHEI M DCCVIII.*

FIG. 60. Georg Ernst Stahl (1659–1734) from the portrait in his famous work and its title page. (Courtesy of the Biomedical Library, University of California, Los Angeles.)

juice. Hoffmann, too, believed this refined force circulated the material particles in the nervous juice and propelled them to the fibers of the muscles, evoking a tonus when at rest and a contraction during activity. This concept of necessity accepted tubular nerve structure, allowing for spirits to be brought from the cerebrum for voluntary movements and from the cerebellum for involuntary and unconscious ones. All tissues and all organs were under the control of these powerful animal spirits. Throughout the process, aether was essential for it extracted these important particles from the food and controlled their circulation. Even the soul, the "anima sensitiva," although God-given, depended on this medium whose activities provided it with sensations.[7] Hoffmann also believed in a "sensus communis" where all sensations met. Unwilling to accept Descartes' location of this in the pineal, Hoffmann opted for the centrum ovale.

As with all these early philosophies, we find hovering between mind and brain, the ghost of the soul. This is less confusing for English speakers for they have a noun for "mind," which is distinct from "soul" or "spirit." The French do not (which raises problems concerning Descartes' intended meanings) and neither do the Russians, a difficulty which caused some of the disagreement between Sherrington and Pavlov in the next century. Hoffmann's intention is clear. He used the Latin term "mens" to differentiate between the soul and the circulating (material) spirits which had such a prominent role in nerve and muscle interaction.[8]

[7]"Subtilissimae aethereae elasticae particulae."

[8]*Fundamenta medicinae.* Vol. I. Huebner, Halle, 1695.

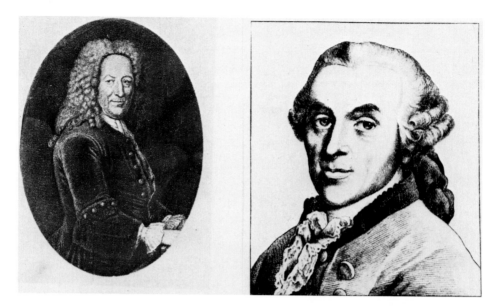

FIG. 61. **Left:** Friedrich Hoffmann (1660–1742). Professor of Medicine at the University of Halle. Portrait by Anton Pesne (frontispiece to his *Opera Omnia Physico-Medica*). **Right:** Johann August Unzer (1721–1799), staunch supporter of Stahl and Professor at Halle following Hoffmann.

To man, but not to brutes, he gave his immaterial "mens," bringing with it the God-given power to think and to reason.

Hoffmann therefore stands astride the positions taken by the true vitalists and the mechanists. His influence was great, especially in the clinical field in which he was a prominent and prolific writer. Following the format used by Boerhaave, Hoffmann wrote his *Fundamentals of Medicine* in the form of *Institutes*, focusing on the physics and chemistry of the body in health and disease. He traveled to England where his influence was seen later in the works of Cullen. Honored by many, he was elected a member of the Berlin Academy of Sciences, the Academy of Sciences in St. Petersburg, and a foreign member of the Royal Society. He died in 1742 at the age of 82.

Johann August Unzer (1727–1799)

The teachings of Stahl in Halle were passed down to Johann August Unzer, who was born in that town and received his doctorate in medicine there in 1748. Later, he set up his medical practice in Altona, a town on the Elbe near Hamburg. He was absorbed with the conflicts of vitalism and materialism and after several preliminary publications on the influence of the soul on the body,[9] some of which defended Stahl's theories,[10] he produced his major work.[11] Here, he revealed his reluctance to dethrone the soul in the management of the nerves and of muscle movement while still acknowledging some of the mechanistic

[9]*Gedanken vom Einflusse der Seele in ihren Körper.* 1746. (Thoughts on the Influence of the Soul on the Body.)

[10]Betrachtungen über Stahl's theoretischen Grundsatz. (Reflections on the Fundamental Principle of Stahl's Theory.) *Hamburg Magazine*, Vol. 10, 1768.

[11]*Erste Grunde einer Physiologie der eigentlichen thierischen Natur thierischer Körper.* Weidmanns, Leipzig, 1771.

views of his times. He proceeded to divide the phenomena he observed among the various levels of the animal kingdom. He denied a soul to some animals, while granting it to others. In this dichotomy of "beseelte" and "unbeseelte" animals (to some of the latter he also denied a brain), he explained neuromuscular actions as being of three types: voluntary, involuntary, and unconscious. In considering the third category, he came close to describing reflexes. In experiments to demonstrate his third category of brainless, soulless animals he decapitated frogs and produced movement by external stimulation of the nerves.

Unzer's concepts were little known until 50 years after his death when his treatise: *Erste Gründe einer Physiologie der eigentlichen thierischen Natur thierischer Körper* was chosen by the Sydenham Society of London for translation into English.[12] The Sydenham Society had been formed in 1843 with the goal of publishing important medical works not accessible in the English language. Thomas Laycock (1812–1876), a Yorkshireman educated in London, Paris, and Göttingen (later, Professor of Medicine at Edinburgh—an unusual post for an Englishman) undertook the translation from the German of Unzer's long work. In enthusiastic support of the concept of reflex action, he also translated from Latin the great work of Jiri Prockaska.[13] Thus, it was only in the 19th century that general knowledge of these two classics existed.

Unzer dissociated himself from the teachings of Stahl who held that, although the soul was unaware of them, all movements were indeed actions of the soul. He turned to the arguments of those who were concerned with the specific role of the soul in neuromuscular movements and focused his attention on its location. Because it was generally accepted that the soul was located in the head, experiments with decapitated animals were crucial to his work. However, devout vitalists such as Robert Whytt had felt impelled to propose that the soul pervaded the whole body and thus survived the loss of the head, and the idea that some representation of the soul existed within the spinal cord was used to refute the loss of soul in decapitated animals until the end of the 19th century. Another proponent of the soul being located outside of the head was Pflüger, the founder of the famous Pflüger's Archive.[14] By then the soul had been housed in the heart, ventricles, pineal, stomach, blood, corpus striatum, and medulla spinalis.

From his experiments on decapitated animals Unzer maintained that there were two categories of animal function dependent on a vis nervosa (Nervenkräfte) which he equated with animal spirits: one involved the brain, and the other was capable of evoking a muscular movement without sensation reaching the brain. The latter was the case in decapitated animals and was dependent on the property of irritability (Hallerian irritability) in the muscle. He also insisted that his decapitated animals must still be alive—that they must still have animal spirits persisting in their nerves. He explained the difficulty in demonstrating this with higher animals by their profuse bleeding on decapitation. So he worked with worms, butterflies, birds, and most of all, frogs. Evoking movement after removal of the head confirmed for Unzer that neuromuscular motion could take place without awareness. Both conscious voluntary movement and unconscious movement, such as a decapitated frog withdrawing its foot when pinched, were effected by the "vis nervosa." There were two distinct motor

---

[12]English translation by Thomas Laycock: *The Principles of a Physiology of the Proper Animal Nature of the Animal Organism*. Sydenham Society, London, 1851.

[13]Jiri Prockaska (1759–1820). *De Structura Nervorum*, 3 vols. Gerle, Prague, 1789–1794. (English translation by Thomas Laycock for the Sydenham Society. *Dissertation on the Functions of the Nervous System*, London, 1851.)

[14]Eduard Friedrich Wilhelm Pflüger (1829–1910). *Die sensorischen Functionen des Rückenmarks der Wirbelthiere nebst einer neuen Lehre über die Leitungsgesetze der Reflexionen*. Hirschwald, Berlin, 1853.

systems with which, Unzer said, "the animal machines are mysteriously and inscrutably endowed by the Creator." This led him to concede that there might be two kinds of "vis nervosa."

In conscious movements, Unzer believed "the brain secretes the vital spirits from the blood, and distributes them to the nervous system." In explaining movements of headless animals, he surmised that there is an ample store of the "vis nervosa," originally derived from the brain, in the peripheral nerves and possibly in the ganglions and plexuses, where an incoming flow of vital spirits could be turned back (reflektiert) to the muscle without going to the brain. He drew the comparison with a flower that lasts for some time after the stem is cut, and an animal that survives temporarily after being deprived of food.

At the time when Unzer was speculating on the possible role of the ganglions, the Bishop of Carlisle sent a communication to the Royal Society from an English doctor named James Johnstone.[15] Johnstone commented that ever since Fallopius had discovered the ganglions of the intercostal nerves, their role in the nervous system had not been understood.[16] He stated that Lancisi thought them to be muscles "sui generis" which were capable of contractions to propel the nervous spirits to the peripheral muscles to effect contraction.[17] Johnstone scorned this theory as well as Winslow's idea that the ganglions were "little brains."[18] He noted that several nerves met in the ganglions and were enriched by a good blood supply.

After pointing out the location and the destination of the nerves exiting from the intercostal ganglia he emphasized that all of the resulting functions were involuntary, a conclusion leading to his final thesis that they represented a system of nervous control independent of the soul. He restricted this notion of mechanistic independence, however, to the ganglia Winslow named (and we still call) the sympathetic ganglia. He conceded that the spinal roots each have ganglions which connect with the intercostals but which, in addition, have "other fibres fit and free for the commands of the will, as in fact many of them are distributed to muscles under its power and direction."

Unzer was a confirmed deist and throughout his life often referred causes to the Deity. Even animal instincts were for "the satisfaction and will of the Creator" and therefore had great importance. Referring quite frequently to Haller's physiology, he granted that all organs of the body, except for the brain and nerves, were indeed animal machines but the brain was the seat of the soul and the "laboratory" of the vital spirits.

Unzer was a clinician, not an experimentalist, so he made no tests of his theories. He marks an era when purely vitalistic explanations of our bodies were becoming untenable. A prolific writer, he continued to publish medical texts until his death at the end of the century.

Robert Whytt (1714–1766)

Across the English channel an attack on the Hallerian theory of irritability was launched by Robert Whytt. A Scot, who worked on experiments fundamental to modern physiology,

[15]James Johnstone, M.D. Essay on the use of the ganglions of the nerves. *Phil. Trans. roy. Soc.*, 54:177–184 (1764).

[16]Gabrielle Fallopius (1523–1562). *Observationes anatomicae*. Venice, 1564.

[17]Giovanni Maria Lancisi (1654–1720). Quoted in G. B. Morgagni (1682–1771). *Adversaria anatomica*. Padua, 1702–1719.

[18]J. B. Winslow (1669–1760). *Exposition anatomique de la structure du corps humain*, 4 vols. Duprée and Dessesartz, Paris, 1732.

his descriptions of them are often cloaked by his terminology. He made a special study of involuntary movements of the voluntary muscle systems in decapitated animals. The movement of animals after their heads had been severed had attracted the attention of scientists since Leonardo's day. In the previous century Robert Boyle had recognized the implications of this phenomenon in an essay he wrote on "experimental philosophy."[19] Boyle wrote that this phenomenon "may be of great concernment in reference to the common doctrine of the necessity of increasing influence from the brain, being so requisite to sense and motion." Boyle's curiosity about the brain and its workings was interwoven with his great interest in theology, although his views on the latter did not please his contemporaries. Dean Swift was moved to parody his fellow Irishman in a satire called "A Pious Meditation upon a Broomstick in the Style of the Honourable Mr. Boyle."

Robert Whytt was also concerned with the implications for theology. Born in Edinburgh in 1714, he trained at its University in medicine, though his first medical degree was from Rheims in France. When he returned to Scotland the University of St. Andrews awarded him their MD. He became Professor of Medicine, still maintaining a clinical practice which led to his appointment in 1761 as one of King George III's physicians. In 1763 he was elected President of the Royal College of Physicians of Edinburgh which was founded in 1681.

The lectures he had heard from his teachers, Alexander Monro in Edinburgh and Boerhaave in Leyden,[20] were at the root of his problem with reconciling the movements of decapitated animals with a belief in the dominance of the soul. He dissociated himself from mechanistic explanations, insisting that there was a "sentient principle" in all animal movements, a concept first launched by him in a lecture given to the Philosophical Society of Edinburgh in 1745. Some modern neurophysiologists have proposed that Whytt's sentient principle represents the central component of what is now known as the reflex arc.

Interaction among the nerves was "sympathy," a term frequently used by anatomists such as Winslow, and still in use today. Whytt believed that all interaction was due to the action of the soul which had sites in the spinal cord as well as in the brain. He also included the spinal marrow as a place for the soul in order to explain the movements of decapitated animals and the fact that a pithed frog did not move its limbs (an observation that had been recorded by Leonardo two centuries before).[21] Whytt used other arguments to support his concept of the soul in the spinal marrow. "If the soul," he wrote, "were confined to the brain, as many have believed, whence is it that a pigeon not only lives for several hours after being deprived of its brain but also flies from one place to another...."[22] He drew other examples from decapitated snakes and even a tortoise. The notion of a seat of the soul in the spinal cord lingered on for a hundred years, its last champion being Pflüger in his Rückenmarksseele.[23]

One of Whytt's tenets was that nerves had no branches but were continuous from their roots in the brain or spinal cord and therefore sympathy (i.e. interaction) could not take place in ganglia or plexuses. He was working in an era when belief in a nervous fluid had

[19]Robert Boyle (1627–1691). *Considerations Touching on the Usefulness of Experimental Philosophy*. London, 1663.

[20]First editions of Boerhaave's *Institutiones Medicae* (1708) are preserved in the Edinburgh University Library.

[21]*The Notebooks of Leonardo da Vinci*. McCurdy, London, 1938.

[22]"Nor do we know certainly whether this fluid serves only for the support and nourishment of the nerves or whether it be not the medium by which all their actions are performed."

[23]E. F. W. Pflüger (1829–1910). *Die sensorischen Functionen des Rüchenmarks der Wirbelthiere nebst einer neuen Lehre über die Leitungsgesetze der Reflexionen*. Hirchwald, Berlin, 1853.

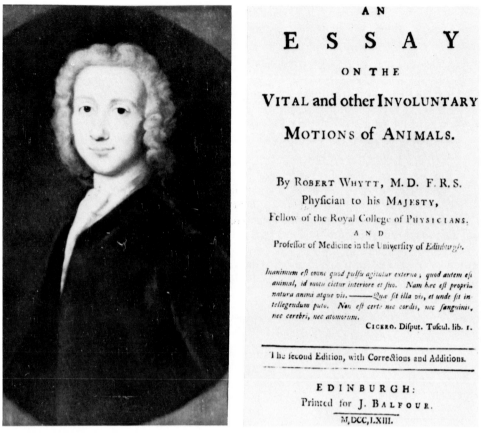

A N

E S S A Y

ON THE

VITAL and other INVOLUNTARY

MOTIONS of ANIMALS.

By ROBERT WHYTT, M.D. F.R.S.
Physician to his MAJESTY,
Fellow of the Royal College of PHYSICIANS,
A N D
Professor of Medicine in the University of *Edinburgh*.

*Inanimum eſt omne quod pulſu agitatur externo ; quod autem eſt
animal, id motu cietur interiore et ſuo.   Nam hæc eſt propria
natura animæ atque vis. ——— Quæ ſit illa vis, et unde ſit in-
tellegendum puto.   Non eſt certe nec cordis, nec ſanguinis,
nec cerebri, nec atomorum.*

CICERO. Diſput. Tuſcul. lib. 1.

The ſecond Edition, with Corrections and Additions.

EDINBURGH:
Printed for J. BALFOUR.
M,DCC,LXIII.

FIG. 62. Left: Robert Whytt (1714–1766). After a painting made in 1738 by Antonio Belluci. (Courtesy of the Royal College of Physicians, Edinburgh.) **Right:** Title page, 2nd edition of Whytt's famous essay first published in 1751.

not been disproved. Whytt accepted the demonstrations from the previous century that muscles are not inflated by nervous fluid,[24] but he was uncertain whether or not it existed in the nerves, either as a nutrient or as an active principle.[25]

Whytt's ideas were to bring him into an argument with Haller that lasted nearly 10 years. The initial criticism from Haller came as soon as he read Whytt's *Essay*.[26] He insisted that contractility was a property of the muscle itself and not dependent on the soul or the "essential principle" of Whytt. "Nothing," he wrote, "is more specious than to derive all motions from the soul."

According to Whytt, all movements were sentient but not necessarily conscious. And had he not been so insistent on control by the soul, he might have been the discoverer of reflex. His work with pupillary dilation in the eye was named by a later generation "Whytt's reflex,"

[24]". . . the extraordinary smallness of the nerves and the very slow secretion and motion of their fluid makes it improbable that muscular motion is owing to the distension of the fibres of the muscle by a sudden influx of that fluid."

[25]"Nor do we know certainly whether this fluid serves only for the support and nourishment of the nerves or whether it be not the medium by which all their actions are performed."

[26]*Essay on the Vital and other Involuntary Motions of Animals*. Balfour, Edinburgh, 1751.

though his observations closely resembled those of Fontana whose explanations were more mechanistic. Whytt's observations of the pupil were drawn mostly from his patients and led him to insist once again that sentience had a central role. He wrote:

> Since the optic nerves and those of the *uvea* arise from different parts of the brain, and have no communication with each other in their course to the eye, it seems evident, that light affecting the *retina* cannot excite the *sphincter* of the pupil into contraction by any immediate mechanical change which it produces, either in the muscle itself, or in the nerves which actuate it; but the uneasy sensation occasioned in the *retina* by the admission of too much light into the eye, may so affect the sentient principle which is present and ready to act wherever the nerves have their origin, as to excite it to contract the orbicular muscle of the *uvea*, in order to lessen the pupil, and exclude the offending cause.

Such a clear declaration of Whytt's unshaken belief in control of the nervous system by the elusive power of the mind was an irritant to Haller. Whytt and Haller disagreed on both sensibility and irritability. Haller denied sensibility to many tissues, such as the tendons, marrow, and cornea.[27] In every case his testing point was the evident evocation of pain. Concerning irritability, Haller felt it was an inherent property of the muscle (a vis insita). This was partially accepted by Whytt but he insisted on control by his "sentient principle." The argument represented a confrontation between vitalism and mechanism and it is not surprising that both protagonists remained convinced of their own theories. Their altercations form a kind of watershed between vitalism and materialism, not to be settled in the 18th century.

BIBLIOGRAPHY

Georg Ernst Stahl (1659–1734)

Selected Writings

Dissertatio Inauguralis Medica de Medicina Medicinae Curiosae. Halle, 1714.

Negotium Otiosum, seu Skiamachia. Halle, 1720.

Theoria Medica Vera Physiologiam et Pathologiam. Halle, 1737.

Secondary Sources

Daremberg, C. *Histoire des Sciences Médicales*, Vol. 2. pp. 1020–1060. 1870.

Gottlieb, B. J. Bedeutung und Auswirkungen des Hallischen Professors Georg Ernst Stahl auf den Vitalismus des XVII Jahrhunderts. *Nova Acta Leopoldina*, 12:502 (1943).

King, L. S. Stahl and Hoffmann: a study in eighteenth century animism. *J. Hist. Med.*, 19:118–130 (1964).

Rather, J. J. G. E. Stahl's psychological physiology. *Bull. Hist. Med.*, 35:37–49 (1961).

Sudhoff's Classics of Medicine, Vol. 36. Barth, Leipzig, 1961.

---

[27]Experiments published by Haller in his *Mémoires sur les parties sensibles et irritables du corps animal.* D'Arnay, Lausanne, 1760.

Friedrich Hoffmann (1669–1742)

Selected Writings

Medicinae Rationalis Systematicae, 2 vols. Halle, 1718, 1720. (French translation: *La Médecine Raisonné*. J-J Bruhier d'Albaincourt, Paris, 1739.)

Opera Omnia Physico-Medica, 6 vols. De Tournes, Geneva, 1741–1750.

Fundamenta Medicinae ex Principiis Naturae Mechanicis in Usum Philiatrorum Succinte Propositae. Huebner, Halle, 1695. (Translated into English by L. S. King. Macdonald, London, 1971.)

Secondary Sources

Daremberg, C. *Histoire des Sciences Médicales*, Vol. 2, pp. 905–953. Paris, 1879.

King, L. S. *The Growth of Medical Thought*. University of Chicago Press, Chicago, 1963.

King, L. S. Medicine in 1695: Friedrich Hoffmann's Fundamenta Medicinae. *Bull. Hist. Med.*, 43:17–29 (1969).

Rothschuh, K. E. *History of Physiology* (translated by G. B. Risse). Krieger, New York, 1973.

Johann August Unzer (1727–1799)

Selected Writings

Gedanken von Einflusse der Seele in ihren Körper (Thoughts on the Influence of the Soul on the Body). 1746.

Betrachtungen über Stahl's theoretischen Grundsatz (Reflections on the fundamental principle of Stahl's theory). *Hamburg Magazine*, Vol. 10, 1786.

Erste Grunde einer Physiologie der eigentlichen thierischen Natur thierischer Körper. Wiedmann, Leipzig, 1771. (Translated by Thomas Laycock: *The Principles of Physiology*. Sydenham Society, 1851.)

Secondary Sources

Canguilhem, G. *La Formation du Concept de Réflexe aux XVIIᵉ et XVIIIᵉ Siècles*. Presses Universitaires de France, 1955.

Robert Whytt (1714–1766)

Selected Writings

An Essay on the Vital and Other Involuntary Motions of the Animal. Hamilton, Balfour, and Neill, Edinburgh, 1751.

Observations on the Nature, Causes and Cure of those Disorders which are Commonly Called Nervous, Hypochondriac, or Hysteric, to which are Prefixed some Remarks on the Sympathy of the Nerves. Balfour, Edinburgh, 1765.

Physiological Essays. Hamilton, Balfour, and Neill, Edinburgh, 1755.

The Works of Robert Whytt (published by his son). Becket and Deffondt, London and Balfour, Edinburgh, 1768. Includes: An essay on the vital and other involuntary motions of animals, 1751.

Observations on the Sensibility and Irritability of Parts of Man and Other Animals. Balfour, Edinburgh, 1755.

Observations on the Nature, Causes and Cure of Those Disorders which are Commonly called Nervous, Hypochondriac or Hysteric. Balfour, Edinburgh, 1764.

Secondary Sources

French, R. K. *Robert Whytt, the Soul and Medicine*. Wellcome Institute of the History of Medicine, London, 1969.

Spillane, J. D. *The Doctrine of the Nerves*. Oxford University Press, 1981.

CHAPTER X

The Great Italian Schools

Leopoldo MarcAntonio Caldani (1725–1813)

Leopoldo MarcAntonio Caldani, a Bolognese born in 1725, began to study medicine at the age of 16 at the University of Bologna where later he became a professor. Essentially an anatomist, he was convinced that dissection could reveal the organization responsible for observed phenomena. A great admirer of Haller, he initiated many experiments to test irritability. His procedure was to trigger convulsions by stimulation of tissues. He used electricity from a frictional machine to stimulate tissues in many kinds of animals, mostly frogs, goats, dogs, and sheep, but an appointment during his training to the hospital of Santa Maria della Morte gave him the opportunity to work on humans. Caldani demonstrated his experiments to the Istituto delle Scienze in Bologna and later wrote about them to Haller who, after translating them into French, published them four years later. One of his descriptions follows:

> We uncovered the crural nerves of a frog and cut them close to their exit from the vertebra, placed them on a board so that they formed four curves. An electrified rod was brought within one, two or three inches of them, and we always saw the muscles of the lower extremity make a movement. However, this took place solely by influence of the electrical matter and without a spark being evoked. At the end of about fifty minutes we found the nerves empty and almost entirely dried up. At this time we were no longer able to produce the same effect in them, neither with needles nor with our finger, but when the electrified wire was brought near them, the same movements could be observed, although they were much weaker.[1]

[1]Leopoldo Caldani. Letter to Haller, 1756. In: A. Haller. *Mémoires sur les parties sensibles et irritables du corps animal*, Vol. 3, pp. 143–144. Lausanne, 1760.

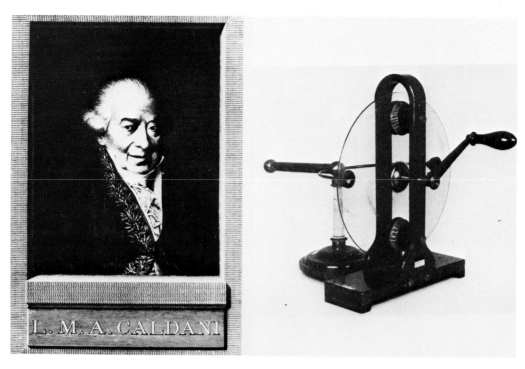

FIG. 63. Left: Leopoldo MarcAntonio Caldani (1725–1813), Professor of Medicine at Bologna, from the engraving by Gaetano Bozia after the portrait by Schiavoni. (Courtesy of the Wellcome Institute of History of Medicine, London.) **Right:** The electrostatic machine made by Dolland in London and used by Caldani and Fontana in their stimulating experiments to study irritability of tissues (Istituto delle Scienze, Bologna.)

In 1755 the University of Bologna appointed him to the chair of Medicine and he was joined by Felice Fontana who also had an interest in Hallerian irritability. These experiments came close to, but did not reach, the discovery that the nerve impulse was electrical in nature. They only suspected that movements caused by stimulation of other parts of the body traveled to the muscles along the nerves. Galvani also worked at the same university. His research led to the theory that the nerves themselves produced electricity.

Haller's criterion for irritability was that the tissue stimulated must contract. Caldani was unable to establish this for nerves. A large number of the experiments reported by Caldani concern his and Fontana's search for irritability in the dura mater. They looked for this not only in animals, but in conscious man during trepanization. They were astonished at their failure to evoke signs of pain when they pinched the dura mater. At that time collections of lymph or pus on the dura mater were regarded as the main cause, by irritation, of spasms and epileptic convulsions. They were able to produce convulsions by pressure on the brain, but not by irritation of the dura mater.

Caldani was especially interested in the experimental production of seizures. He attempted to confirm in animals, observations made during autopsies on man. In particular, he wished to show that hemiplegic signs appeared on the opposite side of the body to the brain lesion.

Their findings, that convulsions were caused by lesions of the brain, were puzzling in the light of accepted doctrine that the brain was insensitive. Irritability, excitability, contractility, elasticity, sensibility, and sensation were not yet clearly differentiated, and trans-

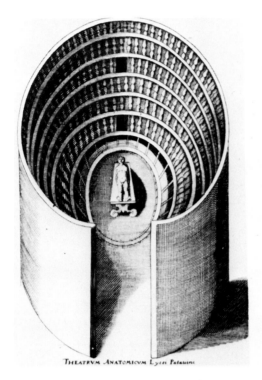
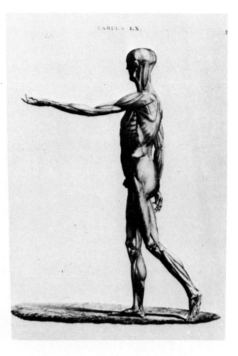

THEATRVM ANATOMICVM Lycei Patauini

FIG. 64. **Left:** The famous anatomical theatre at Padua where Caldani taught after succeeding Morgagni as Professor of Anatomy. **Right:** A plate from the folio of anatomical drawings prepared by Caldani and his nephew, Floriano, and published by Picotti in the 9-volume *Icones Anatomiae*, Venice, 1801–1814.

mission through nerves still not understood. A cloud of confusion enveloped 18th century physiological thinking.

In 1760, while teaching anatomy in Bologna, Caldani met so much opposition to his Hallerian views, that he decided to move to Venice. In 1764, he was appointed professor of theoretical medicine at Padua where he taught the methods of Boerhaave, and wrote his *Institutiones*. Documents in the archives at Bologna tell us that during carnival time, when everyone else took vacation, he had the opportunity to give a public lecture in the great Anatomical Theatre in Padua.

In 1771 he achieved his goal of succeeding his friend Morgagni, in the chair of anatomy at Padua. Morgagni had taught anatomy from illustrations in books but Caldani insisted on demonstrating with cadavers. There was, however, much less opportunity for experiment in Padua than in Bologna. In addition, there was compulsory publication of all lectures. So he turned to writing his *Institutiones* and, with the help of his nephew, prepared the Elephant Folios of anatomy, five volumes of text that are his legacy to science. Caldani died in 1813, a year before the final volume went to press. Honors had come to him, including the presidency of the newly formed Accademia di Padova, which he had been instrumental in creating.

Felice Gaspar Ferdinand Fontana (1730–1805)

Felice Gaspar Ferdinand Fontana was born in Pomarolo, a village in the Tyrol near Rovereto. The Tyrol was a bishopric, and the young Fontana trained there for the church.

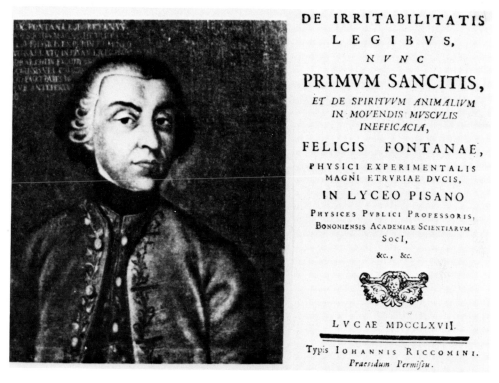

DE IRRITABILITATIS
LEGIBVS,
NVNC
PRIMVM SANCITIS,
ET DE SPIRITVVM ANIMALIVM
IN MOVENDIS MVSCVLIS
INEFFICACIA,

FELICIS FONTANAE,
PHYSICI EXPERIMENTALIS
MAGNI ETRVRIAE DVCIS,

IN LYCEO PISANO

PHYSICES PVBLICI PROFESSORIS,
BONONIENSIS ACADEMIAE SCIENTIARVM
SocI,

&c., &c.

LVCAE MDCCLXVII.

Typis IOHANNIS RICCOMINI.
Praesidum Permissu.

FIG. 65. Left: Felice Fontana (1730–1805), from a portrait in the Accademia degli Agiati at Rovereto. (Courtesy of the late Dr. Luigi Belloni.) Right: Title page of Fontana's treatise on the laws of irritability, published when he was at Bologna.

Although he never engaged in religious activities, he always wore the garments of his rank as lay abbot. His memory is kept alive at his birthplace where a portrait, painted long after his death, hangs in the town hall. After his education in Verona, he went to the university at Parma which had been founded in 1502.

From there he moved to Bologna, where he came under the influence of Caldani and his theory of irritability. Fontana's experiments followed the same procedure as those of Caldani and Haller. He surveyed the reaction of various animal tissues to stimulation by acids, needles, and electricity. The latter was produced by a frictional machine which is preserved in the Istituto delle Scienze in Bologna. His own treatise on the subject, however, was not published until after he had moved to Pisa on his appointment there as Professor of Logic.[2]

Fontana's period in Bologna was at the height of the interest in irritability, partly due to the eminence of Haller but also because no plausible hypothesis of muscle movement had yet been promulgated to replace the old concept of nervous fluids flowing into the muscles. The 17th century explorers on their move toward experimentally established fact has passed on to the 18th the legacy of some classic experimental findings. Outstanding among these were: Swammerdam's demonstration that muscle did not increase in volume on contraction when the nerve was stimulated (the first laboratory experiment ever made on neuromuscular transmission); the cruder experiment of Borelli's in which he disproved the concept of a gaseous spirit coming from the nerve by slitting the muscles of an animal struggling under

[2]*De irritabilitatis legibus nunc primum sancitis.* Dissertatio in tres partes distributa. Pisa, 1767.

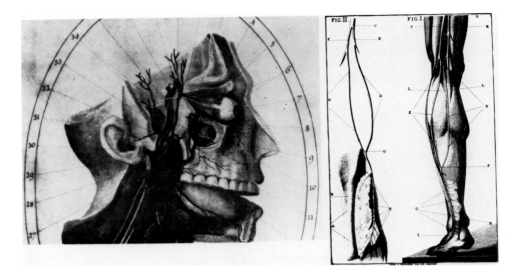

FIG. 66. **Left:** Susini's model of dissected head and neck showing the branches of the 'intercostal' nerve the distribution of which was sought by Fontana to settle a controversy. (Specimen in the Josephenum Museum in Vienna.) **Right:** Urbain Tossetti's drawings of the branches (G) of the sural nerve to the membranes surrounding the Achilles tendon (H) but failing to innervate it, thus confirming Fontana's insistence that tendons are insensitive. (From: Haller: *Mémoires sur les parties sensibles et irritables du corps animal*, Vol. 2, pp. 423–500, 1760.)

water (no bubbles resulted), and the equally cruder experiment of Goddard that a man's arm did not increase in volume when he clenched his fist (see Part I of this volume).

In a dissertation given in Bologna in 1757, Fontana refuted the theories of his colleague, Laghi, who was an opponent of the Hallerian doctrine of irritability. The dissertation was addressed as a letter to Tossetti in Rome and published three years later by Haller.[3] His argument was against Laghi's claim that the tendons were sensitive. Tommaso Laghi was for many years a teacher of anatomy at Bologna. He gathered a group around him for discussions at his house and formed a little "academy."[4] Laghi insisted that he had demonstrated sensibility to stimulation (by a hot wire) of the periosteum, the dura mater, and the tendons. This raised questions as to whether or not these tissues were innervated. Vieussens was quoted as finding nerves in the Achilles tendon, while Leeuwenhoek was quoted as failing to find them with his microscope. Fontana's contention was that the animal's reacting with pain was due to the innervation of overlying skin and not to the irritation of the tendon itself. Tossetti's own work is found in several letters in support of Fontana, the fourth of which is illustrated by drawings of the innervation of the lower limb (Fig. 66).[5] Urbain Tossetti, himself a prolific experimenter, was a Reverend Father and lecturer in philosphy and mathematics at the College of Nazareth in Rome. All of his letters denied sensitivity to the tendon.

Fontana proceeded to report 174 experiments which he summarized as follows. "Tendons are insensitive, so is the dura mater, both in man and beasts, as are also the arteries." Other tissues which he found to be insensitive were the periosteum, the pleura, and the peritoneum.

[3]Albrecht Haller. *Mémoires sur les parties sensibles et irritables du corps animal*, Vol. 3, pp. 159–243. D'Arnay, Lausanne, 1760.

[4]Salvatore di Renzi. *Storia della medicina in Italia*. Filiatre-Sebezio, Naples, 1848.

[5]Albrecht Haller. *Mémoires sur les parties sensibles et irritables du corps animal*, Vol. 2, pp. 155–172, 175–215, 246–277, 425–500.

His experiments on the heart led him to state that irritation of its nerves neither accelerated nor slowed its beat.

As had Caldani, Fontana reported his results to Haller who translated them into French and published them in 1760 in his *Mémoires*.[6] Fontana continued to send reports to Haller although they were frequently not in agreement with the master. In a private letter, Haller commented that Fontana's dissertation, based on his experiments, was "pleine de subtilité italienne."[7]

Seven years later Fontana produced his own treatise on the subject. He opened his work with a lightly worded phrase in which he noted that Hallerian irritability had raised so much dissension among Italian scientists, that it might well be called "an irritation to all Italy."[8] He also made the claim that "the reward of my effort has been to read the animal Spirits out of office for ever. . . ."

Fontana, in fact, did not agree with Haller who viewed irritability and contractility as identical. His work with heart muscle convinced him that contraction did not always follow stimulation. Haller's concept of the stimulus to heart muscle was not acceptable. He felt that it was the action of the blood as it flowed first into the auricle and then into the ventricle.[9] Fontana disagreed.[10] He argued, that there is always blood in the ventricle, even when not in diastole, so that contraction should never cease. Fontana also ridiculed those who, in opposition to Haller, explained the rhythm of the heart by the animal spirits within the muscle fibers. His own explanation was that irritability is reduced by repetitive stimulation and that muscles resume their passive shape by elasticity. The period of relaxation envisaged by Fontana as necessary before another contraction can be elicited has been named by modern scientists "the refractory period."[11] Fontana first formulated his views for heart muscle but later extended the concept to skeletal muscle. He pointed out that the muscle itself could fail from fatigue.

So great was the influence of Haller in Europe that the suggestion, from many sources, that the mysterious power of electricity might yield the answer to the action of nerves and muscles, was largely ignored by the mainstream researchers. The concept of electricity existing in the tissues had not been conceived by Caldani or Fontana. It was a young student in the University of Bologna, Galvani, who brought this concept into prominence at the end of the century.

Fontana's experiments on electrical stimulation of animal tissues did not stir much attention until after Galvani's *Commentary* appeared. In 1793, attention was drawn to a letter by Fontana, in the *Journal de Physique*, describing experiments on cardiac muscle in which he demonstrated acceleration of the heartbeat.[12] His technique was to place the excised heart between two plates of different metals, zinc and antimony. He showed that this had an effect on the tissue, recording similar contractions in worms, insects, and denervated, headless

[6]Albrecht Haller. *Mémoires sur les parties sensibles et irritables du corps animal*, Vol. 3, pp. 159–243. D'Arnay, Lausanne, 1760.

[7]Haller: Letter to Tissot. 3 April 1758. In: *Albrecht von Haller an August Tissot, 1754–1777*. Huber, Berne, 1977.

[8]*De irritabilitatis legibus nunc primum sancitis*. Dissertatio in tres partes distributa. Roccomini, Lucca, 1767.

[9]Albrecht Haller. *Deux mémoires sur le mouvement du sang et sur les effets de la saignée*. (Translation A. Tissot.) Bousquet, Paris, 1756.

[10]"Si donc il y a toujours du sang dans la cavité des ventricules, la cause de la systole existera donc toujours, et la contraction ne devra jamais cesser." Letter to Tossetti published by Haller in *Mémoires sur les parties sensibles et irritables du corps animal*, Vol. 3, p. 235.

[11]H. E. Hoff. The history of the refractory period. *Yale J. Biol. Med.*, 14:635–672 (1941–2).

[12]*Journal de Physique*, 42:238 (1793). (This letter is reproduced in Sue's *Histoire de Galvanisme*, Vol. I, pp. 63–64.)

animals. In his letter Fontana promised to publish a work on "the new principle of muscular movement." He shared the common reluctance to accept that animal tissue could itself produce electricity. The promise to publish was never fulfilled, possibly because of Volta's discovery of bimetallic electricity, i.e., the flow of current between two dissimilar metals.

Fontana reported that irritation of the vagus nerves had no effect on the heart. He also found no irritability in the intestines and lungs, and was uncertain whether the dura mater reacted to stimulation. Most of his observations were made while working with Caldani in Bologna, but when he moved to Pisa he expanded his research to include work on dilation of the pupil caused by light falling on the retina.[13] To previous descriptions by Caldani, Haller, and Whytt, he added the observation that, in a state of fear or excitement, the pupils remained dilated in spite of light reaching the eye.[14] He used his pet cat to explore this phenomenon, suspending it over a flame to frighten it. The same domestic cat was the subject of an observation, familiar to modern researchers, on sleep and wakefulness. He held the eyelids open for a very long period and noted that when the animal finally slept, the pupils became extremely narrow, narrower even than when awake in the light. He also noted the convulsive jerks of the animal when in the stage of sleep he called "sonno profundo," thus anticipating today's recognized stages of sleep. Another contribution from this distinguished cat was Fontana's observation that the separate illumination of one eye produced a reduction of pupillary diameter in both eyes.[15] Fontana sent his work to Haller who praised it without comment in a letter to Tissot in 1766.[16] While working with the iris Fontana found the ciliary duct, a discovery which brought him a request from the professor of anatomy at Uppsala to publish it in the *Acta* of the Academy of Uppsala. Fontana sent the following reply.

> I send you the drawings of the new duct which I discovered in the eye, only because you asked me to. Do with them whatever you wish. I feel completely indifferent to them. I do not care much about this old discovery; in fact, I call it a discovery only because you like to call it that.

Fontana had been appointed in 1765 to the Chair of Logic in Pisa. While there, he republished part of his dissertation, this time in Italian.[17] The treatise, which is more philosophical in style than his earlier version, gives a more mature view of the problem of muscle contraction. In it, he claimed that the notion of nervous fluid being the active cause of muscular motion had been disproved forever.

In 1775 Fontana was called by the Grand Duke of Tuscany to create, at the Pitti Palace in Florence, a Cabinet of Physics and Natural History, and in 1776, he was appointed to the Chair of Physics at the University. He spent 30 years in Florence, traveling to England and France to add to the collections of his museum. He also constructed some instruments of his own design, including a thermometer and a barometer. The latter has survived and can be seen in the Museum of the History of Science, in Florence, together with some instruments from the times of Galileo and the Accademia del Cimento.

Fontana is remembered in many museums throughout Europe for the wax (and some wooden) figures which he encouraged to be made for the teaching of anatomy. Some of these are of the full figure, elegantly dressed and coifed with only the area for study fully

[13]Felice G. F. Fontana. *Dei moti dell'iride*. Riccomini, Lucca, 1765.

[14]Robert Whytt. *Essay on the Vital and Other Involuntary Motions of Animals*. Hamilton, Balfour, Neill, Edinburgh, 1751.

[15]G. Bilancione. Felice Fontana Trentino. *Archeion*, 12:296–362 (1930).

[16]Letters. 5 July 1766. In: *Albrecht von Haller's Briefe an August Tissot (1754–1777)*, edited by E. Hintzsche Huber, Berne, 1977.

[17]*Richerche filosofiche sopra la fisica animale*. Cambiagi, Florence, 1775.

exposed and dramatically colored. An outstanding collection of these is in Josephenum, the historical museum and library in Vienna, housed in the old building of the Emperor Joseph's Academy of Medicine and Surgery. Others are found in Montpellier (donated by Fontana in gratitude to Napoleon), Bologna, Florence, and Pavia.[18]

The collection made by Fontana, on instructions from the Grand Duke of Tuscany, for the Cabinet of Natural History in Florence was seen by Emperor Joseph II of Austria who immediately recognized both its beauty and didactic value. He asked Fontana to have some figures made for the Military Medical Academy which he had founded in 1786 in Vienna. In due time they were delivered by mule over the Alps in 40 cases. Joseph paid 30,000 florins for them. A description of the negotiation is in the State Archives.

When one sees these amazing waxworks, laid out in room after room of the Josephinum in Vienna, where they are now housed, one is surprised that such delicate work could survive the journey.[19]

> The preparations are set up in caskets of rosewood with gilt edges and walls of the finest glass. In this way they are protected from dust, without being obscured from the eye of the observer. The caskets may be opened for study. The wax preparations are surrounded by drapery of white silk and pillows of blue satin decorated with silver fringes, and with curtains of green silk which serve partially for decoration and partially for conservation. Over each preparation hang framed colored drawings with labels in Latin and in Italian. The drawers beneath the caskets contain the descriptions of the preparations in German and in Italian.

For students of the nervous system, one of the most interesting figures is the dissected head showing the cervical sympathetic. It was made at a time of controversy over cranial involvement with the "intercostal" nerve, now known as the sympathetic. This wax model is now in Florence, in the Museum La Specola, with an accompanying drawing showing the nerve branches.[20]

Of Fontana's many experiments, the best known were those on the properties of gases.[21] His research also focused on poisons and venoms, including those in the vegetable family. It was in vegetable matter that he saw, with his microscope, a "body" within the cell, presumably the nucleus—another original finding. He discussed this in his *Treatise on the venom of the viper*, written partially in Italian while he was at Pisa and published in French in 1781.[22] Here, Fontana also discussed his work with the microscope, and his structural analysis of the nerve. His observations on the action of snake venom, as well as his many experiments on frogs and birds, led him to conclude that the action was not conveyed by the nervous system. He found that a snake bite to a denervated limb produced the usual reaction, a result that caused him to investigate the role of blood, and the destruction by the venom of its ability to coagulate. In the 18th century, however, Fontana's most important work was in toxicology, including his demonstration that a parasite was responsible for the devastating blight on grain that plagued his country.

In his microscopic studies of the nerve fiber, Fontana described and illustrated the axis cylinder (see Fig. 67) and depicted the spiral bands which had puzzled many observers with

---

[18]A fine example of a wax figure from Florence is in the Science Museum in London as part of the Wellcome Museum of the History of Medicine.

[19]M. Jantsch. Zur Geschichte der Wiener anatomischen Wachspräparatensammlung. *Wien. med. Wsch.*, 101:753–754 (1951).

[20]P. K. Knoeffel. Florentine anatomical models in wax and wood. *Medicina nei Secoli*, 3:329–340 (1978).

[21]*Recherches physiques sur la nature de l'air nitreux et de l'air déphlogistique.* Nyon, Paris, 1776.

[22]*Traité sur le venin de la vipère sur les poisons américains, sur le laurier-cerise et sur quelques autres poisons végétaux.* Florence, 1781.

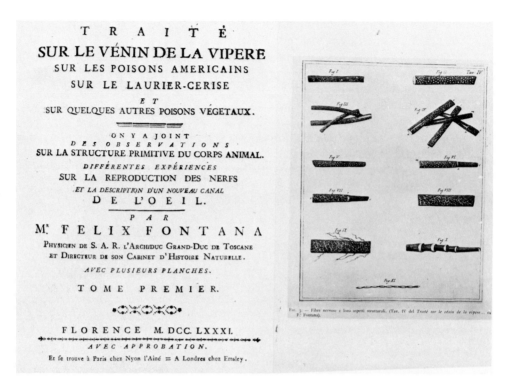

FIG. 67. Left: Fontana's famous treatise on the venom of the viper, to the end of which is appended his observations on nerves. **Right:** Fontana's drawing of nerve fibers with a core interpreted as axis cylinders.

more primitive lenses.[23] Fontana's conclusions on the question of the character and contents of the nerve are more clearly expressed in private correspondence than in his published works. In a letter written in 1782 to a friend in Provence, he described in great detail some experiments he made on nerve filaments teased out from what he described as the nerve cylinders.[24] He stripped off the sheath and examined the fibrils between two fine magnifying lenses through which he could see the structure of the nerve and what happened when he squeezed the two lenses together. This was a technique which he had used for some years. When he applied pressure to the fine nerve tendrils he found that "une matière glutineuse, élastique, transparente" came out of the cut end. This glutinous material was insoluble in water and when compressed proved to be granular, the grains being 4 or 5 times smaller in diameter than blood corpuscles. He repeated this observation in many species, including humans. He was apparently unaware that his fellow countryman, Borelli, had made a similar observation in the previous century.[25]

His observations led him to conclude that the nerve cylinders were true canals, containing an elastic, glutinous and graniform material. In his letter he said, rather provocatively, that he did not know whether or not physiologists would choose to regard the grains he had found as animal spirits. He pointed out that animal movements were too rapid for a flow

[23]*Osservazioni sopra la ruggine del grano.* Riccominni, Lucca, 1767.

[24]*Journal de Physique,* 24:417–421 (1784). (Lettre de M. l'Abbé Fontana à M. Gibelin, à Aix-en-Provence, datée de Florence du Juillet, 1782.)

[25]G. A. Borelli. *De motu animalium,* Vol. 2. Bernado, Rome, 1680.

of this viscous material to be the agent but he noted that it was elastic and therefore could perhaps vibrate in place, without any flow taking place. He ended with a criticism of the many theories being proposed without proofs. In fact, in *Treatise on the Venom of the Viper* he reported experiments in which he examined nerve "cylinders" under the microscope and could detect no vibration and no movement. He felt that his observations made the explanation of vibrations in the nerve fibers untenable and left the privilege of imagining the invisible to the metaphysicians. He added that the failure to explain muscular movements forced him to look for some other principle—if not ordinary electricity, then something analogous to it, such as what one saw in the electric fish.[26] His achievements are remarkable, for microscopes in his day were not achromatic, nor had they any correction for spherical aberration.

Fontana's instructions from the Grand Duke of Tuscany to travel to London and Paris to seek objects for his museum took him to a Europe in ferment. The Age of Enlightenment had brought concern for the rights of man, and 1776, the year of Fontana's first voyage, was in this respect an annus mirabile. In England Gibbon's first volume had stressed the happiness of the people of the Roman Empire, during the time of Marcus Aurelius. It was [27] "the only period of history," he wrote, "in which the happiness of a great people was the sole object of government," and that when this concern for the people died, so did the Empire. Thomas Paine's *Common Sense*,[28] and the American Declaration of Independence also embodied the philosophy of Enlightenment. Both the French Declaration des Droits de l'Homme and the American Revolution had their three word clarion call declaring their goals, though they shared only one word in common: Life, Liberty, and the Pursuit of Happiness; Liberté, Egalité, et Fraternité.

After Fontana's death some of the structures he had been first to note were accredited to later scientists, but the leading physiologists of the next century paid him tribute. Müller recognized him as the first to achieve the correct view of the fine structure of the nerves, and Henle pointed out that Remak was, in fact, repeating the description given by Fontana 50 years earlier.

Fontana had lived to see the publication of Galvani's claim for animal electricity. Galvani brought this out in 1791, and before Fontana died he had learned of the conflict with Volta. He referred to this without taking sides though Galvani's nephew, Aldini, claimed that he had made experiments with Fontana in Florence. Aldini in his book published the year before Fontana died, claimed that:[29]

> About two years ago I made several experiments at Florence with the celebrated professor Felix Fontana, and we saw that a 100 plaques of zinc and silver, after having been submerged together in water, gave a very strong action. He tells me in his letters that he has done the same experiment in several ways and always with the same result.

Half a century later, Emil Du Bois-Reymond (who claimed to have proved the existence of electricity in nerve) gave great credit to Fontana. His flowery tribute was that "Spallanzani and Fontana, in the second half of the 18th century, shone in Italy like twin stars."[30] No mention here of Galvani.

Fontana died in 1805 and was honored by burial in Santa Croce, the pantheon of Florence.

[26]*Traite sur le venin de la vipère*, Vol. 2, p. 244.

[27]Edward Gibbon (1737–1794). *Decline and Fall of the Roman Empire*, Vol. I. 1776.

[28]Thomas Paine. *Common Sense*. Bell, 1776.

[29]Giovanni Aldini (1762–1834). *Essai théorique et expérimental sur le galvanisme*, Vol. I., p. 13, p. 45. Fournier, Paris, 1804.

[30]Emil Du Bois-Reymond (1818–1896). *Untersuchungen über thierische Electricität*, 2 vols. Reimer, Berlin, 1848, 1849.

BIBLIOGRAPHY

Leopoldo MarcAntonio Caldani (1725–1813)

Selected Writings

Sull' Insensitività ed Irritabilità di Alcune Parti degli Animali. Two letters to Haller. 1757.

Sopra l'Irritabilità e Sensitivita Halleriana. Letter to Haller 1759. (Both the above translated into French and published by Haller in his *Memoires sur les Parties Sensibles et Irritables du Corps Animal.* D'Arnay, Lausanne, 1760.)

Institutiones Pathologiae. Padua, 1772.

Institutiones Physiologiae. Padua, 1773.

Institutiones Anatomicae. Venice, 1787.

Sui Fenomeni che Accadono ai Muscoli di Alcuni Animali di Sangue Freddo Tagliati Attraverso, Irritando Inappresso la Midolla Spinale. 1763. (Translated into French and published in Vol. 5 of *Correspondence de Haller.* Berne, 1763.)

Icones Anatomicae, quotquot sunt Celebriores, Ex Optimis Neotericorum Operibus summa Diligentia Depromtae et Collectae (with Floriano Caldani), 9 vols. Picotti, Venice, 1801–1814.

Secondary Sources

Dezeimeris, O., and Raige, D. *Dictionnaire historique de la médécine ancienne et moderne.* Béchet, Paris, 1831.

Hintzsche, E. (Ed.). *Albrecht von Haller–MarcAntonio Caldani. Briefwechsel. 1756–1776.* Bern, 1966.

Felice Fontana (1730–1805)

Selected Writings

Richerche Filosofiche Sopra il Veleno della Vipèra. Riccomini, Lucca, 1767.

De Irritabilitatis Legibus nunc primum Sancitis. Dissertatio in tres partes distributa. Riccomini, Lucca, 1767. [English translation by J. F. Marchand and H. E. Hoff. *J. Hist. Med.,* 10 (1955).]

Richerche Filosofiche Sopra la Fisica Animale di Felice Fontana. Cambiagi, Florence, 1775.

Recherches Physiques sur la Nature de l'Air Nitreux et de l'Air Déphlogistique. Paris, 1776.

Dei Moti dell'Iride. Riccomini, Lucca, 1765. [Translated into French. *J. de Physique,* 10:25–104 (1777).]

Traité sur le Venin de la Vipère, sur les Poisons Américains, sur le Laurier-Cerise, et Quelque Autres Poisons Vegetaux, 2 vols. Florence, 1781. (English translation by J. Skinner. London, 1787.)

[Tissot, A.] Letter from Fontana to Tosetti in: *Albrecht von Haller's Briefe an Auguste Tissot, 1754–1777.* Huber, Berne, 1977.

Secondary Sources

Belloni, Luigi. Anatomica plastica. *Ciba Symposium,* 7:229–333 (1959); Ibid., 8:84–87, 129–132 (1960).

Bilancioni, G. Felice Fontana Trentino. *Archeion,* 12:296–362 (1930).

Clarke, E., and Bearn, J. G. The spiral nerve bands of Fontana. *Brain,* 95:1–20 (1972).

Earles, M. P. The experimental investigation of viper venom by Felice Fontana (1730–1805). *Ann. Sci.*, 16:255–268 (1960).

Hoff, H. E. The history of the refractory period. *Yale J. Biol. Med.*, 14:635–672 (1941–2).

Jantsch, M. Zur Geschichte der Wiener anatomischen Wachspräparatensammlung. *Wien. med. Wschr.*, 101:753–754 (1951).

Knoefel, P. K. Felice Fontana (1780–1805). Works unpublished and works unwritten. *Physis*, 18:(2) 185–197 (1976).

Knoefel, P. K. Florentine anatomical models in wax and wood. *Medicina nei Secoli*, 3:329–338 (1978).

Knoefel, P. K. *Felice Fontana (1730–1805). An annotated bibliography*. Trento, 1980.

CHAPTER XI

The Age of Enlightenment

In the 18th century a great intellectual movement swept across Europe and left its name in history as the Age of Enlightenment. This movement affected all theories of the mind, the brain, and the nervous system. In this period a line was drawn between science and theology, thus preparing the way for acceptance in the following century of reflex action and a theory of nervous action that excluded the soul. Deism was excluded but in its place there was Nature, though the two were not to be confused. Man was not identical to a machine, and more important for science, a hypothesis was not a fact.[1] The Enlightenment had its core in France, and a legacy from Descartes: Its followers became known as the *philosophes*. Essentially a development in ideology, it affected current concepts of the nervous system, and what emerged was a conflict between experimental procedure and hypothetical deduction.

Denis Diderot (1713–1784)

A prominent leader of the movement was Denis Diderot who published his views quite widely and was immediately attacked for placing ultimate power in an autonomous Nature rather than a recognized Deity. Born in 1713 and schooled by the Jesuits, he never persevered in any one profession other than writing. His works were considered inflammatory and dangerous. In one of his earlier works, *Lettre sur les aveugles à usage de ceux qui voyent*, he recited the case of the English mathematician, Saunderson, blind from childhood, who declared that if he was to believe in the existence of God he must be allowed to touch him.[2]

---

[1]"Aie toujours présent à esprit que la nature n'est pas Dieu, qu'un homme n'est pas une machine, qu'une hypothèse n'est pas un fait." Diderot. *Pensées sur l'interprétation de la nature*.

[2]Denis Diderot. *Lettre sur les Aveugles à usage de ceux qui voyent*. Paris, 1749.

This essay caused Diderot to be sent to Vincennes, the great prison on the east side of Paris—such was the power of the Church. Yet, when one reads the "Letter" one recognizes, not atheism, but agnosticism.

Diderot also attempted a treatise called *Éléments de physiologie* but never brought it to fruition.[3] He had had some brief scientific training in the laboratory of Rouelle, who also taught Lavoisier.[4] Unlike Descartes, who had visited slaughterhouses and to whom he owed so many of his ideas, Diderot made no anatomical search of the nervous system to find mechanisms to support his views. Even in the contemplation of the evolution of animals and man from chaos, Descartes had insisted that Nature was fully competent to develop the "nerves, veins, bones and other parts of an animal... in every case according to the precise laws of mechanics." As he was writing to a priest, he added that "God imposed these laws on Nature."[5]

One of the more practical outcomes of the movement of the Enlightenment was the publication of the *Encyclopedia* of Diderot and D'Alembert.[6] The first attempt of its kind to bring together the arts and the pure and applied sciences, both theoretical and practical, it came out in installments over a period of fourteen years. Not all sections were written by the two protagonists. The section on Cartesianism was written, for example, by the Abbé Pestre, and Jean-Jacques Rosseau wrote on music. Several parts were written by d'Holbach and the article on "Memory" is by Condillac. At Diderot's invitation, two articles were written by Nicolas Demerest ("Fontaine" and "Geographie Physique"). Demerest had made a name for himself, and won a prize for his study of the land bridge that once existed between England and France.[7] In spite of the many contributors, Diderot's philosophy is prevalent throughout all of the volumes. The section on Genius is written by himself, a theme he further developed in the *Neveu de Rameau*. He held that genius was an intrinsic quality and could not be acquired. As D'Alembert wrote in the introduction, the *Encyclopedia* was to be "a sanctuary where man's knowledge is protected from time and from revolutions."[8]

The *Encyclopedia* was originally conceived as a dictionary that explains its alphabetical format, but Diderot's goal grew more ambitious. The series, 17 volumes of text and 11 volumes of illustrations, was designed to give not only factual scientific information but to encourage progress toward the betterment of the "condition humaine." Later, four supplementary volumes were published without the participation of Diderot. The *Encyclopedia* encountered not only attacks from the Church but, in the later volumes, some articles were mutilated by the printer, Le Breton, who was subsequently sent to the Bastille. The four supplementary volumes with which Diderot was not involved were printed in Holland. By 1758 there had been a quarrel and a break between Diderot and his closest collaborator, D'Alembert, whose name after the 7th volume is no longer associated with the *Encyclopedia*. D'Alembert was a brilliant mathematician, and an admirer of Newton, though unrestrained by his theological tenets.

The strength of the *Encyclopedia*, for all experimental sciences, was its emphasis on the detailed description of current technology and its excellent diagrams of the instruments and

---

[3]Manuscript in the Public Library in Leningrad.

[4]Guillaume François Rouelle (1703–1770), chemist and lecturer at the Jardin du Roi.

[5]René Descartes. Letter to Marin Mersenne. February 20, 1639.

[6]*Encyclopédie, ou Dictionnaire raisonné des sciences, des arts et des métiers.* Le Breton, Paris, 1751–65.

[7]Nicolas Demerest. Dissertation sur l'ancienne junction de l'Angleterre et de la France. Académie d'Amiens, 1753.

[8]Jean-le-Rond D'Alembert. Discours préliminaire. In: *l'Encyclopédie*. Paris, 1751.

how they worked. For students of the nervous system, the most interesting sections are those by Diderot on fibers, and his notes on Haller in the supplement.[9] In the alphabetized *Encyclopedia*, in sections written by Pierre Tarin, a Paris physician, we find Haller's anatomy listed under "A" and his physiology under "P," including a striking plate of Haller's drawings of the brain.

The *Encyclopedia* appeared during the years when Haller's theory of irritability was dominant. In a long article in Volume 15 (1765), Henri Fouquet from the Faculty of Medicine at Montpellier launched a long and pungent attack on Haller. This was placed under the heading of "Sensibilité" but covered the concept of irritability which, contrary to what Tissot claimed, he felt was not a concept original to Haller.[10] Fouquet then went into the confusion surrounding the terms irritability, contractility, sensibility, excitability, and sensation. He was clearly antagonistic to Haller, commenting on the cruelty of his experiments and "les tourmens d'un nombre infini d'animaux." In addition, he specifically called Haller in error in denying irritability to cellular tissue.

In the supplements, published after the *Encyclopedia*, there are also articles on irritability and sensibility that were either written or inspired by Haller, though not signed by him.[11] These short pieces ignore Fouquet's attacks, and concern the sensibility of tendons. One section, without mentioning Willis, attacks the prominence given to the corpus callosum.[12]

Diderot's own views on the nervous system are clear. He placed great importance on the fiber, associating nervous conduction and muscular contraction with a continuous tension critical for life. We find this view developed most fully in the section entitled *Fibre* in the *Encyclopedia*, and in his (posthumously published) *Eléments de physiologie*. The concepts of "tension" and "elasticity" are used throughout Diderot's long discussion of fibers, and his "mouvement tonique" presages the idea of tonus. "Toute *fibre*," he said, "dans quelque partie du corps humain que ce soit, est douée plus ou moins d'une force élastique..."

For Diderot the fibers were themselves sentient and animate, constituting most of the tissues of the body. The bundles of nerve fibers were believed to merge into the muscle, where they became muscular fibers. His view included elements of the ideas of Boerhaave, Haller, Baglivi, and even de Gorter who had stressed the role of transverse fibers which divided the gross fiber into vesicles. These, said Diderot, were inflated during contraction by animal spirits.[13]

Diderot's opinions on the brain are found in his *Eléments de physiologie*, and his *Oeuvres complètes*.[14] He described its overall structure, pointing out that the cortical part was mushy, hardening with age until it could scarcely be cut, while the subcortical part was firmer, more dense, and with "une pulpe uniforme." He must have handled a freshly excised brain for he made the same observation, of a kind of stratification that Gennari was to emphasize some years later.[15] But Diderot's writings on science reveal, not his own discoveries, but the breadth of his reading and his assessment of current concepts.

[9]*Encyclopédie*, Vol. 6, pp. 661–675.

[10]*Encyclopédie*, Vol. 15, pp. 38–52, 1765.

[11]*Supplement 3*, pp. 663–665 and *4*, pp. 776–779, 1777.

[12]"Rien prouve qui le corps calleux ait le moindre prérogative sur les autres parties de encéphale."

[13]"On suppose qu'alors les fibrilles transversales qui forment dans l'état de repos des reseaux lâches et parallèles autour des grosses *fibres*, se tendent, resserent ces *fibres* en différents points, et y produisent des vésicules qu'enflent les esprits animaux." (*Encyclopédie*, Vol. 6, p. 662.)

[14]*Oeuvres complètes de Diderot*, Vol. 9, edited by Assezat and Tourneux, p. 310. Paris, 1875–1877.

[15]F. Gennari. *De peculiari structura cerebri nonnullis que ejus morbis*. Parma, 1782.

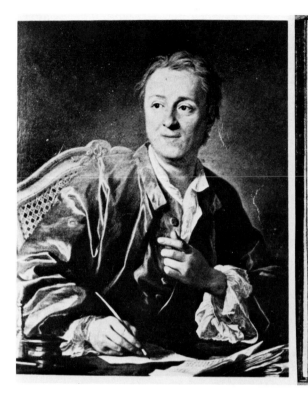

(46)

perſuadés, qui vivent comme s'ils l'étoient, *ce ſont les
fanfarons du parti.* Je déteſte
les fanfarons, ils ſont faux :
je plains les vrais Athées,
toute conſolation me ſemble
morte pour eux ; *& je prie
Dieu* pour les Sceptiques, ils
manquent de lumieres.

XXIII.

Le Déiſte *aſſure* l'exiſ-
tence d'un Dieu, l'immor-
talité de l'ame & ſes ſuites :
le Sceptique n'eſt point déci-
dé ſur ces articles : l'Athée

*beaucoup de Deistes n'admettent point
l'immortalité de l'ame.*

FIG. 68. **Left:** Portrait of Diderot painted by Louis-Michel Van Loo in 1767 and given by his descendants to the Louvre. **Right:** Page from Diderot's *Pensées philosophiques* with handwritten comment by Voltaire in the copy in his collection now in Leningrad. (Courtesy of V. Merkulov, Leningrad.)

Diderot's statue surveys the busy Boulevard St. Germain in Paris, near the house where he lived. There are many portraits of him, including the well-known work by Louis-Michel Van Loo in the Louvre. This portrait was not entirely pleasing to Diderot who commented that it was "trop jeune, tête trop petite, joli comme une femme, lorgnant, souriant, mignard, faisant le petit bec, la bouche en coeur...."[16]

After his death in 1784 his works, and those of Voltaire, were brought to St. Petersburg by Catherine the Great who had purchased them from him during a brief visit in 1773 when he had acted as her librarian. Upon her death, Diderot's works were scattered. Voltaire's works, however, are intact in the Saltykov-Shchedrin building of the Public Library in Leningrad. There are nearly 7,000 items, including Voltaire's collection of Diderot material with a first edition of the *Lettre sur les aveugles*, some pages torn from the *Encyclopedia*, and much correspondence. Voltaire's copies are especially interesting for he wrote many notes in the margins. For example, in his copy of *Pensées philosophiques*, where Diderot described three categories of atheists and their disbelief in an afterlife, Voltaire noted that "Beaucoup de déistes n'admettent point l'immortalité de l'âme" and added some caustic remarks about Diderot and d'Alembert, whom he called "philosophes prétendus."[17]

[16]Diderot. Salon de 1767. In: *Oeuvres Esthétiques*. Garnier, Paris, 1956.

[17]Catalogue No. 1037. Saltykov-Shchedrin State Public Library, Leningrad.

Microfilms of some of the letters of Voltaire in the Leningrad collection are in the Vendeul Archives in the Bibliothèque Nationale in Paris, together with some of his original manuscripts which he had bequeathed to his daughter, Mme. de Vendeul.[18] These are mostly his criticisms of art and artists such as Chardin, Boucher, and Fragonard, the last of whom had painted his portrait. There are also essays on drama and the manuscript of his provocative novel *La Religieuse*.

The second volume of the *Encyclopedia* (1752) is on art, written anonymously but most certainly by Diderot. He had many artist friends, among them the sculptor, Falconet, whom he successfully recommended to Catherine for design of the equestrian statue of Peter the Great on the banks of the Neva River. The spirited steed represents Mother Russia and under its hoofs is a snake, symbolizing the forces of ignorance and evil.

Diderot did not live to see the French Revolution since he died (of gallstones)[19] in 1784. He was buried in the church of Saint Roch in Paris where the register lists him as a member of the Academies of Berlin, Stockholm, and St. Petersburg, and names his occupation as librarian to Catherine the Great. All of Voltaire's efforts to have Diderot elected a member of the French Académie des Sciences failed. Here, also, is the grave of d'Holbach who contributed no less than 375 articles to the famous *Encyclopedia* to which Diderot had given 25 years of his life.

Both Voltaire and Rousseau had been refused Christian burial in Paris, but after the Revolution their remains were brought back to the city, there to experience nearly as turbulent an existence as in life. An elaborate procession bore Voltaire's coffin (and a replica of Houdon's statue) to the Pantheon. This ancient church, named for Sainte-Geneviève, and standing on the hill of her name, had been returned to sanctity by Louis XV, but in the Revolution was converted into a Pantheon whose crypt was to be the burial place for the famous sons of France. Three years after Voltaire's reburial, Rousseau's remains were brought to Paris, again with pomp, and accompanied by a statue of him in a Roman toga. However, neither they nor the Pantheon was left in peace. On restoration of the monarchy, the Pantheon became a church once more. Louis XVIII ordered the coffins of these two famous dissidents removed from the sacred crypt and placed below in unhallowed caves. Nor was this their last resting place for in 1897 the coffins were again brought up, opened, examined, and restored to the gallery of the famous where they now lie. A rumor that Rousseau, who had died in poverty, had shot himself was laid to rest, for his skull was intact. Voltaire's bones were in a jumbled pile from their many journeys.

Jean-le-Rond d'Alembert (1717-1783)

Diderot's colleague and associate on the *Encyclopedia* was of distinguished heritage but of illegitimate and secret birth. Until 1748 the Church required baptism by immersion, and behind Notre Dame was a small chapel for this purpose, called Saint-Jean-le-Rond. It was on the steps of this chapel that the abandoned infant, who took its name, was found. He became one of France's outstanding mathematicians. Brought up by a foster mother, d'Alembert was recognized by his father, an army officer, and given a sound education at the Collège de Quatre Nations. This college, a Jansenist school, was founded by Cardinal Mazarin[20] for the education of pupils drawn from the four provinces joined to France, by

---

[18]H. Dieckmann. *Inventaire du Fonds Vendeul et inédits de Diderot.* Droz, Geneva, 1951.

[19]Letter from N.C. de Vendeul to his brother. August 1784. Archives de la Haute-Marne.

[20]Jules Mazarin (1602–1661).

the treaty of Westphalia, at the end of the Thirty Years War (Piedmont, Alsace, Flanders, and Artois). The college opened for classes in 1688 but after the French Revolution was suppressed by the Convention in 1793. The building, on the Seine, now houses the five academies of the Institut National, and an immense library where there is a collection of books seized from private libraries during the Revolution. The college provided a high level of education, especially in mathematics, which was d'Alembert's chosen field.

D'Alembert made no direct contribution to the experimental science of physiology. His concept of a unifying principle, derived from the mechanistic approach and seeded by Descartes, was not recognized until the 20th century. His abilities, however, were recognized while he was quite young. At the age of 24 he was elected to the Académie Royale des Sciences, and much later in 1772 was honored by a seat among the "immortals" in the Académie Française, of which he became the "secrétaire perpétuel." The Académie des Sciences was class structured in a way that evoked protest from the more enlightened members, including d'Alembert, whose attempt at reform failed. A visit to the Prussian Academy of Sciences in Berlin brought d'Alembert an offer from Frederick the Great to succeed Malupertius as its president, but he refused.

His view of the nervous system followed John Locke's basis of sensationalism: that all knowledge was derived from sense experience; hence the sciences should be based on actual perception—a view that no one would challenge today. He tended to support the corpuscular theory of matter that had appeared in the previous century.[21] His fame derived largely from the introduction he wrote for the *Encyclopedia*, in which he claimed to define the goals of human knowledge. For his friends, his break with Diderot was tragic. Meetings with Diderot, Condillac, and Rousseau in small Paris cafes[22] had turned into rich social events in the Paris salons of Mme. du Deffand and Mlle. Lepinasse.[23] The salons of 18th century France were the centers for intellectual exchange.

D'Alembert is also known for his contribution to the first seven volumes of the *Encyclopedia*, but his ruling interest was mathematics. D'Alembert continued the exploration of the laws of motion and the physical laws of the universe while Diderot, Voltaire, Rousseau, and others were turning to human experience and perception, rather than mathematics, as the source of knowledge. This move was spurred by the appearance in 1770 of d'Holbach's *Système de la Nature*, and aroused widespread protest. For example, the English poet William Blake was much disturbed by the movement, which he was convinced must fail.[24] Later, the French Revolution inspired him to write a poem in 7 books vividly describing its horrors.[25]

The group eventually broke up. Voltaire and Jean-Jacques Rousseau died in 1778, both in exile from Paris, d'Alembert died in 1783, and Diderot the following year. The torch was left with d'Holbach who had by this time quarreled with them all.

Paul-Henri Thiry d'Holbach (1723–1789)

One of the most prolific contributors to the *Encyclopedia* was d'Holbach, born in the Palatinate on the frontier of the Rhine. After education at the University of Leyden, followed by travels to England, he settled in 1749 in Paris where he met Diderot and Rousseau, and

[21]*Traité de dynamique*, 1743.

[22]Jean-Jacques Rousseau (1669–1740). *Confessions*, Book 7.

[23]M. Glotz and M. Maire. *Salons du XVIIIe Siècle*. Hachette, Paris, 1945.

[24]William Blake (1757–1827): "Mock on, Mock on Voltaire, Rousseau:/Mock on, Mock on: t'is all in vain!/ You throw the sand against the wind,/And the wind blows it back again."

[25]*The French Revolution*, a poem in seven books. 1791.

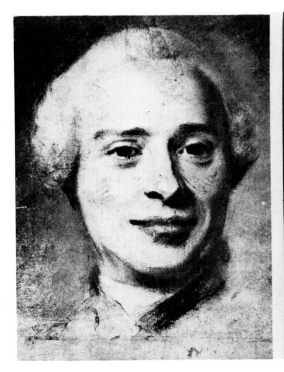
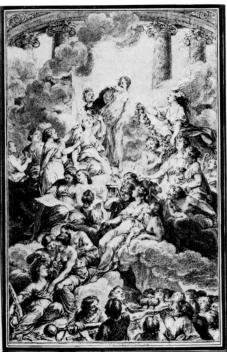

FIG. 69. Left: Portrait of d'Alembert painted by Quentin Latour (Musée de Saint-Quentin). **Right:** Frontispiece to the *Encyclopedia* designed by Charles-Nicholas Conchin in 1764. According to Diderot, the design shows Truth being uncovered by Reason. The original is in a private collection in Baltimore.

being himself a convinced materialist, he joined the ferment of free thought that surrounded them. Within a year of his arrival he was involved in the design of the *Encyclopedia*. He planned to undertake all sections related to metallurgy, mineralogy, and geology. This he did, contributing 375 articles, but his interest in psychology led him to work with the brain and sensory nervous system. From this grew his most famous book, *Système de la Nature*.

Strongly materialistic, and more atheistic than Diderot, d'Holbach gave the brain all of the characteristics previously claimed for the soul. "C'est à l'aide de cet organe intérieur que se font toutes les opérations que l'on attribue à l'âme."[26] All actions, interactions, and influences within the animal body and brain operated by infinitely small movements within the organs. It was the great variety of movement within the brain that he claimed constituted the intellectual faculties. Through these internal movements, the brain not only received perceptions and sensations but acted immediately upon them. It also had storage capacity which was the basis of thought. The inflow to the brain from all sections of the body was subject to modification, comparison, and combination, to form the thinking process—the process that was responsible for memory, intelligence, and will. The means by which this was achieved were mechanistic but the brain had choice. Regarding the ramifications of nerves spreading throughout the body, d'Holbach drew the analogy of the spider at the center of its web reacting immediately to change in motion anywhere in its domain.[27]

[26]*Système de la Nature, ou des lois du monde physique et du monde moral*. Paris, 1770.

[27]Diderot had made the same analogy when protesting current concepts of the brain as cream cheese. Salon, 1767.

In pursuing his concept that all information was brought to the brain by movement of some material agent, d'Holbach concluded that to be effective this movement must be more rapid than any that could be conveyed by a nervous fluid. He proposed that the agent was electricity.[28]

> D'ailleurs je serais assez tenté de croire que ce que les médecins nomment le fluide nerveux, ou cette matière si mobile qui avertit si promptement le cerveau de tout ce qui passe en nous, n'est autre chose que la matière électrique. . . .

D'Holbach produced works on mineralogy and metallurgy but many are on his philosophy, which was strongly atheistic. His position on religion brought him great trouble with the courts and many of his works were suppressed, some even in the 19th century. He himself felt it prudent to leave the country occasionally to avoid persecution.

D'Holbach had inherited the title of Baron from his uncle who had been enobled by Louis XIV. He also inherited an ample fortune that enabled him to devote time to writing and the lavish salon that he set up in his house, which still stands on the Rue des Moulins. The "thinkers" of his time met there, among them Diderot, Helvetius, and, some years later, the aging Benjamin Franklin. It is possible that this meeting caused d'Holbach to suggest that electricity might be the agent in the nervous system, though Franklin did not share this conception.

D'Holbach died in January 1789. He was buried in Saint-Roch, where Diderot had preceded him. He had achieved membership in the Academies of St. Petersburg and Berlin but his atheistic views were too controversial for the Academy of France, which had also refused Diderot.

BIBLIOGRAPHY

Denis Diderot (1712–1785)

Selected Writings

Lettre sur les Aveugles, à Usage de Ceux qui Voyent. Paris, 1749.

Encyclopédie, ou Dictionaire Raisonneé, des Sciences des Arts et des Métiers. 17 + 11 volumes. Paris, 1751–1765.

Lettres sur les Sourds et Muets. London, 1757.

La Rêve d'Alembert (posthumous). First published in Germany in a translation made by Goethe, 1805. (First French publication, 1821.)

Oeuvres Philosophiques (collected works), 6 vols. Rey, Amsterdam, 1772. Edited by P. Vernière. Garnier, Paris, 1961.

Le Neveu de Rameau. Paris, 1772–1773.

Oeuvres Complètes de Diderot, edited by Assezat and Tourneux. Paris, 1875–1877.

Oeuvres Esthétiques (collected works), edited by Paul Vernière. Garnier, Paris, 1956.

[28]*Système de la Nature.*

Secondary Sources

Crocker, G. L. *Two Diderot Studies: Ethics and Esthetics.* Johns Hopkins Press, Baltimore, 1952.

Dieckmann, H. Diderot's conception of genius. *J. Hist. Ideas*, 11:151–182 (1941).

Kemp, J. *Diderot, Interpreter of Nature* (English translation of Selected Writings). International Publishers, New York, 1943.

Morley, J. *Diderot.* Chapman and Hall, London, 1880.

Vexler, Felix. *Studies in Diderot's Esthetic Naturalism.* Columbia University Press, New York, 1922.

Wilson, A. M. *Diderot: the Testing Years.* Oxford University Press, 1957.

Jean-le-Rond d'Alembert (1717–1783)

Selected Writings

Traité de Dynamique. David, Paris, 1743.

Preliminary Discourse (to the Encyclopedia), 1751.

Opuscules Mathématiques, 8 vols. David, Paris, 1761–1780.

Mélanges de Litterature, d'Histoire, et de Philosophie, 5 vols. Chatelain, Amsterdam, 1770.

Secondary Sources

Briggs, J. M. *D'Alembert: Philosophy and Mechanics in the Eighteenth Century.* University of Colorado Press, 1964.

Hankins, T. L. *Jean d'Alembert. Science and the Enlightenment.* Clarendon Press, Oxford, 1970.

Paul-Henri Thiry d'Holbach (1723–1789)

Selected Writings

Encyclopédie, ou Dictionnaire raisonné des Sciences, des Arts et des Métiers (Diderot and d'Alembert). 375 articles with d'Holbach's signature in volumes II to XVII. Paris, 1751–1780.

Système de la Nature ou des Loix du Monde Physique et du Monde Morale (published under the name "Mirabaud"), 2 vols. London, 1770.

Discours Préliminaire. Privately printed, London, 1770.

Le Bon Sens, ou Idées Naturelles Opposées aux Idées Surnaturelles. London, 1772.

Secondary Sources

Naville, P. *D'Holbach et la Philosophie Scientifique au XVIIIᵉ Siècle*, 2nd edn. Gallimard, Paris, 1967.

Topazio, V. W. D'Holbach's conception of nature. *Modern Language Notes.* 1964.

Willey, R. *The Eighteenth Century Background.* London, 1940.

CHAPTER XII

Development of Research on the Spinal Cord

In the early 18th century there was doubt as to whether the brain was a simple outgrowth of the spinal cord or the spinal cord a mere elongation of the brain. What did these two systems have in common? Were the long fibers of the spinal cord connected with the brain? Were they bearing messages to the brain or from the brain or could the same nerve tracts do both? And what was the role of the liquid found in the ventricles and in the subarachnoid space? Was this a common irrigation system, an excretory system, or a nutrient system?

The ancients had attached much importance to the ventricles, not only as reservoirs of fluid but also as the seat of mental functions and man's soul. As late as 1796 this belief lingered on. Soemmering proposed that the soul-force (Seelenkraft) exerted its action at the locus where the fluid from the ventricles met the terminals of the nerves.[1]

Domenico Felice Antonio Cotugno (1736–1822)

One of the first important contributions to research on spinal fluids was made by Domenico Cotugno who, in 1764, demonstrated the continuity of the ventricular and spinal fluids as well as their origin from the blood vessels. The idea had been surmised but not proven by earlier writers such as Willis,[2] a century before, and Haller.[3]

---

[1]"Wäre dieses richtig: so—dünkt mich—liessen sich auch manche Erscheinungen bei der Rückwirkung *(Reactio)* des Hirns durch die Spontaneität der Seelenkraft näher erläutern." S. T. Soemmering (1755–1830). *Über das Organ der Seele*, p. 59. Nicolovius, Königsberg, 1796.

[2]T. Willis. *De Cerebri Anatome*. Martyn and Allestry, London, 1664.

[3]Albrecht Haller, *De Partibus Corporis Humani Sensibilibus et Irritabilibus*. Göttingen Gesellschaft der Wissenschaften, Göttingen, 1752.

The structure of the meninges and the pia mater is vascular; the fluid surrounding these two was a target of Cotugno's research. He found that the fluid was always present in the subarachnoid space in the spinal cord and that it was in constant circulation with the fluid of the ventricles, a fact denied by Haller. Unfortunately, Cotugno's discoveries lay buried in a small book on the role of the nerves in sciatica.[4] Little attention was paid to it until the following century when Magendie made claim to the discovery but later not only acknowledged Cotugno but reprinted Cotugno's book in his own journal.[5] Cotugno's Cartesian concept that the pineal gland acted as a valve-like controller for the opening did not survive.

Domenico Felice Antonio Cotugno, born in a village on the heel of Italy, was a physician trained at the University of Naples and its Hospital for Incurables where he was able to do research on cadavers. He lived in a divided Italy, during the time of the Napoleonic invasion. Cotugno pursued his research, rising in the esteem of his colleagues, and became physician of the King. He died in 1822, leaving behind his superb library, a catalog of which is in the Biblioteca Nazionale in Naples.

Domenico Mistichelli (1675–1715)

In the early 18th century a critical discovery was that the long descending fiber tracts of the spinal cord crossed at the level of the pyramids. At this time, Domenico Mistichelli published a text on apoplexy.[6] He was a Pisan by birth, and later Professor of Medicine at its University. In this tract Mistichelli described and depicted (Fig. 70) a crossing of the meninges fibers covering the medulla oblongata but not those of the medulla itself, whose fibers he was unable to identify with his primitive microscope. These findings led him to believe that nerves originated there, and also that they carried animal spirits. His description follows.[7]

> ... what I have recently observed, that is, that the medulla oblongata externally is interwoven with fibres that have the closest resemblance to a woman's [plaited] tresses. Whence it occurs that many nerves that spread out on one side have their roots on the other; so for example, those that extend to the right arm, through such plaiting, can readily have their roots in the left fibres of the meninges. The same may be understood of those on the left proceeding from the right; and so one may go on describing many, if not all the other nerves, that have their origin immediately from the spinal cord.

Mistichelli was trying to explain how a brain lesion on one side caused paralysis of the limbs on the other side. In the year following the appearance of Mistichelli's tract, a clearer explanation was published in a small book of letters, written by François Pourfour du Petit.[8]

François Pourfour du Petit (1644–1741)

A pupil of Duverney at the Jardin du Roi in Paris, with a degree in medicine from Montpellier, Pourfour du Petit was a surgeon in the French army during the wars of the Spanish Succession, wars fought by Louis XIV in Flanders and the Low Countries against

[4]Domenico F. A. Cotugno (1736–1822). *De Ischiade Nervosa Commentarius*. Simonii, Naples, 1764.

[5]F. J. Magendie. Mémoire sur un liquide que se trouve dans le crâne et de canal vertébral de l'homme et des animaux mammifères. *J. Physiol. Exper. Pathol.*, 5:27–37 (1825).

[6]*Trattato dell'Apoplessia*. Rossi, Rome, 1709.

[7]Translation by C. D. O'Malley. In: *The Human Brain and Spinal Cord*, pp. 282–283. University of California Press, Berkeley, 1968.

[8]*Lettres d'un Médecin des Hôpitaux du Roy à un autre Médecin de ses Amis*. Albert, Namur, 1710.

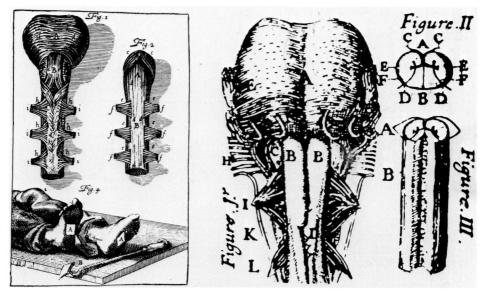

FIG. 70. **Left:** The first depiction of the decussation of the pyramidal tracts. (From: D. Mistichelli. *Tractato dell'Apoplessia*. Rome, 1709.) **Right:** Pourfour du Petit's illustration of the crossing of fibers within the cord (marked D) to effect the contralateral damage he found in his experiments on the dog. (From Pourfour du Petit. *Trois Lettres d'un Médecin des Hôpitaux du Roy*. 1710. From the copy in the Bibliothèque Nationale. Reproduction by courtesy of the late Dr. August Tournay.)

formidable opponents such as Marlborough and the Prince Eugène. The French surgeon made his observations on the decussation of the pyramids while in the army. He drew his conclusions from observations of victims of brain abcesses resulting from head injuries and from experimenting on dogs, while working in a military hospital in Namur, south of Brussels.

He dissected the spinal cord and pyramids more carefully than had Mistichelli and came closer to identifying and illustrating the fiber systems which decussate within the cord. He also drew cross sections to depict the precise level where they appeared. His contribution was more important to anatomy than to neurophysiology for he, like Mistichelli, interpreted the function as being that of animal spirits crossing from one side to the other.

In Pourfour du Petit's first letter he described in detail observations of soldiers with head wounds and stated the need to follow these up with experiments. By today's standards, the technique used in his experiments was crude. He made a small hole over the right parietal region of a dog and drove a steel probe through it, driving it down to touch bone. The immediate result was loss of movement in the left legs but, strangely enough, on the fourth day the dog "walked easily on his four feet."

On the 8th day, however, the dog had a convulsion and died. Upon opening the skull he found the wound covered by membrane and some infection in the dura mater. Pourfour du Petit wrote to a friend that here was proof that the animal spirits crossed from one side to the other.[9] He also believed he had discovered how this crossing came about. Each pyramidal body, he wrote, divided at its inferior part into two large bundles of fibers. Those on the right passed to the left, and those on the left, to the right. He depicted this in a drawing which he sent with the letter (Fig. 70).

[9]"Voilà, je crois, Monsieur, des preuves convaingnantes du changement des esprits animaux d'un côté à l'autre."

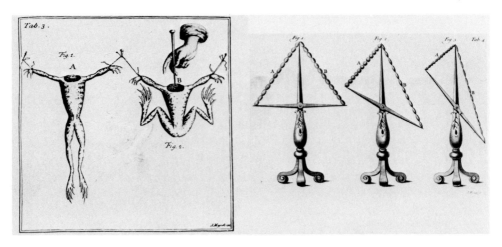

FIG. 71. Illustrations from Alexander Stuart's *Dissertatio de Structura et Motu Musculari*, 1738.   **Left:** Contractions obtained by pressure on the spinal cord in a decapitated frog.   **Right:** Stuart's model of vesicles in the muscle changing shape when it contracts.

Pourfour du Petit continued research on the nervous system and the pathways followed by the "animal spirits" until his death. His work received recognition, bringing him membership in 1725 in the Académie des Sciences. Some of his findings were forgotten, only to be discovered again in the next generation. For example, his demonstration that the sympathetic nerve was not a branch of a cranial nerve was demonstrated by Fontana half a century later.

The identification of the spinal columns, and their direction of conduction, remained uncertain for several years after Pourfour du Petit's reports but in 1741 the two dorsal columns and the two ventral columns were clearly differentiated by Huber. Johann Jacob Huber, from Switzerland, had studied with Haller and obtained a doctorate at Basel. He was Professor of Anatomy and Surgery at the Collegium Carolinum in Cassel, a city on the Nesser River. In his work, illustrated with fine drawings, he pointed out "four filaments," describing their contrasting positions, anterior and posterior, in the spinal marrow.[10] This anatomical contribution, however, did not supply the neurophysiological function of these tracts. Understanding of their mode of action was delayed by the persistent belief that every nerve in the body had a canal within it leading directly from the brain, which served as a pipeline bearing the animal spirits essential for all nervous action. The spinal cord was seen as bundles of nerve fibers grouped into columns.

Alexander Stuart (1673–1742)

The relationship of the brain to the spinal cord was studied by the Scotsman Alexander Stuart, who had obtained his medical degree from Leyden in 1709, studying under the great Boerhaave. Interested in the relationship of nerve to muscle, he believed that a nervous fluid was essential to muscular motion and developed an ingenious hydraulic and mechanical model. He described his theory in detail in his *Dissertatio de Structura et Motu Musculari*[11]

[10]Johann Jacob Huber (1707–1778). *De Medulla Spinali Speciatim de Nervis ab ea Provenienibus Commentatio cum Adjunctis Iconibus.* Vanderhoek, Göttingen, 1741.

[11]*Dissertatio de Structura et Motu Musculari.* Richardson, London, 1738.

and in one of the Croonian Lectures to the Royal Society.[12] His thesis was that "the structure of a muscular fibre is supposed vesicular, with a reticular plexus of blood-vessels invading each vesicle." He drew diagrams (Fig. 71) to illustrate the change in shape of these "vesicles" when squeezed by the pressure of the muscle's contraction. Stuart supported his thesis by an experiment on a decapitated frog.

> This experiment is performed by suspending a live Frog by the fore legs in a frame . . . When having cut off the head from the first vertebre of the neck with a pair of scissors, a small probe, the button at its extremity being first filed flat, is to be pushed very gently down upon the upper extremity of the medulla spinalis, in the first vertebre of the neck; upon which the inferior limbs, which hung down loose, will be immediately contracted. . . . The same probe pushed gently through the hole of the occiput of the scull on the medulla oblongata, will make the eyes move, and sometimes the mouth open.

Stuart did not illustrate these effects on the head but drew a striking picture of the contracting legs. He recorded that this effect could not be repeated indefinitely, and held that an interval "seems to be necessary for recovering the equality of the circulation, which was disturbed by the immediate preceding convulsion, as it throws the blood violently out of the muscles in the time of their contraction or systole, which cannot be restored immediately in such a languid state of circulation, as this Experiment must bring on."

Stuart was not the first to make such observations on decapitated frogs, but his concept of muscular contraction was novel. He invoked the power of expanding and contracting blood vessels in the mechanism of contraction, relegating the nervous fluid to the role of trigger, "as the quantity of animal spirits propelled into the muscles must be supposed to be very small." He explored, with a microscope, the structure of the blood vessels in the muscles and the nerve endings. This was a hydraulic process in which "a very strong muscular motion may be easily exerted by a very slight impulse through the nerves."

Stuart received many honors including election as a Fellow of the Royal Society and membership of the French Académie des Sciences.

James Johnstone (1730–1802)

The relationship of the brain to the spinal cord was a puzzle in the 18th century; the function of the structure of the roots leaving the cord at all levels was unknown. The enlargements on the nerve tracts connected to the cord could be seen even by the naked eye, and there was uncertainty as to whether these were motor or sensory in function. Galen had thought that the presence of a ganglion indicated that the nerve was motor. Alexander Monro, the great Scottish physician who had trained with Boerhaave, noted that these ganglia lay on the posterior roots and that their coalescence with the anterior roots was peripheral to the swellings.[13] But, like Galen, he thought they were concerned with what he called "muscular nerves," and defended them as such against the suggestion of James Johnstone that their action was to cut off sensation.[14] Johnstone wrote about his concept to the Royal Society who published it in the *Philosophical Transactions* in 1765. He took to task Lancisi's

---

[12]Lecture III of the Croonian Lectures. *Proc. roy. Soc. London*, 40:36–48 (1739).

[13]Alexander Monro (1733–1817). *Observations on the Structure and Functions of the Nervous System.* Elliot, Edinburgh, 1783.

[14]James Johnstone (1730–1802). Essay on the use of the ganglions of nerves. *Phil. Trans. roy. Soc.*, 54:177–184 (1764).

theory that the ganglions were themselves muscles, capable of contractions,[15] and Winslow's that they were "little brains."[16] This idea he ridiculed.

> The brain needs no muscular force to impress motion upon the animal spirits; and granting Ganglions to be, as is ingeniously conjectured by Lancisi and Winslow, subsidiary brains, or analogous to the brain in their office, neither will they need any such muscular apparatus and force. A power, in fine, no less than chimerical, as it supposes the force of muscles of the greatest exertion and effect, to be derived from those of least bulk and strength (which must be in some proportion to the quantity of muscle fibers); and would be a single instance of a mechanical force producing another infinitely greater than itself.

Johnstone pressed his opinion that the ganglia are involved with involuntary movements.

> May we not then, reasonably conclude, that Ganglions are to be the instruments, by which the motions of the heart and intestines are, from the earliest to the last periods of animal life, rendered uniformly involuntary; and that to answer this purpose is their use, which they subserve by a structure unknown to us, no less than that of the brain, though it seems not improbable the first may be analogous to the last?

Johnstone was a practicing physician who had trained under Robert Whytt. He had a lifelong interest in the nervous system and followed up his communication to the Royal Society with a book entitled *The Use of the Ganglions of the Nerves*.[17] In this text he wrote that the ganglions were both sensory and motor.

Before the concept of spinal reflexes was born, the function of ganglia on the spinal roots continued to be a mystery. One suggestion came from a prominent anatomist in Paris.

Jacques-Bénigne Winslow (1669–1760)

Jacob Winslow was born in the Danish town of Odense and educated at the University of Copenhagen. After working there as a teacher of anatomy he moved in 1698 to Paris where he spent the rest of his life. The following year, as his relative Nicholas Steno had done before him, he joined the Catholic Church, a move that made future appointments in protestant Denmark impossible. Winslow changed his name to Jacques-Bénigne and began training with Duverney at the Jardin des Plantes, where he was appointed Professor of Anatomy and Surgery. The Jardin des Plantes, its name meaning garden of plants (which it is indeed today), was one of the most important centers for research in the medical sciences. Founded in 1620 with four chairs—medicine, surgery, anatomy, and botany—it was the major teaching center in Paris, the gardens providing medicinal plants rather than floral displays.

Joseph Guichard Duverney was one of the outstanding teachers of the time and a great experimenter but he published little, though long before Galvani's famous *Commentary* we find reports of his demonstrations.

One of his early public demonstrations showed the stimulation of muscle through irritation of its nerve. It was made before the Académie Royale de Sciences in Paris in 1700, and it was reported that:[18]

---

[15]Giovanni Maria Lancisi (1654–1720). *Tabulae Anatomicae Clarissimi Viri B. Eustachius*. Rome, 1714.

[16]Jacques-Bénigne Winslow (1668–1760). *Exposition Anatomique de la Structure du Corps Humain*, Part VI. [Illustrated by plates from Bartelemeo Eustachius (1520–1574).] Duprez and Desessartz, Paris, 1732. (English translation by G. Douglas: *An Anatomical Exposition of the Human Body*, 2 vols. Donaldson and Elliot, Edinburgh, 1772.)

[17]James Johnstone (1730–1802). *The Use of the Ganglions of the Nerves*. Shrewsbury, 1771.

[18]*History and Memoirs of the Roy. Acad. Sci., Paris*, p. 187. Translated and abridged by John Martyn and Ephraim Chambers. Knapton, London, 1742.

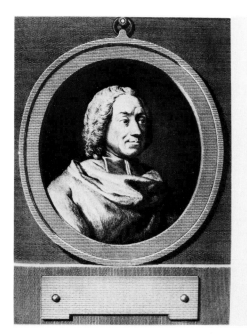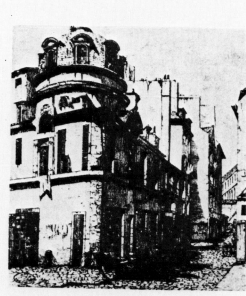

FIG. 72. **Left:** Jacques-Bénigne Winslow (1669–1760), the great teacher of anatomy. **Right:** The first amphitheatre for the teaching of anatomy built for this purpose in Paris. Still standing but used for administrative purposes.

M. Duverney showed a frog just dead, which in taking the nerves of the belly of this animal which go to the thighs and legs, and irritating them a little with a scalpel, trembled and suffered a sort of convulsion. Afterwards he cut these nerves in the belly, and holding them a little stretched with his hand, he made them do so again by the same motion of the scalpel. If the frog has been longer dead this would not have happened, in all probability there yet remained some liquor in these nerves, the undulation of which caused the trembling of the parts where they corresponded, and consequently the nerves are only pipes, the effect whereof depends upon the liquor which they contain.

Upon the death of Duverney, Winslow succeeded him to the principal chair in anatomy. Nearly all the great French anatomists of this period were associated with the Jardin du Roi: Humand, Ferrem, Petit, Vicq d'Azyr, and Winslow. In addition to the most brilliant names in botany, there were appointments in chemistry, numerology, and zoology. Among the last was Lamarck who had moved away from his interest in botany, which had brought him membership in the Académie Royale des Sciences. The latter was destroyed in 1793, during the Terror. The Jardin du Roi was renamed the Musée Nationale d'Histoire Naturelle, and Lamarck became a Professor of Zoology, in charge of insects and worms.[19] The second professorship in zoology was at the same time given to Geoffray Saint-Hillaire who worked on vertebrate animals.

Lamarck's theory of evolution was used in the next century, and a statue to him was placed at the main entrance of the Jardin des Plantes. On the back of the statue there is a rather strange plaque showing a young girl with her hand on his shoulder assuring him, in

[19]Jean Baptiste Pierre Antoine Lamarck (1744–1829). *Physiologie Zoologique*, Vol. 1. Dentu Libraire, Paris, 1809.

———. *Histoire Naturelle des Animaux sans Vertébrés*. Verdière Libraire, Paris, 1815.

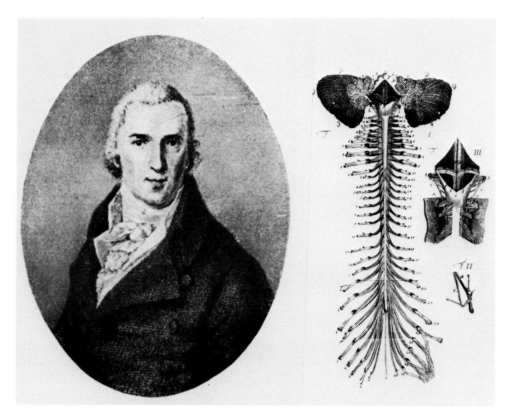

FIG. 73. **Left:** Jiri Prochaska (1749–1820) of Prague. Proponent of automatic reflection in the medulla and spinal cord. **Right:** Prochaska's illustration of the spinal roots and their ganglia. (*De Structura Nervorum*, 3 vols. Gerbe, Prague, 1780–83.)

French, that "Posterity will admire you: it will avenge you, my father." Her prophecy has not been fulfilled.

Winslow's work in Paris was studied in the homes of anatomists and surgeons, for there was no center for such instruction. Paris, with one of the oldest universities of the world, the Sorbonne, had no school of medicine. It was not until 1472 that a Faculty of Medicine was established in a building of its own on the rue des Rats, whose name was later changed to honor Louis XIV's adviser, Colbert. When the ban on dissection of cadavers was revoked a new anatomical theater was built at the expense of Parisian physicians. Under its fine dome Winslow gave his demonstrations of dissection but the Revolution brought an end to these activities once again. The beautiful building remains to this day, preserved by the administration of the City of Paris and bearing on its walls a plaque honoring Winslow.

It is in his most important publication, *L'Exposition Anatomique de la Structure du Corps Humain*, that we find his views on the nervous system, including a discussion of the spinal cord and the ganglions on the roots. These he believed to play a very important part in mediation of involuntary movements. There was much interest in what was called "the sympathy of parts" for here was a mechanism for the integration of body parts that eluded nervous influence flowing from the brain. Some suggested an interaction took place peripherally in a plexus, or, as Willis had suggested, an anastomosis of sensory and motor endings. Winslow introduced the concept that the ganglia of the chain, lying along the spinal

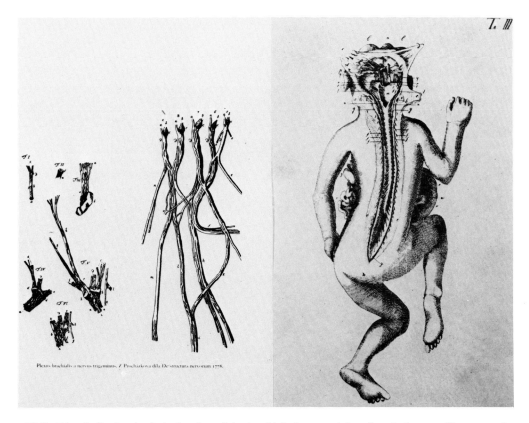

FIG. 74. **Left:** Prochaska's drawing of the brachial plexus and the trigeminal nerve. He proposed a similar relation between the spinal roots and their ganglia. **Right:** Prochaska's drawing of the spinal cord of an ancephalic monster. (From *De Structura Nervorum*. Prague, 1780.)

cord, were "small brains." These he envisaged as centers where intercommunication between nerves could take place, effecting "sympathy" between various visceral organs. "These ganglions," he wrote, "differ more or less from each other in size, colour and consistence, and may be looked upon as so many origins or germina dispersed through this great pair of nerves and consequently as so many small brains." This ingenious theory of the sympathy of parts has left its name on the structures: the sympathetic chain.

Winslow's theories were followed by those of Unzer, of Halle, and his pupil Prochaska in Prague. Unzer, the pupil of Stahl, postulated several sites where impressions might be turned back. These included the brain, the ganglia, bifurcations of nerves, and the plexuses. Only in the case of the brain was there conscious awareness of the impression that had caused the reflection.[20]

Jiri Prochaska (1749–1820)

Born in Moravia (now Czechoslovakia), Prochaska became interested in the nervous system while he was a student at the University of Vienna, where he gained his degree in 1776. In 1778 he went to Prague where he remained for the rest of his life, rising to become

[20]The Sydenham Society in England gave Unzer's book and that of Prochaska to the same translator, Thomas Laycock, teacher of Hughlings Jackson, and through him the word "reflection" became an accepted English term.

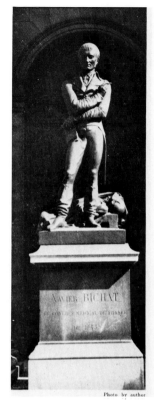

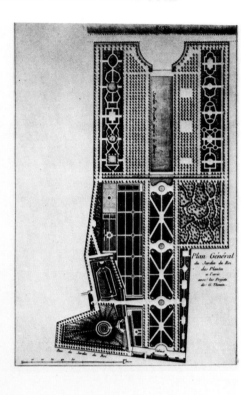

FIG. 75.   Left: Marie-François Bichat (1771–1802). Brilliant young pathologist whose training in philosophy merged into his teaching of medicine. His statue in the courtyard of the old Ecole de Médecine.   **Right:** Before Paris established a school of medicine the most important locus of teaching in medicine, anatomy, surgery, and botany was the Jardin du Roi where the medicinal plants were grown. (From the engraving by George du Rouge who sent a copy to Thomas Jefferson.)

Professor of Anatomy, Physiology, and Ophthalmology. His most important work on the nervous system was, however, written soon after he arrived in Prague (*De Structura Nervorum,* 1769). Prochaska believed in a "sensorium commune" where an automatic turn-around took place. He thought this might be located in the medulla or in the cord itself, but he did not agree with Unzer that this could be in the ganglia. However, he did agree that the nerves themselves might have an intrinsic life force, a "vis insita," that enabled them to function in isolation from the brain. He supported this argument by citing the movements of ancephalic monsters.

In the 18th century, the concept of "reflex action" raised not one problem but two. In addition to the question of how this could be effected, there was the question of teleology, the significance of movements over which the soul of man had no control.

Prochaska's teacher, Unzer, had demanded a teleological significance for involuntary movement at a level higher than the organism itself. He transferred purpose from the individual to the Creator, and made a synthesis between the most machine-like characteristics of man's body and a divine omnipotence. Prochaska was more down to earth, proposing that the purpose of unconsciously initiated movements was preservation of the individual. At the close of the century the problem of reflex action was still unsolved.

Marie-François Xavier Bichat (1771–1802)

That the ganglia have an even greater and more mysterious role was argued by Bichat, the brilliant young French pathologist. For him, all sympathetic ganglia were the nervous representation of the involuntary, unconscious, or, as he called it, "the organic life." He noted the difference between sympathetic and spinal ganglia, observing that irritation of the latter caused muscular convulsions, indicating some motor role.[21]

Bichat studied pathology after a training in philosophy which later permeated his writings. He had leanings toward the teachings of Stahl and the vitalistic position of the animists at Montpellier. These are detected in his best known work, *La Vie et la Mort*. His contributions to anatomy and physiology are found in a textbook published just before his early death in 1802.[22] This work reflects his pursuit of the meaning of structures, first from dissection of cadavers and later from experiments on living animals. And it is in this work that one finds his concepts of nervous function in ganglia.

BIBLIOGRAPHY

Domenico Cotugno (1736–1822)

Selected Writings

De Aquaeductibus Auris Humanae Internae Disertatio. Aquinae, Naples, 1761.

De Ischiade Nervosa Commentarius. Simonii, Naples, 1764.

Secondary Sources

Belloni, L. L'opera nevrologica di Domenico Cotugno. In: *Essays on the History of Italian Neurology*. Istituto di Storia della Medicina, Università degli Studi, Milano, 1963.

Levinson, A. Domenico Cotugno. In: *The Founders of Neurology*, pp. 19–23. Charles Thomas, Springfield, Ill., 1953.

Viets, H. Domenico Cotugno: his description of the cerebrospinal fluid. *Bull. Inst. Hist. Med.*, 3:701–738 (1935).

François Pourfour du Petit (1664–1741)

Selected Writings

Trois Lettres d'un Médecin des Hopitaux du Roy. Albert, Namur, 1710. Mémoire dans lequel il est demonstré que les nerfs intercostaux fournissent des rameaux que portent des esprits dans les yeus. *Mémoires Acad. Roy. de Sci.*, 26:262–272 (1772).

Secondary Sources

Best, A. E. Pourfour du Petit's experiments on the origin of the sympathetic nerve. *Med. Hist.*, 13:154–174 (1969).

---

[21]". . . tout irritation d'un filet venant des ganglions vertébraux produit tout de suite des convulsions dans les muscles correspondants."

[22]Marie-François Xavier Bichat (1771–1802). *Anatomie Générale, Appliquée à la Physiologie et à la Médecine*, 2 vols. Brosson, Paris, 1802.

Clarke, E., and O'Malley, C. D. *The Human Brain and Spinal Cord*. University of California Press, 1968.

Alexander Stuart (1673–1742)

Selected Writings

Experiments to prove the existence of fluid in the nerves. *Proc. roy. Soc.*, 37:327–331 (1731).

Dissertatio de Structura et Motu Musculari. Richardson, London, 1738.

Three Lectures on Muscular Motion Read Before the Royal Society. Woodward, London, 1739.

Jacques-Bénigne Winslow (1669–1760)

Selected Writings

L'Exposition Anatomique de la Structure du Corps Humain. Desprez, Paris, 1732.

Secondary Source

Snorrason, E. *L'Anatomiste J-B. Winslow 1669–1760*. Copenhagen, 1969.

Jiri Prochaska (1749–1820)

Selected Writings

De Structura Nervorum, 3 vols. Graefer, Prague, 1780–1783.

De Functionibus Systemis Nervosa et Observationes Anatomico-pathologicae. Gerbe, Prague, 1784. (English translation by T. Laycock. *A Dissertation on the Functions of the Nervous System*. Sydenham Society, London, 1851.)

Adnotationum Academicarum. Gerbe, Prague, 1784.

De Carne Musculorum. Graefer, Vienna, 1778.

Controversae Questiones Physiologicae. Graefer, Vienna, 1778.

Secondary Sources

Kruta, M. V. *Med. Dr. Jiri Prochaska 1749–1820* (in Czech). Nakladatelství (Czechoslovak Academy), Prague, 1956.

Kruta, M. V. G. Prochaska's and J. E. Purkinje's contributions to neurophysiology. In: *Von Boerhaave bis Berger*, edited by K. Rothschuh. Fischer, Stuttgart, 1964.

Gutmann, E. Jiri Prochaska a reflexni theorie. *Czecholov Fisiol.*, 1:1–8 (1952).

Neuberger, M. Die Physiologue Georg Prochaska, in Vorlaufer Purkinjes. *Vienna med. Woch.*, 1155–1157 (1937).

Gutmann, E. *Uvaha O Funkich Nervove Soustavy* (in Latin), Nakladatelství (Czechoslovak Academy), Prague, 1954.

Marie-François Xavier Bichat (1771–1802)

Selected Writings

Recherches Physiologique sur la Vie et la Mort. Paris, 1800. (English translation by F. Gold, with notes by F. Magendie. Richardson and Lord, Boston, 1827.)

Anatomie Générale Appliquée à la Physiologie et à la Médecine, 4 vols. Brasson, Gaban, Paris, 1801.

Secondary Sources

Allbury, W. R. Experiment and explanation in the physiology of Bichat and Magendie. *Studies in the History of Biology*, 1:47–131 (1977).

[Centenary Volume on Bichat] *Bull. Soc. Français d'Histoire de la Médecine.* 1902.

Lain, E. P. Sensualism and vitalism in Bichat's Anatomie générale. *J. Hist. Med. and All. Sci.*, 3:47–64 (1948).

CHAPTER XIII

Beginnings of Electrophysiology

When the 18th century opened, electricity and nervous conduction were still mysterious powers. Could they be related? Other explanations were failing, one by one. In a period impressed by Harvey's discovery, there was interest in the possible function of blood in neuromuscular action. Blood had played a role in Descartes' afferent system, bringing particles to the brain to stimulate the pineal, but he had not proposed an efferent role for the nerves that went to the muscles. Willis, however, had given the cerebral blood vessels the function of distilling the blood to extract the animal spirits[1] and Mayow had invoked fermentation in the blood of his "nitro-aerial spirit" as having "the chief part in the origination of animal motions."[2] Borelli had recognized two agents as necessary for muscular contraction. One came from the nerve to react with another from the blood, already in the muscle, thus forming an "ebulliton" or fermentation.[3]

Another candidate for the principal role in neuromuscular contraction that also failed was vibration. This notion had also occurred to Borelli and was a variation of the pulsation theory of Baglivi who believed the dura mater continuously pulsated and transmitted an oscillation to the motor nerves.[4] Croone also considered it a possible agent for moving the spirits down the nerve.[5] In the following century, the idea would reach its zenith in David Hartley's book.[6] Even Fontana had given it passing consid-

[1] J. Willis, *The Anatomy of the Brain*, p. 88. Pordage translation, 1684.

[2] J. Mayow. *Tractatus Quinque*. Sheldonian, Oxford, 1674.

[3] G. A. Borelli. *De motu animalium*, Vol. 2. Bernado, Rome, 1681.

[4] G. Baglivi. *De fibra motrice et morbosa*. Perugia, 1700.

[5] W. Croone. *De ratione motus musculorum*, Section 26. (Bound with T. Willis' *Opera Omnia*. Dring, Harper & Leigh, London, 1664.)

[6] David Hartley, *Observations on Man, His Frame, His Duty, and His Expectations*. London, 1749.

eration in a letter to a friend.[7] However, an experiment was performed by an English country clergyman, Stephen Hales, that denied the force of blood the role of agent in muscular contraction.

Stephen Hales (1677–1761)

Educated at Cambridge University, with degrees in natural philosophy and theology, Hales was also exposed to electrical experiments, hydrostatics, and the dissection of animals. He learned techniques which he took with him to the rectory in Teddington, then a country village on the Thames, outside London. His initial research, pursued between the duties of tending his parochial flock, was in the hydrostatics of plants. His book *Vegetable Staticks* was an immediate success.[8] It was translated into French by the botanist Buffon, director for many years of the Jardin du Roi where his statue by Pajou now stands.[9] Hales's studies later turned to experiments on the "haemastaticks" of the blood.

In the second volume, he tells us how the idea came to him:[10]

> It may not be improper here to take notice that being the unsatisfactory conjectures of several, about the cause of muscular motion, it occurred to me, that by fixing tubes to the arteries of animals, I might find pretty nearly, whether the blood, by its mere hydraulic energy, could have a sufficient force, by dilating the fibres of the acting muscles, and thereby shortening their lengths, to produce the great effects of muscular motion. And hence it was, as I mentioned in the preface to Vol. I, that I was insensibly led on from time to time into this large field of statical and other experiments.

In this work he was the pioneer in the measurement of blood pressure. By inserting cannulae he determined arterial and venous pressures in many animals including a horse. This he strapped on its back to the picket fence of his garden while making his measurements.

These measurements led him to an important conclusion:

> From this very small Force of the arterial Blood among the muscular Fibres we may with good reason conclude, how short this Force is of producing so great an Effect, as that of muscular Motion, which wonderful and hitherto inexplicable Mystery of Nature, must therefore be owing to some more vigorous and active Energy, whose Force is regulated by the Nerves; but whether it be confined in Canals within the Nerves, or acts along their surfaces like electrical Powers, is not easy to determine.

Again the suggestion of a role for electricity crops up. Charleton had called electricity and magnetism the "occult qualities" and, in the 17th century, murmurs had been heard that perhaps electricity was related to nervous conduction. Hales admired Newton and must have been familiar with the *Opticks*, for he had been elected a Fellow of the Royal Society in 1718 when Newton was its president. In 1753, he was elected to the Académie royale des Sciences of Paris.

The ingenuity of Hales did not stop with measurements of blood pressure. He was convinced of the importance of fresh air and designed methods of ventilating prisons and holds of ships. He calculated the amount of air needed in the lungs from his observations of blood pressure, and tested a ventilating device in a boat outside his house on the Thames. Hales died in 1761 and was buried, at his wish, in Teddington churchyard. Later a monument was raised to him in Westminster Abbey.

[7]F. Fontana, Lettre de M. l'Abbé Fontana à M. Gibelin à Aix-en-Provence, datée de Florence du Juillet 1782. *Journal de Physique*, 24:417–421 (1784).

[8]*Vegetable Staticks.* Innys and Woodward, London, 1727.

[9]G. L. Leclerc, *Compte de Buffon: La statique des végétaux, et l'analyse de l'air.* 1735.

[10]*Statickal Essays: Containing Haemastaticks.* Innys, Manby, and Woodward, London, 1733.

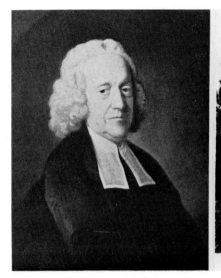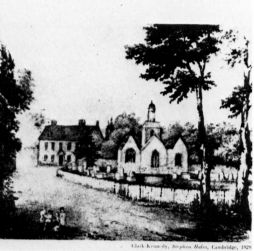

FIG. 76.   Left: Stephen Hales (1677–1761). (From the portrait by Thomas Hudson in the National Portrait Gallery, London.)   **Right:** The parish church at Teddington with the picket fence to which Hales tied his animals while measuring their blood pressure with a cannula in the artery.

Isaac Newton (1642–1727)

Whatever the agent was in the nervous system, it was invisible and extremely speedy in its action. This led Newton to write the following passage in the last paragraph of the *General Scholium.*

> And now we might add something concerning a certain most subtle spirit, which pervades and lies hid in all gross bodies, by the force and action of which spirit, particles of bodies attract one another at near distances as well as attracting the neighbouring corpuscles; and light is emitted, reflected, refracted, inflected, and heats bodies; and all sensation is excited, and the members of the animal body are moved at the command of the will, namely by the vibrations of this spirit mutually propagated along the solid filaments of the nerves, from the outward organs of sense to the brain and from the brain into the muscles. But these are things that cannot be explained in a few words, nor are we furnished with that sufficiency of experiments which is required to an accurate determination and demonstration of the laws by which this electric and elastic spirit operates.[11]

This concept embraces both vibrations and electricity though one notes that, as a true scientist, he asks for supporting experiment.

Newton's reference to vibrations echoes an early comment he had made in the first edition of *Opticks*. In Query 12 he wrote, "Do not the Rays of Light in falling upon the bottom of the Eye excite Vibrations in the *Tunica Retina*? Which Vibrations, being propagated along the solid Fibres of the optick Nerves into the Brain, cause the Sense of seeing." He continues, "...the Vibrations of their parts are of a lasting nature, and therefore may be propagated along solid Fibres of uniform dense Matter to a great distance, for conveying to the Brain the impressions made upon all the Organs of Sense."

[11]Isaac Newton. General scholium. *Principia Mathematica*, Vol. 2, p. 393. London, 1713. (Andrew Motte's translation, London, 1729.)

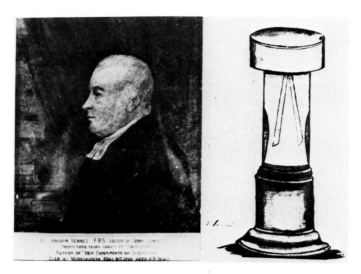

FIG. 77. The portrait of Abraham Bennet that hangs in the vestry of the church of Wirksworth in Derbyshire. It has been suggested that this may be the work of Joseph Wright, but it is certainly more primitive in treatment than most of this painter's works. In the original, written on one of the pile of books, can be seen the title: *Experiments in Electricity*, and on a scroll: Rev. Abm. Bennet F.R.S. On the right is one of his electroscopes. (The author is indebted for the photograph to the Reverend G. Busby, Rural Dean of Wirksworth.)

In the second edition of *Opticks*, Newton added more queries and extended the concept of vibration to include the motor nervous system. In the 24th Query he wrote:[12]

> Is not Animal Motion perform'd by the Vibrations of this Medium, excited in the Brain by the Power of the Will, and propagated from thence through the solid, pellucid, and uniform Capillamenta of the Nerves and the Muscles, for contracting and dilating them? I suppose that the Capillamenta of the Nerves are each of them solid and uniform, that the vibrating Motion of the Aetherial Medium may be propagated along them from one End to the other uniformly, and without interruption.

But the leading figures in the physiology of the time would accept neither "aether" nor electricity. The powerful Haller, who still believed in nervous fluid, stated it to be "more gross than fire, or aether or electrical or magnetic matter, since it can be retained in channels."

One disadvantage of early experimenters was the lack of instrumentation for measuring very small currents of biological origin. Up to the time of Volta the most sensitive instrument available was the modification of Cavallo's electrometer, perfected by the curate of a rural parish in Derbyshire, England.

The Reverend Abraham Bennet of Wirksworth, a village on the Derwent, designed and constructed the delicate instrument that carries his name. He replaced the silver wires used by Cavallo and the gilded straws of Cavendish with strips of gold leaf. It was the movement of these strips, when charged, that made Newton sceptical of the prevalent theory of electricity. It was believed that electricity drawn from a charged body was an emanation or effluvium produced by that body. This appeared to contradict the law of gravitation, for there was no loss of weight.

[12]Isaac Newton. *Opticks: or a Treatise of the Reflections, Refractions, Inflections and Colours of Light* (in English), 2nd edn, Query 24. London, 1717.

In the little medieval church where he spent so many of his years there hangs a small portrait of the Rev. Bennet. The portrait is not by a very skilled hand which makes unlikely the suggestion that it is by Joseph Wright (a friend of Bennet's and a purchaser of his book). Bennet's famous book, *New Experiments in Electricity*, appeared in 1789. A copy was bought for his local scientific society (the Derby Philosophical Society) in two installments of two shillings and sixpence each, one made before publication and one after, the payments being authorized by Erasmus Darwin. Some interesting and unpublished manuscripts by Bennet are in the Derby Public Library.

Long before the work of Galvani and his concept that electricity was produced within the animal body, many experimenters, charmed with the power of frictional machines, had been enjoying themselves with bizarre demonstrations of the effect of electrifying people under various conditions. They had little understanding of what was happening but the results were spectacular and drew much attention. The best planned experiments of this kind were those of Stephen Gray in England.

Stephen Gray (1666?–1736)

Stephen Gray, whose birth date is unknown and of whom no portrait has been found, died as a charity pensioner at Charterhouse, which had been a monastery since the 14th century, before Henry VIII converted it into a home for aged pensioners and a boys' school. In the 19th century, long after Gray lived there, this school became one of England's outstanding public schools where the boys still proudly wear their 16th century uniforms.

Gray, the pensioner, had powerful friends. One of these was the competent scientist Jean Theophilus Desaguliers, born in 1683 in the same city as Réaumur, La Rochelle, a port on the Bay of Biscay made famous by the experiments there of John Walsh on electric fish. Two years after the birth of Desaguliers, Louis XIV revoked the Edict of Nantes and religious freedom in France ended. Desaguliers' family joined the exodus of Huguenots to England. Desaguliers was educated at Oxford, where he met Newton and became a member of the Royal Society. He was one of Stephen Gray's most staunch supporters. Another friend of Gray was Granville Wheeler, who let him experiment at his country house, Otterden Place in Kent. It was already known that the human body could be charged electrically if it was insulated from the ground. At first it was thought that a layer of air had to be present between the subject and the ground. The characteristics of conductors and nonconductors were only beginning to be understood.

Gray, through his eminent friends, had the opportunity to communicate his experiments to the Royal Society in the form of letters to the Secretary. The first series of these, however, was not on electrifying the human body but on telescopy and his astronomical observations.[13] It is in 1731 that we first learn of such an attempt.

Further on in the series, Gray wrote the following letter.

> April 8, 1730. I made the following Experiment on a Boy between eight and nine Years of Age. His Weight, with his Cloaths on, was forty-seven Pounds ten Ounces. I suspended him in a horizontal Position, by two Hair-Lines, such as Cloaths are dried on: They were about thirteen Feet long, with loops at each End. . . . Then the Leaf-Brass was placed under the Feet, his Shoes and Stockings being on, and the Tube held near his Head, his Feet attracted, but not altogether at so great a Hight as his Head . . .

[13]Stephen Gray (1666?–1736). A letter to Cromwell Mortimer, M.D., Sec. R.S. containing several experiments concerning electricity. *Phil. Trans. roy. Soc.*, 37:18–44 (1731).

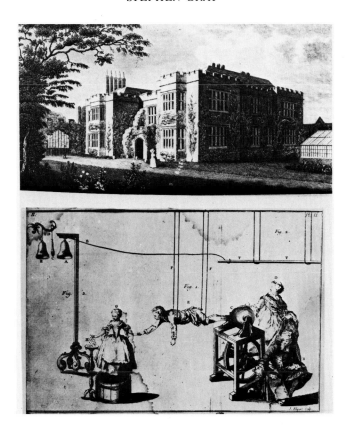

FIG. 78. Granville Wheeler's house, Ottenden Place in Kent, where the classic experiments of Stephen Gray were mostly performed. No illustrations of his were published but many other workers repeated them and provided charming illustrations such as this from Winkler, Professor of Greek and Latin at Leipzig. (From *Essai sur la Nature. Les Effets et les Causes avec Description de deux nouvelles Machines à Électricité.* Torry, Paris, 1748.)

Gray's source of electricity was the "electric virtue" he produced by the rubbing of various substances, usually a glass tube, and his indicator of reaction was the movement of his Leaf-Brass electroscope. Most of Gray's experiments were on the little understood phenomenon of electrical conduction. He stated, "By these Experiments we see that Animals receive a greater Quantity of Electrick Effluvia..." The tendency was to explain his demonstrations in terms of attraction and repulsion being properties of the body itself.

In pursuit of evidence that the mysterious power might be electricity a great deal of knowledge had to be acquired about this elusive agent itself. In order to study it, more advanced methods of producing it had to be developed. When this was accomplished, the need arose to study its action on the animal body—to determine if the effects of electrical stimulation on muscle and nerve were in any way similar to natural movements. Finally, if animal tissues themselves produced electricity, very delicate instruments had to be designed in order to detect it. The means for measuring electrical current in animal tissue were provided by two gentlemen of the 18th century, André Marie Ampère and Alessandro Volta.

The first step toward using electricity as an instrument in examining the nervous system was its differentiation from another power, magnetism. The attractive power of amber, when rubbed, was known to the Greeks at least 600 years BC. Thales described it by saying "amber is endowed with a soul and attracts to it light objects."[14]

Two thousand years later a differentiation was made between electricity and magnetism. The differentiation was made by William Gilbert in a publication entitled *De Arte Magnetica*,[15] followed two years later by the classic *De Magnete*.[16] Gilbert, physician to Queen Elizabeth, did not write of animal electricity but recognized the difference between the attractive force of frictional electricity and the magnetism of the lodestone, a naturally occurring magnetic ore. His work influenced the thinking of all those who tried to explain the earliest recognized form of biological electricity, found in the electric fish.

The first stimulators for what we would now call electrophysiology were all based on the development of a spark produced by friction. The 17th century was on the threshold of discovering a source of friction when von Guericke demonstrated that a rotated sulphur globe on being rubbed by hand attracted light objects.[17] The spark, the desired proof of electricity, was not achieved until the 18th century.

Frictional machines, usually using glass, were the source of discharge used to stimulate both man and animals. Hauksbee had designed a globe generator by which he could evoke a glow in an evacuated tube.[18] A demonstration to the Royal Society led to the identification of the phenomenon as an effluvium and sure evidence of a spark. The Hauksbee generator received immediate recognition in many countries and examples of it can be found in museums throughout the world (e.g. in Leningrad, Leipzig, Leyden, London, Paris). Still, there was no effective way of storing this electricity. A storage technique was developed, almost accidentally and simultaneously, in two different countries, thirty years after Hauksbee's death. This development was achieved by Ewald George von Kleist in Pomerania and Petrus van Musschenbroek in Leyden.

Von Kleist is little known to the world of physics.[19] A description of his invention came to us from the writings of others. He was Dean of the Cathedral in Kamin, a city in the Baltic duchy of Brandenburg which later became part of Prussia and is now part of Poland. The first mention of it is by Krüger, an advocate of electrical stimulation in cases of muscular paralysis. Later it was included in a textbook written by Gralath.[19a] His invention brought him election to the Berlin Academy of Sciences. A tablet on the wall of his house in Kamin declares him to be the inventer of "elektrische Verstärkungsflasche" (Kleistsche Flasche) and gives the date as 1745. The discovery had been quite accidental.

Petrus van Musschenbroek (1692–1761)

More immediate credit was given to a prominent physicist, a Professor of Physics at Leyden, Petrus van Musschenbroek. It is of interest that von Kleist had been a student at

[14]Thales (625 BC–546 BC). Quoted in M. Sirok: *Historique de l'Electricité en Générale et de l'Electricité Médicale*. Vigot, Paris.

[15]William Gilbert (1544–1603). *De Arte Magnetica*. 1598.

[16]William Gilbert. *De Magnete, Magnetisque Corporibus, et de Magno Magnete Tellure*. Peter Short, London, 1600.

[17]O. von Guericke (1602–1686). *Experimenta Nova* (ut vocantur) *Magdeburgica de Vacuo Spatio*, Book IV. Amsterdam, 1672.

[18]Francis Hawksbee (1666–1713). *Physico-Mechanical Experiments*. Printed by the author, London, 1709. Some experiments made on the attraction of bodies in vacuo. *Phil. Trans. roy. Soc.*, 24:2165–2175 (1705).

[19]Ewald George von Kleist (1700–1748). Letter to J. G. Krüger. In: J. C. Krüger, *Geschichte der Erde*, pp. 177–181. Hemmerde, Halle, 1746.

[19a]D. Gralath. Geschichte der Elektricität. *Versuche und Abhandlungen der naturforschenden Gesellschaft zu Danzig*, 2:402–411 (1754).

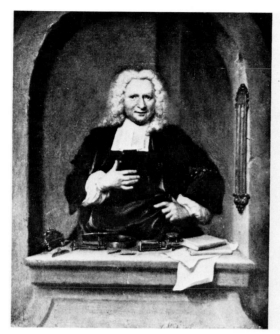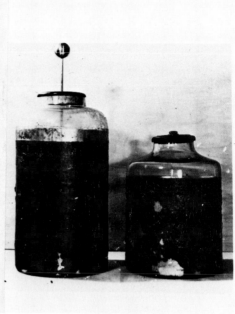

FIG. 79. Left: Petrus van Musschenbroek (1692–1761) from the portrait by J. M. Quinkhard, depicting him among his physical instruments including a compass, a pyrometer, a barometer, and a lodestone. (From the Boerhaave Museum, Leyden.) **Right:** Two early Leyden jars in the same collection. (Photograph by courtesy of the Boerhaave Museum.)

Leyden and perhaps experienced the search for a possible means of strong electricity. Both Musschenbroek's and von Kleist's achievements were accidental but their importance cannot be exaggerated. They discovered, for the first time, a technique for storing an electric charge. A method for producing a constant flow of direct current was discovered by Volta[20] at the beginning of the next century, and Nikola Tesla came up with alternating current in 1884.[21]

Petrus van Musschenbroek, born in Leyden in 1692, came from a family of instrument makers, which stood him in good stead when he became interested in the instruments being used in research on animal electricity. He graduated in medicine, in 1715, from the University of Leyden and, in 1719, received a doctorate in philosophy and gained his first professorship at the University of Duisberg on the Rhine.

Musschenbroek moved on to Utrecht and then back to Leyden where he became one of the great teachers of this distinguished university. Eventually he inherited the chair of Gravesande, the prominent physicist. Musschenbroek's role in any story of the development of electrophysiology centers on his almost accidental invention of the famous Leyden jar, later used by all eighteenth century investigators of animal electricity, including Galvani.

There are several accounts of his initial experiment, derived from contemporary letters. One of these was sent to the eminent physicist Réaumur, who gave the letter to Nollet. Nollet, a great publicist, reported its contents to the Académie des Sciences in 1746.[22]

[20]A. Volta (1745–1827). On electricity excited by the contact of conducting substances of different kinds. *Phil. Trans. roy. Soc.*, 90:403–431 (1800).

[21]Nikola Tesla (1856–1943). Selection of his notes and correspondence. In: *Nikola Tesla 1856–1943*, edited by L. I. Anderson. Belgrade, 1950.

[22]J. A. Nollet. *Mémoires de l'Académie Royale des Sciences*, pp. 1–25. Paris, 1746.

The experiment that was described apparently took place while Musschenbroek was striving to conserve electricity in a conductor and delay the loss of its charge in air. He used water as a conductor, insulating it from air in a nonconducting glass jar. However, when he charged the water with a wire leading from an electrostatic machine, he found the electricity dissipated as quickly as ever. His assistant, Andreas Cuneus, holding a jar containing charged water, accidently touched the inserted wire with his hand and got a shock. His hand had formed one "plate," the charged water, another, and the glass jar, the intervening dielectric. A condenser was born.

Musschenbroek's description of the experience which was reported in Latin to Réaumur, was spread by Nollet. "I want to tell you of a new but terrible experiment which I advise you never to attempt yourself . . . the arm and the whole body was affected in so terrible a manner that I cannot express: in a word I thought it was the end of me."[23]

It was Nollet who coined the name "Leyden jar" though supporters of von Kleist remained faithful to the name "Kleistsch Flasche." It became the principal source of stimulation gradually supplanting the frictional machine, for here was a device for storing electricity. Musschenbroek went on to explore more extensively the physics of the Leyden jar and included in his teaching course instructions on what to expect from this experiment.[24]

> The spark will be the red color of fire, will be very violent: it will cause a very strong commotion in the hand, in the arm, in the chest and, in a word, in the whole body of the experimenter; it is sometimes so terrible, that it can wound the person holding it: it can even cause a high fever, a hemorrhage or some other sickness.

Nollet, with his flair for publicizing, designed spectacular demonstrations of the power of electricity. He lined up, hand-in-hand, 180 soldiers in the Gallery at Versailles to demonstrate to the King that when the men at each end of the chain touched the poles of a Leyden jar, the whole line of men leapt into the air. He repeated the experiment for some monks at Chartreuse, using a chain of men 3 kilometers in length.

Jean-Antoine Nollet (1700–1770)

Jean-Antoine Nollet, who reported to the world the experiences of Musschenbroek with the Leyden jar, was one of the most fascinating characters in this period of science. Born in the opening year of the century near Compiègne in the Ile-de-France, the area between Picardy and Flanders, he was trained for the Church, a career for which the top scholars among the schoolboys of the time were usually destined, and progressed through the sequence of steps to a deaconate. He continued to wear the Geneva bands and was always addressed as Abbé Nollet.

This was as far as he went in the Church. Another interest superseded theology and to this, the study of the physical sciences, he devoted the rest of his intellectual life. It began as a hobby when he took up enamel work and learned to manipulate materials by changing their physical state. His manual dexterity led to his making many ingenious articles of a mechanical nature. These had some didactic value and attracted the attention of Louis XIV's grandson, the Comte de Clermont, who invited Nollet to join the "Society of Arts," a group particularly interested in the mechanical arts and which met from time to time in his house. This royal patronage was one of the most powerful influences on Nollet.

[23]J. A. Nollet. *Essai sur l'Electricité du Corps*. Guérin, Paris, 1746.

[24]*Institutiones Physicae*. Leyden, 1748.

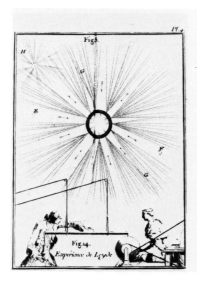
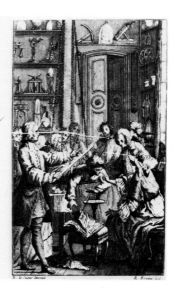

FIG. 80. **Left:** Nollet's reproduction of the experiment by Musschenbroek in which shorting the condenser made by a Leyden jar produced an alarming shock. **Right:** Nollet demonstrating to an audience at the Court of Versailles the experiments of Stephen Gray. (From *Essai sur l'Electricité du Corps Humain.* 1746.)

Nollet became friend and pupil of the physicist Cisternai DuFay[25] and with him became intensely interested in the properties of electricity that were being revealed by scientists in England. These included Hauksbee who improved the electrostatic machine and demonstrated luminescence in an evacuated tube. But the experiments that seized the imagination of du Fay and Nollet were those of Stephen Gray which demonstrated the phenomenon of static electricity. The replication of one of Gray's experiments became one of Nollet's more popular demonstrations. In this century, Nollet was not the only scientist impressed by this experiment, which showed that in some mysterious way the human body could function as a vehicle for the transmission of static electricity. Experimenters in many countries repeated the procedure and confirmed the result. Consequently there are several illustrations in books of that period to depict it. Nollet, himself, in his *Essai sur l'Electricité des Corps*, used an engraving of this experiment as his frontispiece.

DuFay lived in Tremblay, just outside Paris, and in his garden he and Nollet tried out and confirmed many of Gray's initial findings on electricity, including its transmission through a great length of wire and the drawing of a spark from a charged human body. This they tried on themselves before demonstrating it in public. One of DuFay's discoveries, which led to some controversy with Benjamin Franklin, was the concept of two sorts of electricity, vitreous and resinous, which repelled each other. The so-called vitreous was obtained from rubbing glass, quartz, animal fur, and precious stones. Resinous electricity came from rubbing amber, silk, and paper.

The opportunity for the first of Nollet's many foreign travels came when he was 34 and the occasion was a visit to England where he was able to observe the popular course in experimental physics that had been organized so successfully by Desaguliers, Newton's

[25]Charles du Cisternay DuFay (1698–1739). Quatrième mémoire sur l'électricité. *Mémoires de l'Académie Royale des Sciences*, pp. 457–476. Paris, 1735.

demonstrator.[26] This experience was instrumental in the formulation of Nollet's later projects, but the crowning event at the time was his election as a foreign member of the Royal Society.

In Paris, Nollet had another powerful advocate. The famous Réaumur, impressed by his manual dexterity, engaged him in the development of an improved thermometer, and it was through another interest of Réaumur that Nollet made his first excursion into biology. The problem of fertilization of frog spawn at that time was still a mystery. Nollet attempted but failed to collect male frog seminal fluid, but this did not lessen his enthusiasm for Spallanzani's success forty years later. Spallanzani not only collected the fluid but succeeded in fertilizing some spawn; this was the first recorded example of artificial insemination in the laboratory. Réaumur himself entered the controversy over animal electricity when he studied electric fish, though his own conclusion was that the shock was merely a muscular grip.

Another biological problem which Nollet approached in an experimental fashion was whether or not sound traveled through water. Scientists had raised the question as to whether or not fish could hear. The Abbé proceeded to sink a mooring in the Seine and then dived in and held on to it. He trained himself to stay for longer and longer periods under water without breathing until eventually he could stay long enough for experiments to be made. He found he could hear, though feebly, a pistol shot, a bell, a whistle, and the sound of a human voice. Nollet followed this up with a laboratory experiment in which he used water from which all the air had been removed, and proved that the transmission of sound was not carried by dissolved air.

His most original contribution to science, and one of importance for concepts of a nervous system acting through fluids, was his discovery of the semipermeability of animal tissues. In the experiment in which he made the discovery, he filled a cylindrical phial with spirits of wine and sealed the end with a piece of mesentery. The whole was then immersed in water. To his surprise, five hours later he found the phial so full of liquid that the mesentery sealing on the top was bulging out. On pricking this with a pin, he released a jet of liquid a foot high. At first he thought the effect must be due to differences in temperature between the water and the alcohol, but a control experiment soon dismissed this explanation. He then reversed the experiment putting water in the flask and alcohol outside and found then the mesentery was drawn into the bottle and the amount of liquid contained diminished. He also noticed that for the experiment to succeed, both fluids had to come in contact with the mesentery. In an era when the chief agent for neuromuscular action was thought to be a "nervous fluid," the question of osmosis through membranes was one that had not been faced. Diffusion of water through tissues was already known but preferential direction of passage was a new finding. Nollet followed this up by applying one of his vacuum pumps to pull water through a membrane and established that an equal negative pressure did not extract any alcohol. These observations laid the foundation for our modern knowledge of osmosis.

In 1738, four years after his visit to Desaguliers in London, Nollet published his first scientific work, *Programme ou idée générale d'un cours de physique expérimentale avec un catalogue raisonné des instruments que servent aux expériences*. This book was the fruit of the experiences Nollet had in teaching an experimental course for four years.

It was a practical course in which the students, many of whom were women of fashion, were drawn from the lay public. With their own eyes they saw the apparatus and experiments that demonstrated the physical laws they were learning. So successful was this nonacademic

[26]Jean Theophile Desaguliers (1683–1744). *A Dissertation Concerning Electricity*. Innys and Longman, London, 1742.

educational program, that it had great influence on the teaching of science in the schools and colleges. The experimental approach began to replace the didactic, philosophical, and logical treatment previously used and laboratory science began to come into its own.

Success of this course was not Nollet's only reward. In 1739, still young for such an honor, he was elected to the Académie Royale des Sciences. This was followed by a summons to give his course at the Royal Court at Versailles where the Dauphin was one of his pupils. So successful was he that the following year he was asked to repeat the course for the young Dauphine, the new wife of the Dauphin.

The course brought him fame and demands for exhibitions elsewhere. In 1740 he gave the course at the court of the King of Sardinia in Turin, where some of his apparatus is still preserved, and in Bordeaux by invitation of Montesquieu.[27] Montesquieu, although not a scientist, had a great interest in scientific theories, supplying some himself. (For example, he thought that the weather was responsible for the English temperament.) He also decided to buy a cabinet of instruments and invited Nollet, in 1741, to teach a course in experimental physics. Other centers followed suit, and what was essentially the physics of Newton was established in Cartesian France, though Nollet himself paid tribute to both great men. Nollet's pupils during his many years of teaching were distinguished not only for their social rank. One of the most famous was Lavoisier.

His course and his publication, which was scarcely more than a list of experiments and apparatus, were an established success and Nollet proceeded to expand his "Programme" into a more detailed form. In 1743 the first two volumes of a 6-volume series, *Leçons de Physique Expérimentale*, were published.

Nollet's books were not intended for physicists but for the instruction of the less scientifically educated. He selected the most interesting items from any particular field, along with the latest discoveries, choosing especially those that could be easily proven by an experiment. Some of the lessons crossed from physics into biology, for instance, those on the use of the microscope, and the section on the physics of sound which elaborated the anatomy of the ear. The physics of heat and steam was of continued interest to the Abbé, and some of his steam pumps have been preserved to this day in several museums, among them, the Conservatoire des Arts et Métiers in Paris. These he used to study the properties of a vacuum and rarified gases.

New editions of the first two volumes of the "Leçons" were brought out to meet the great demand, and other volumes were added. The fifth of these was devoted to the study of light and detailed many experiments with mirrors and prisms. Again biological interests were included; the anatomy and physiology of the eye were described with an explanation of myopia and presbyopia.

As a means of meeting dissension, Nollet published his *Lettres sur l'Electricité*. These appeared in parts over a period of 14 years. The Abbé was well established in royal favor; not only was he appointed to the newly created Chair in Experimental Physics at the Collège de Navarre but he was one of the fortunate few to be granted living quarters in the Galeries du Louvre. These rooms were a gift of the King by Letters Patent dating back to 1608 when Henry IV designated them for the use of artists and savants. They were where the "petits cabinets du sud" of the great art gallery are now located, and had a view of the Seine. Here the Abbé lived until his death in 1770, surrounded by artists, two of whom left us portraits of him—Pigalle, the sculptor, a bust, and Quentin La Tour, the pastelist, a portrait. An oil portrait of him by Jacques La Joue hangs in the Musée Carnavalet.

[27]Charles-Louis de Secondat Montesquieu. *De l'Esprit des Loix*. Barillot, Geneva, 1748.

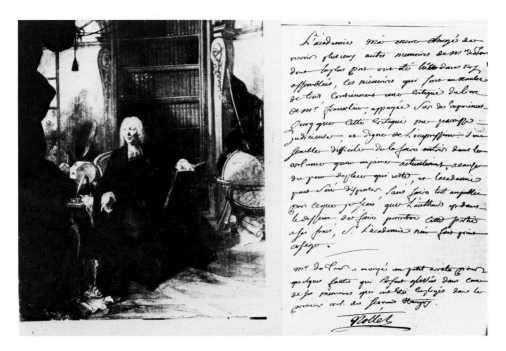

FIG. 81. **Left:** The Abbé Nollet (1700–1770) in his study at La Muette and surrounded by instruments. From the oil painting by Jacques La Joue that hangs in the Musée Carnavalet in Paris. **Right:** Nollet was a prolific writer and many of his manuscripts survive. (Courtesy of the Archives de l'Académie des Sciences, Paris.)

BIBLIOGRAPHY

Stephen Hales (1677–1761)

Selected Writings

Vegetable Staticks: or An Account of some Statical Experiments on the Sap in Vegetables: being an Essay towards a Natural History of Vegetation. Innys and Woodward, London, 1727.

Statical Essays: Containing Haemastaticks: or an Account of some Hydraulick and Hydrostatical Experiments made on the Blood and Blood Vessels of Animals. Innys, Manby and Woodward, London, 1733.

Secondary Sources

Allan, D. G. C., and Schofield, R. E. *Stephen Hales: Scientist and Philanthropist*. Scolar Press, London, 1970.

Clark-Kennedy, A. E. *Stephen Hales, D.D. F. R. S. An Eighteenth Century Biography*. Cambridge University Press, 1929.

Burget, G. E. Stephen Hales. *Ann. Med. Hist.*, 7:109–116 (1925).

Foster, M. *Lectures on the History of Physiology*. Cambridge University Press, 1901.

Stephen Gray (1666?–1736)

Selected Writings

A letter to Cromwell Mortimer, M.D., Sec. R.S. containing several experiments concerning electricity by Mr. Stephen Gray. *Phil. Trans. roy. Soc.*, 37:18–44 (1731).

Two letters from Mr. Stephen Gray, F.R.S. to C. Mortimer, M.D., Sec. R.S. containing further accounts of his experiments concerning electricity. *Phil. Trans. roy. Soc.*, 37:391–404 (1732).

A letter from Mr. Stephen Gray, F.R.S. to Dr. Mortimer, Sec. R.S. containing some experiments relating to electricity. *Phil. Trans. roy. Soc.*, 39:401–403 (1735).

Secondary Sources

Cohen, I. B. Neglected sources for the life of Stephen Gray. *Isis*, 45:41–50 (1954).

Corrigan, J. F. Stephen Gray: an early electrical experimenter. *Science Progress*, 19:102–114 (1934).

DuFay, C. A letter from Mons. du Fay, F.R.S. and of the Royal Academy of Sciences at Paris to his Grace Charles Duke of Richmond and Lenox concerning electricity. *Phil. Trans. roy. Soc.*, 37:258–265 (1732).

Hackman, W. D. *Electricity from Glass.* Sijthoff and Noordhoff, Alphen, 1978.

Walker, W. C. On the detection and evaluation of electrical charges in the eighteenth century. *Am. Sci.*, 1:66–100 (1936).

Jean-Antoine Nollet (1700–1770)

Selected Writings

Leçons de Physique Expérimentale, 6 vols. Guerin, Paris, 1743–64.

Conjectures sur l'électricité des corps. *Memoires de l'Académie des Sciences*, 44:107 (1745).

Essai sur l'Electricité des Corps. Guerin, Paris, 1746.

Expériences de l'électricité appliquée à des paralytiques. *Mémoires de l'Académie des Sciences*, 11:28 (1749).

Lettres sur l'Electricité, Part I, 1753. Part II, 1760. Guerin, Paris.

Secondary Sources

Levy, E. *Le Cabinet de Physique des Enfants de France.* Didot, Mesnil, 1937.

Torlais, J. *L'Abbé Nollet.* Sipuco, Paris, 1954.

Quegnon, H. *L'Abbé Nollet Physicien.* Paris, 1925.

Petrus van Musschenbroek (1692–1761) and Jean-Antoine Nollet (1700–1770)

Secondary Sources

Dorsman, C., and Grommelin, C. A. The invention of the Leyden jar. *Janus*, 46:275–280 (1957).

Heilbron, J. L. A propos de l'invention de bouteille de Leyde. *Rev. Hist. des Sciences*, 19:135–142 (1966).

Hackmann, W. D. *Electricity from Glass.* Sijthoff and Noordhoff, Alphen, 1978.

Roller, D., and Roller, D. H. D. *The Development of the Concept of Electric Charge*. Harvard University Press, 1954.

Swezey, K. M. Nikola Tesla. *Science*, 127:1147–1159 (1958).

Torlais, J. *L'Abbé Nollet. Un Physicien au Siècle des Lumieres*. Sipuco, Paris, 1954.

Suggested Readings for Electrotherapy

Bartelon, P. *L'Électricité du Corps Humain dans l'Etat de Sante et de Malade*, 2 vols. Croulebois, Paris, 1784.

Boissier de la Croix de Sauvages, F. *Mémoires Historiques sur les Effets de l'Electricité dans la Cure des Rhumatisms Sciatiques et autres Douleurs*. Martee, Montpellier, 1752.

Dulieu, L. Les debuts de l'electrologie médicale a Montpellier. *Montpeliensis Hippocrates*, 42:21–30 (1968).

Jallabert, J. *Experiences sur l'Électricité avec Quelques Conjectures sur la Cause de ses Effets*. Barrillot, Geneva, 1748.

Mangin, L'Abbe de. *Histoire Generale et Particuliere de l'Électricité ou ce qu'on dit de Curieux et d'Amusant quelques Physiciens de l'Europe*, 3 vols. Rollin, Paris, 1752.

Nollet, J.-A. *Recherches sur les Causes Particulières des Phénomènes Électriques*. Guerin, Paris, 1749.

CHAPTER XIV

Attempts at Electrotherapy

A more serious presentation which he called "électricité foudroyante" was presented by Nollet to the Académie des Sciences in 1746, under the title *Quelques nouveaux phénomènes d'électricité*. In this communication the Abbé suggested that the movements of the body evoked by electricity might be utilized in the treatment of paralytics. Nollet with the help of two physicians attempted the electrification of two paralyzed patients. One reported feeling tingling in his arms, a sensation he had not had for years. Nollet then tried to resuscitate a dead bird. On failing, he did an autopsy and found petechial hemorrhages.

Nevertheless, the idea that electrification might have therapeutic value caught on and swept across Europe, giving rise not only to serious studies but to many preposterous claims as the method fell into the hands of quacks. The Abbé himself brought out a volume called *Essai sur l'Electricité des Corps* in which he described in detail his method for producing and applying frictional electricity. He explored the influence of electricity not only in animals, but in plants.

The nervous ailments that Nollet attempted to cure with his electrification were commonly ascribed, by the physicians of the day, to a slowing down of animal spirits in the nerve canals or to an engorgement of these canals. Nollet, in his laboratory, tested the effect of electrification on the flow of liquids in capillary tubes, and convinced himself that it was accelerated. This was, in fact, not an original observation. A German physician, Boze, had previously made similar experiments with the same results.

But it was not plain sailing for those who espoused electrotherapy. A member of the Académie des Sciences, Antoine Louis, was the first to attack. He had failed to alleviate the paralysis of the patients on whom he had used electrotherapy and he stated that "not only had it not succeeded, but it was clear as day from all that was known of animal physiology, of disease and of the powers of electricity, that far from being a cure it only hurt the poor patients who had agreed to submit to these tests."[1]

But the possibilities of electrotherapy remained a burning question. Little or no differentiation was made by the physicians of the time between the various causes of paralysis of a limb. Consequently many brilliant "cures" were reported as well as many failures. In addition, the details of the technique varied among the practitioners. Nollet's procedure was to have the patient, completely naked, placed in a kind of swing, insulated from earth by being suspended from the ceiling with silk ropes. Nollet's feet rested on a block of resin. Electricity was transmitted to the patient from a frictional machine through an iron wire wrapped around his body. From time to time sparks were drawn off from the paralyzed limb by bringing a bar of iron close to it. The derivation of this procedure from Stephen Gray's famous experiment is obvious. This treatment was followed up with 5 or 6 electric shocks from a Leyden jar in a manner similar to that used by Musschenbroek.

Not surprisingly, it was impossible to reinstate voluntary movement in the case of paralysis caused by head wounds, and involuntary movements depended on what part was stimulated, or, as we would say now, on the motor point. Nollet reached some wise conclusions as a result of his foray into the field of electrotherapy. He said, "I have electrified some soldiers whose paralysis resulted from wounds. This is perhaps a cause that renders the paralysis incurable and my efforts useless...posterity, better informed, will perhaps laugh at our attempts, but she can hardly blame the motive that led us to explore the possibilities of electricity."

Where most experimenters had focused their attention on the startling sensation produced by electric shock, one of the first to note the contraction of muscle was Krüger, one of Stahl's successors at the University of Halle. Johann Gottlieb Krüger, in 1742, wrote the thesis for his medical degree on "sensation" but he had already begun to experiment with electricity and had noted that a movement, "Bewegung," necessarily followed the sensation.[2] He did not question involvement of the nerve, but his observation led to the enormous wave of excitement for the use of electricity in cases of muscular paralysis. His own pupil, Kratzenstein, was prominent among those making claims for electrotherapy.[3]

Using frictional electricity and noting from experiments on himself that electrification of his body caused him to sweat, Kratzenstein advanced the hypothesis that the loss of salt containing fluid could have beneficial medicinal effects. No doubt this proposal stemmed from the concept that bloodletting had therapeutic value.

He based his claims on two cases in which there was restoration of movement in contracted fingers. He also noted the induction of sound sleep, the forerunner of that observed in electrosleep. As the news spread around Europe, attempts at cures were made in many centers, at first mostly in cases of paralysis. The fact that contraction of a muscle could be obtained at the moment of direct stimulation was not considered a cure. The role of innervation was not yet understood.

The rare cases of success anteceded the understanding of hysterical paralysis and encouraged the establishment of many centers for the treatment of paralytic conditions. Among the most famous was the school of Montpellier under the leadership of Boissier de la Croix

[1]Read Nollet's letter to Royal Society, 1746. Translated by Staek.

[2]J. G. Krüger. *Zuschrifft an seine Zuhörer, Worinnen er ihnen seine Gedancken von der Electricität mittheilet und ihnen Zugleich seine künftige Lectionen bekannt macht*. Hemmerde, Halle, 1744.

[3]C. G. Kratzenstein. *Abhandlung dem Nutzen der Electricität in der Arzneywissenshaft*. Hemmerde, Halle, 1744.

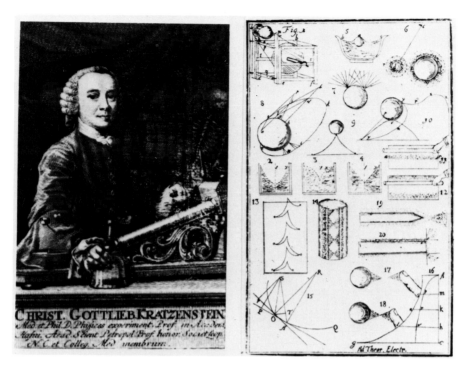

FIG. 82. **Left:** Christian Gottlieb Kratzenstein (1723–1795), pupil of Krüger at Halle and enthusiastic experimenter in electrifying the human body, both in health and disease. **Right:** Illustration from Kratzenstein's *Theoria Electricitatis* (Hemmerde, Halle, 1746) in which he defended his teacher's theory that electricity was a whirl of air caused by the discharge.

de Sauvages. One of de Sauvages' pupils, Deshais, published a thesis entitled *De Hemiplegia per Electricitatem Curanda*. It showed his recognition of the role of the nerve supply, though it was still versed in Galenist terms. Deshais wrote, "paralysis is caused by the arrest of nervous fluid destined to circulate in the brain because it meets an insuperable resistance in the nerve fibers. Thus we must increase the pressure of the nervous fluid when hemiplegia resists ordinary remedies."[4] He added that hemiplegia could be cured or, at any rate, improved by electrification.

Electricity and its effects on the human body were favorite subjects for theses. In the collection of unpublished manuscripts (1750–1760) by Jacques de Romas that is preserved in the City Archives of Bordeaux, there is one on electricity that includes observations on electrification of two paralytic patients. Another example is found in the thesis collection at the University of Montpellier, written in 1750, by Jean Thecla DuFay. He restricted his topic to the electrical nature of the nervous fluid and did not discuss therapy. His thesis did, however, give a useful review of the experiments and knowledge of his time. He concluded his account boldly: "Ergo Fluidum nerveum est Fluidum electricum."[5] Montpellier was a center for studies in electricity. It was there that Boissier de Sauvages endowed a convent hospital solely for electrical therapy (1740–1760). In 1748 de Sauvages received a prize

[4]Jean-Etienne Deshais. *De Hemiplegia per Electricitatem Curanda*. Martel, Montpellier, 1749.

[5]Jean Thecla Felicitas DuFay. *Ad Fluidium Nervum est Fluidam Electricitum*. Martel, Montpellier, 1750.

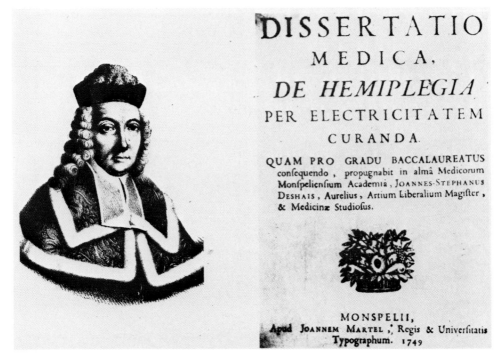

FIG. 83.   Left: François Boissier de la Croix de Sauvages (1706–1767) wearing the distinctive formal costume of a professor at the University of Montpellier. A great believer in electrotherapy, he founded a convent hospital solely for this type of treatment.   **Right:** Thesis by one of his pupils, J. C. Deshais, boldly claiming the cure of hemiplegia by electricity. (By courtesy of the University of Montpellier.)

from the Académie Royale des Sciences at Toulouse for a dissertation on hydrophobia, which was published in 1758.[6]

In this, in what he termed a "Digression sur l'électricité," he championed the existence of animal electricity and evolved a bizarre hypothesis about nerve and muscle activity in hydrophobia: Given that muscular movement was proportional to the force of the nervous fluid, the venom of rabies, on mixing with it, doubled the velocity and the density of the nervous fluid—hence the nerve force and the resultant muscular movement were eight times stronger than normal. By this tortuous reasoning, de Sauvages explained the violent muscular spasma in hydrophobia.

Academies were generous with prizes for discoveries of medical uses of electricity, which no doubt accounts in part for the plethora of such theses. Another prizewinner was Jean Paul Marat who met a violent death in the French Revolution. His essay won a prize from the Paris Academy but drew the rebuke that his criticisms of other workers were too forcefully expressed.[7] Many absurd claims for electrotherapy were made by physicians, which caused much subsequent quackery. A contemporary critic ridiculed many of these claims, but anonymously. However, his gay and witty style betrayed his identity to Nollet as that of

[6]François Boissier de la Croix de Sauvages (1706–1767). *Dissertation sur la Nature et Cause de la Rage.* Forest, Toulouse, 1758.

[7]Jean Paul Marat (1744–1793). *Mémoire sur l'Electricité Médicale.* Meguignon. Paris, 1784.

another gentleman of the Church, the Abbé Mangin.[8] Nollet, who had gathered acclaim through his use of electrotherapy and who had also done his bit to expose the quacks, scolded Mangin. A more efficient source of electricity came to the aid of electrotherapists. A natural one had been used for some years, namely, the shock delivered by the marine torpedo. When applied to the soles of the feet, it was said to relieve the pain of gout. One of the many to espouse the new electrifying technique was the Abbé Bertholon. He traveled widely in Europe, bringing back reports of strange cures and diseases that others could not replicate.[9] He was not alone in the variety of claims he made, for this form of "therapy" had spread widely through Europe. So diverse were the diseases for which cures were being claimed that academies in several countries offered prizes to those who could clarify which diseases were cured solely by electrotherapy. "Quelles sont les maladies que dependent de la plus ou moins de grande quantité de fluid électrique dans le corps humain, et quels sont les moyens de remedier aux unes et aux autres?" This was a spur to many, including Bertholon who, in his two volumes on the electricity of the human body, claimed to examine his cases as to whether electrification was the only ameliorator of the patient's condition or when used in conjunction with other therapies. A great believer in a "latent electricity" within the body, he held that it was manipulation of this inherent electricity that formed the basis of the cures he had noted. This concept was a reworking of "animal spirits." In no way did he foresee the intrinsic electricity of nerve and muscle found (but little understood) by Galvani.

At the turn of the century, books on the history of medical electricity began to appear, for example, Vivenzio's.[10] The early ventures in applying electricity to patients were gradually analyzed and achieved a rational basis, with the elucidation of the relationships between nerve, muscle, spinal cord, and brain. One method, however, for which great claims were made as a treatment has not, even today, reached the first stage of scientific rationale. This is electroconvulsive shock.

These early claims for electrotherapy spawned a rush of publications from all over Europe, many making the most extravagant of claims. As a consequence, controversy broke out as more and more claims could not be confirmed—the one hold-out being the relief of stiffness of rheumatic fingers, the original findings of Kratzenstein. In an era when paralysis due to failure of the nerve supply was not understood, the fact that muscles contracted if the electrical stimulation were applied directly to them lay behind all claims for cures, even to the claim for reanimation of the dead. Some of the most bizarre experiments were made by Galvani's nephew, Aldini.

Therapeutic claims were made by a surprising number of men whose fame lies in other fields: John Wesley, the founder of Methodism, Marat, the activist in the French Revolution, and Oliver Goldsmith, the Irish poet, all made claims. But the main center for electrotherapy was in Montpellier under the leadership of Boissier de Sauvages. The Faculty of Medicine in Montpellier is the oldest in France with statutes dating from 1220. The Faculty of Medicine in Paris followed in 1253 with its formal statutes drawn up in 1274. By the time the Revolution closed all universities in 1792 there were seventeen Faculties of Medicine throughout France.

Many early experimenters, Fontana and Caldani, for example, had noted the convulsions of their frogs when electricity was applied to their brains. ("Si enim conductores non dissectae

[8]l'Abbé de Mangin (died 1772). *Histoire Générale et Particulière de l'Electricité ou ce qu'on dit de Curieux et d'Amusant Quelques Physiciens de l'Europe*, 3 vols. Rollin, Paris, 1752.

[9]Nicole, Bertholon (1742–1800). *De l'Electricité du Corps Humain dans l'Etat de Santé et de Malade*, 2 vols. Croubois, Paris, 1780.

[10]G. Vivenzio. *Istoria dell'Elettricita Medica*. Naples, 1784.

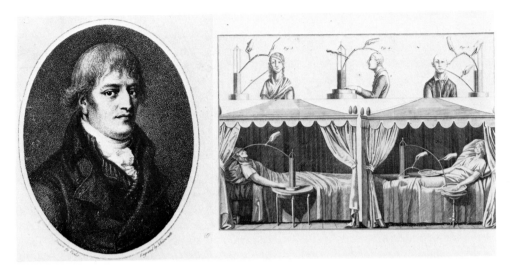

FIG. 84. **Left:** Giovanni Aldini (1762–1834), nephew of Galvani and proponent of electrotherapy. **Right:** Aldini's experiments with electroshock therapy in man. **Above:** Mental patients with the electrodes in various positions connecting to voltaic piles for stimulation. **Below:** Two recently dead patients connected directly, or by saline baths, to voltaic piles. (From: G. Aldini. *Essai Théorique et Expérimental sur Galvanisme.* Fournier, Paris, 1804.)

spinale medullae, aut nervis, ut consuevimus, sed vel cerebro-contractiones vel nullae, vel admodum exiguae sunt.") In the early 19th century, Galvani's nephew Aldini experimented with electroshock in man. Impressed with the muscular contractions he had obtained on stimulating animals and cadavers, he stood close to the guillotine to receive heads of criminals in as fresh a condition as possible. He found that passing a current, through the ear and mouth, or through the exposed brain and mouth, evoked facial grimaces. The fresher the head the more remarkable the grimace. He then applied electrical stimulation from a voltaic pile to the living. His concept was that the contractions were excited by "le développement d'un fluide dans la machine animale" which was conveyed by the nerves to the muscles.[11] We recognize here the explanation popularized by Bertholon.[12]

One of his early experimental techniques reaches into the twentieth century, for Aldini applied his galvanism to the mentally ill. Having experimented on himself with electrodes in both ears, or in one ear and his mouth, or on forehead and nose, he experienced a strong reaction, followed by prolonged insomnia lasting several days. He found the experience very disagreeable but thought the changes it produced in the brain might be salutary in psychoses. Passing the current between the ears produced violent convulsions and pain, but he claimed good results in patients suffering from melancholia.

Attempts to cure paralyzed patients had also been made in Russia where Daniel Bernouilli of the Swiss family of mathematicians had joined the St. Petersburg Academy of Sciences in 1726. As Professor of Physiology, he became interested in muscular movement and published a paper in Latin.[13] On changing to an appointment in mathematics, Bernouilli

[11]Giovanni Aldini. *Essai Théorique et Expérimental sur Galvanisme*, 2 vols. Fournier, Paris, 1804.

[12]Nicole Berthelon (1742–1800). *De l'Electricité du Corps Humain dans l'Etat de Santé et de Malade*, 2 vols. Croubois, Paris, 1780.

[13]Daniel Bernouilli (1700–1782). *Testamenta Nova de Motu Musculorum.* Commentaries of the St. Petersburg Academy of Sciences, pp. 57–62 (1728).

began to explore electricity and attempted to resuscitate drowned birds, and it was a pupil of his, Ilya Gruzinov, who later, on becoming Professor of Physiology at Moscow University, published in 1804 a dissertation, "On Galvanism and Its Application to Medical Practice."[14]

SELECTED WRITINGS ON ELECTROTHERAPY

Berthelon, P. *L'Électricité du Corps Humain dans l'État de Santé et de Malade*, 2 vols. Croubois, Paris, 1784.

Boissier de la Croix de Sauvages, F. *Mémoires Historiques sur les Effets de l'Électricité dans la Cure des Rhumatismes, Sciatiques et autres Douleurs*. Martel, Montpellier, 1752.

Dulieu, L. Les débuts de l'électrologie médicale à Montpellier. *Montpeliensis Hippocrates*, 42:21–30 (1968).

Jallabert, J. *Expériences sur l'Électricité avec Quelques Conjectures sur la Cause de ses Effets*. Barrillot, Geneva, 1748.

[14]Kh. S. Koshtoyants. *Essays on the History of Physiology in Russia*. Acad. Sci. USSR, Leningrad, 1946. (English translation. Amer. Inst. Biol. Sci., Washington, DC, 1964.)

Chapter XV

18th Century Research on Emission of Electricity by Biological Species. The Electric Fish

Before it could be determined how electricity was involved with the nervous system of the animal, evidence that nervous discharge was indeed electrical had to be established. Of the several known species of electric fish there were five principal ones: (1) The *Malopterurus*, or Nile catfish, named by Lacépède, drawings of which appear on Egyptian tombs and many Greek vases.[1] This fish was used by Du Bois Reymond in his research in the 19th century.[2] (2) The *Gymnotus*, electric eel or Anguille tremblante, described by Philippe Fermin in this account of the animals he found on his visit, in 1765, to the Dutch colony of Surinam.[3] He confirmed the observations on electric fish of several earlier travelers in the Dutch colonies of South America. So many had experienced the shock of this "anguille grosse comme la jambe" that two reports were published in 1758 by the journal of the Society of Haarlem.[4] In these it was suggested that the shock was indeed electrical in nature and not just an extremely rapid muscular grip. (3) The electric ray or *Raja*. (4) The *Mormyrus*

---

[1]B-G. de L. Lacépède (1756–1825). *Essai sur l'électricité naturelle et artificielle*, 2 vols. Didot, Paris, 1781.

[2]Emil Du Bois Reymond (1818–1896). Observations and experiments on Malopterurus brought to Berlin alive. *Gesammelte Abhandlungen zur allgemeinen Muskel—und Nerven-physic*, Vol. 2. (Translated into English. Edited by J. Burdon Sanderson. Oxford, 1887. pp. 369–540.)

[3]Philippe Fermin. *Histoire naturelle de la Holland équinoxiale ou description des animaux dans la colonie de Surinam*. Magerius, Amsterdam, 1765.

[4]*Verhandelingen witgegeeven door te Hollandsche Maatschappe der Wetenschappen te Haarlem*, 2:374–377 and 4:87–95 (1758).

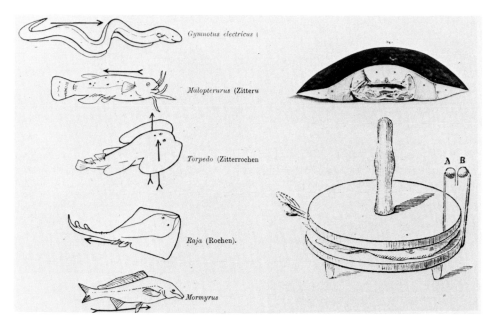

FIG. 85. **Left:** Five kinds of electric fish, the first form of biological electricity to receive attention. **Right:** *Above:* John Hunter's dissection of the marine torpedo showing on the left a nerve trunk. [*Phil. Trans. roy. Soc.*, 63:481–489 (1774)]. This specimen is preserved in the Hunterian Museum. *Below:* Matteucci's experiment, the first to succeed in evoking a spark by the discharge of the fish as evidence of its electrical nature. (*Leçons sur les Phénomènes Physiques des Corps Vivants.* Masson, Paris, 1847.)

or common skate which puzzled Du Bois Reymond half a century later. Though its structure seemed similar to that of the Malopterurus, it failed in his hands to deliver a shock. (5) The marine *Torpedo*, more fully experimented on than any other species.

References to the torpedo are found in the works of all early writers, including Aristotle, Pliny,[5] and Plutarch.[6] The torpedo's power to shock was known to fishermen. Many described its pain and numbing effect, but for centuries no one provided an explanation until Averroes, a 12th century physician, suggested that the effect was like that exerted by a lodestone.[7]

That the phenomenon might be a purely muscular one had occurred to many. Lorenzini (for whom biologists later named the sensory ampullae of the torpedo) was an early observer who concluded that certain muscle fibers in fish were active in the discharge.[8] The physicist Réaumur also was impressed by the muscular structure and deemed this responsible for the numbing effect.

René-Antoine Ferchault de Réaumur was born in 1683 in La Rochelle, where the Atlantic waters were favored for torpedo fishing. During his long career in metallurgy and instru-

[5]Pliny (23–79 A.D.). One of the oldest books in the Natural History Museum in London is a copy of his *Libros Naturalis Historiae*, printed in Venice in 1469. This work has 35 books and in the 32nd is his description of the torpedo and his acknowledgment that the fish had a certain power to shock which he said must be an odor or an emanation from the body.

[6]Plutarch. *On the Instincts of Animals.* Venice, 1469.

[7]Ibn Rushd [Averroes] (1126–1198). Coliget. Tract V, Leaf 10. Bonacosa, Padua, 1255. Arabic manuscripts in Yale University Library.

[8]S. Lorenzini. *Osservazioni interne alle Torpedini.* Florence, 1678.

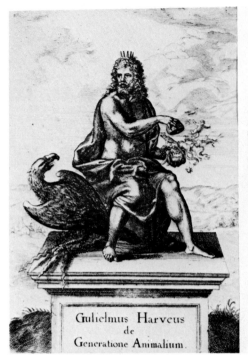
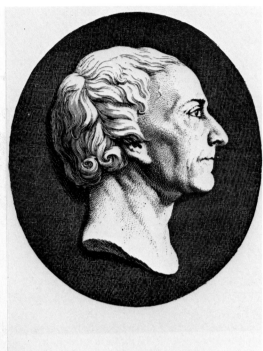

FIG. 86.   Left: The title page to William Harvey's *De generatione animalium* (1651) illustrating his belief that the whole organism is preformed in the egg.   **Right:** Abraham Trembley (1700–1784) whose experiments demonstrating that cut pieces of polyps could regenerate upset all the previous concepts of the generation of animal life. (Portrait by Tardieu.)

mentation, Réaumur was also deeply interested in natural history. He wrote a six-volume work on insects, which included polyps and crustaceans, and a discussion of the conflict between the theories of epigenesis versus preformation.[9]

In the 16th century, William Harvey had written that all parts of the fetus including our brain and nervous system were potentially in the egg. His treatise *On the Generation of Animals* portrayed this idea. In the case of minute organisms, whose ova were invisible, he accepted spontaneous generation. This, he believed, was caused by the Deity, "he takes the right and pious view of the matter who derives all generation from the same eternal and omnipotent Deity, on whose nod the universe itself depends. . . ."[10] Leeuwenhoek had been critical of Harvey and his concept of spontaneous generation. Based on his own discovery of spermatozoa he claimed, "It is exclusively the male semen that forms the fetus, and that all that the woman may contribute only serves to receive the semen and feed it."[11]

In pre-Lamarckian France experiments on fermentation and the "spontaneous generation" of worms from putrefaction caused a storm. These experiments, by an Irishman named Turberville Needham, were published first in English, then in French.[12] Abraham Trembley, a British diplomat working in Holland, found that cut pieces of freshwater polyps could

[9]R-A. F. de Réaumur (1683–1757). *Mémoires pour servir à l'histoire des insectes*, 6 vols. Paris, 1734–1742.

[10]William Harvey (1578–1657). *Exercitationes de generatione animalium*. Pulleyn, London, 1651.

[11]A. Leeuwenhoek (1632–1723). *Phil. Trans. roy. Soc.*, 22:552–560 (1700).

[12]J. T. Needham (1713–1781). *Nouvelles observations microscopiques*. Paris, 1750. (English translation 1747.)

regenerate.[13] Nature was given the prime position in formation of the animal world, displacing Descartes' corporeal soul, which was unable to survive such theories. Descartes believed in the mechanical formation of organisms,[14] but the trend in this period was (with Harvey) toward preformation. Réaumur's loose categorization of polyps as insects added to the controversy; he opposed spontaneous generation. In 1714 Réaumur, returning to his birthplace, performed a long series of experiments on the torpedo, and the conditions under which it would deliver a shock.[15] In a long report to the Académie Royale des Sciences, of which he was a member, he opposed those who considered the shock electrical, describing in detail the movement by which the fish curled its back to bring two strong muscles to give an extremely rapid grip to an exploring hand. Réaumur used an illustration of a dissection showing these muscles. He opposed the suspicions of scientists, such as Fontana, who, when considering the agent involved in the discharge of the electric eel, wrote, "If not ordinary electricity, then something at least strongly analogous to it. The electrical eel and ray, if not actually making it probably at least suggest such a possibility."[16] A less convincing explanation had been proposed in the previous century by Van Helmont, who was influenced by studies in alchemy. He suggested that the discharge of the torpedo was a narcotic ejaculation.[17]

Further examination of the electrophysiology of the phenomenon was done by Matteucci and Du Bois Reymond in the following century. Spallanzani and Galvani also examined the influence of the nerves on the power of the animal to discharge.

The Abbé Lazzaro Spallanzani, whose fame rests firmly on his work in regeneration of animal life and on the natural history of echo-locating bats, was also a collector of marine species. In 1769 he became Professor of Natural History at the University of Pavia in Lombardy (a part of the Hapsburg Empire since 1714 when the Treaty of Rastatt ended the long war of the Spanish Succession), and made several expeditions to collect specimens for the museum at Pavia. During a visit to Rimini on the Adriatic and to Marseille on the Mediterranean, he became interested in the electric fish. In his six-volume account of these travels there are some observations on these animals[18] but his many letters, preserved in various archives, provide more detail.[19] He made many dissections of rays and Torpedoes, studying their anatomy in relation to their power to shock. He became convinced that the shock was electrical ("La scossa si e conosciuta patentemente elettrica").[20]

Many observers had located the electric organs, prominent especially in the marine Torpedo, but few had examined the role played by the nervous system. There was still the possibility that magnetism played a role. Spallanzani disproved this by irritating the fish when insulated by a glass plate. He specifically studied the role, not only of the electric organ itself, but of the muscles and nerves involved.[21] He observed the strong muscles that

[13]A. Trembley (1710–1784). *Mémoires pour servir à l'histoire d'un genre polypes d'eau douce.* Verbeek, Leyden, 1744. (English translation by C. Adams, 1746.)

[14]R. Descartes. *Traité de l'Homme et de la Formation du Foetus.* Angot, Paris, 1664.

[15]R-A. F. de Réaumur. Des effets que produit le poisson appellé en français Torpille, ou Tremble, sur ceux qui le touchent; et de la cause dont ils dépendent. *Mémoires de l'Académie Royale des Sciences,* pp. 344–360 (1714).

[16]F. Fontana. *Traité sur le venin de la vipère,* Vol. 2, p. 244. Florence, 1781.

[17]Johann Baptista Helmont (1579–1644). *Ortus Medicinae.* 1648.

[18]L. Spallanzani (1729–1799). *Viaggi alle due Sicilie e in alcune parti dell-Appennino.* Baldassare Comini, Pavia, 1792–1797. (Translated into English: *Travels in the Two Sicilies and some parts of the Appennines,* 4 vols. Robinson, London, 1798.)

[19]Lazzaro Spallanzani. *Epistolario,* 5 vols. Florence, 1958–1964.

[20]Onoranze a Lazzaro Spallanzani. Reggio Emilia, 1929. (Letter dated July 18, 1782 from Chioggia.)

[21]G. Montalenti, & Lazzaro Spallanzani, *I cursori della Natura,* p. 108. Agnelli, Milano, 1928.

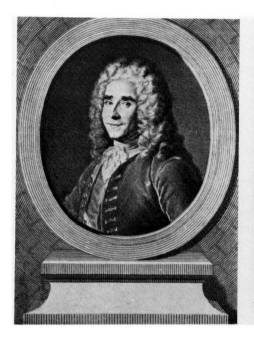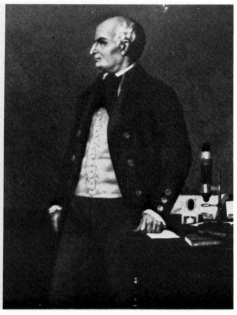

FIG. 87.   Left: René-Antoine Ferchault Réaumur (1683–1757) who was opposed to the suggestion that the numbing effect delivered by the torpedo was electrical in nature, and held that it was caused by a strong muscular grip. (The engraving by Balechon from the original painting by A. S. Belle.) **Right:** The Abbé Lazzaro Spallanzani (1729–1799) who from researches made in his old age concluded that the shock was "obviously" electrical.

had impressed Réaumur but would not accept the suggestion that the attack was mechanical. Among his many correspondents were his friend in Geneva, Charles Bonnet, as well as Caldani, Fontana, Haller, and Galvani.[22] As did everyone at the time, Spallanzani also corresponded with Voltaire.[23]

Spallanzani was supportive of Galvani's views of animal electricity but both men died before a major attack was launched by Volta. Galvani had also contributed to research on the electric fish in the 1780s and 1790s, before the famous *Commentary* was launched. He described his experiments to Spallanzani but did not publish them.[24] However two of his manuscripts on the subject are preserved in the Biblioteca of the Archiginnasio in Bologna.[25]

Galvani went further than other observers of the electric shock from these fish, in his experiments to define the role of the nerves. Other investigators concentrated on the anatomy or the electrical properties but had not designed tests specifically relating the phenomenon to the nervous system. Galvani's work on these fish was done in his later years when, for health reasons, he went to the shores of the Adriatic. He examined both torpedoes and

[22]*Bibliografia delle opere di Lazzaro Spallanzani*. Biblioteca Bibliografica Italica, Florence, 1951.

[23]February 17, 1766: Letter preserved in the Bibliothèque Nationale, Paris. May 31, 1776: Letter preserved in the archives of the Biblioteca municipale in Reggio Emilia.

[24]*Memorie sulla elettricita animale a Lazzaro Spallanzani*, p. 75. 1797. Archives Accad. Sci. Istituto di Bologna.

[25]*Memorie dell'Accademia delle Scienze dell'Istituto di Bologna*, ser. 2, 9:163–176 (1798). Published by S. Gherardi, 1869. Taccuino delle experienze del Galvani sulla Torpedine fatte a Senigaglia ed a Rimini nel 1795. Preserved in the Biblioteca del Archiginnasio, Bologna.

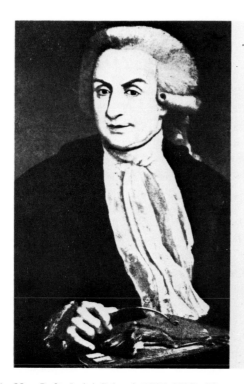

FIG. 88. Left: Luigi Galvani (1737–1798). The contemporary oil painting (probably by Spagnoli) of Galvani that hangs in the University Library of Bologna. Several engravings have been made from this portrait, notably those of Sir Joshua Reynolds' pupil, Marchi. The engravings, however, unfortunately omit the frog. **Right**: Galvani's notes on an experiment he made in 1795 on the marine torpedo. The notes read: "Giorno 16 Maggio, 26. La Rana senza far arco colla superficie della Torpedine fra nervo e muscolo ma toccando coi soli nervi crurali la Torpedina, in qualunque luogo, ma piu col dorso, e o sopra, o in vicinanza de' corpi elettrici cade nelle solite convulsioni a qualunque scossa. . . ." Manuscript preserved in the Biblioteca dell' Archiginnasio di Bologna. (Both photographs are the gift of the late Professor Giulio Pupilli of the University of Bologna.)

rays, and confirmed the French biologist Geoffroy Saint Hillaire's observation that the electric organs in these two species were essentially the same but with their "tubes" differently oriented.[26] Galvani was surprised by the large number of nerves serving the components of the electric organ and he investigated them.[27] He cut the nerve supply to the organs on one side of a torpedo and demonstrated failure of that side to discharge. Severing the head destroyed all discharge which was also independent of the presence of the heart. The mechanism for discharge appeared to be independent of the circulation. With his vast collection of experiments on frog muscle, he was able to compare the contraction evoked by a discharge from a torpedo with that from artificial electrical stimulation. In Figure 88 is a facsimile of Galvani's handwriting on a page of his notes, preserved in the Library of the Archiginnasio di Bologna. Unlike the famous *Commentary* that was prepared for pub-

[26]Etienne Geoffroy Saint-Hillaire (1772–1844). Mémoire sur l'anatomie comparée des organes électriques de la raie, torpille, du gymnote engourdissant, et du silure trembleur. *Ann. Mus. d'Hist. Nat.*, 1:392–407 (1803).

[27]Giovanni Aldini (1762–1834). *Essai théorique et expérimentale sur le galvanisme*, Vol. 2, p. 69. Fournier, Paris, 1804.

lication in Latin, these notes are in Italian. This page records the observation that the frog was convulsed with every discharge from the torpedo when only its crural nerve[28] touched the fish, even though the surface of the torpedo was not making an arc between the nerve and the muscle. Galvani noted that the effect was greatest when the nerve touched the back of the fish and when it was over or close to the electric organ. This animal continued to fascinate biologists in the following century. Many were still uncertain about equating the discharge of the fish with frictional electricity. Even Sir Humphrey Davy, after experimenting on torpedoes, held that the electricity of fishes might be different from ordinary electricity. "I think," he wrote, "it more probable that animal electricity will be found of a distinctive and peculiar kind." He agreed with John Hunter that "The torpedinal organ depends for its powers upon the will of the animal."[29]

Interest was stirred in England by letters written by an English member of Parliament to Benjamin Franklin, in 1772 and 1773. These concerned the reports given to the Academy at La Rochelle, by John Walsh, of his research on torpedoes at La Rochelle and the neighboring Ile de Ré.[30] He described a series of ingenious experiments designed to compare the conditions for discharge by the fish with those of a Leyden jar. As in all early explorations of electricity, one of the tests involved several persons joining hands to become part of the circuit for receiving the shock. But the test, still demanded by many skeptics, of eliciting a spark or deflecting the pith balls of an electrometer, failed. Faraday raised this criticism in his work on Gymnotus half a century later.[31] In none of Walsh's writings did he report success in getting a spark from an electric fish, though later it was claimed that he had demonstrated this with Gymnotus.[32] A discourse on the history and electrical properties of the torpedo, delivered in 1775 to the Royal Society by the eminent Sir John Pringle, mentioned no sparks.[33]

Finally, in the next century, Carlo Matteucci of Pisa demonstrated unequivocally that the discharge could produce a flash and a crackle. In an ingenious experiment, he placed the unfortunate fish (and he said it must be "une torpille très vivace") on an insulated metal plate, while another metal plate held by an insulated handle was lowered over it.[34] Attached to each plate was a wire from which a gold leaf hung. When the fish discharged its shock, the gold leaves moved towards each other and, if separated by exactly the right distance, a spark leaped across the gap.

John Walsh's letters to the *Philosophical Transactions* were followed by drawings of dissections of the torpedo showing the electric organs without a nerve supply. He presumed a "compressed electric fluid" was stored by the fish and emitted with the shock. He noted a movement of the eyes of the fish when discharging, evidence which he thought proved the will of the animal had triggered the discharge.

[28]Electrophysiologists used the term crural nerve presumably by analogy from comparative anatomy, but in the frog it refers to the sciatic nerve.

[29]Humphrey Davy (1778–1829). An account of some experiments on the torpedo. *Phil. Trans. roy. Soc.*, pp. 15–18 (1829).

[30]John Walsh (1725–1795). On the electric property of the torpedo, *Phil. Trans. roy. Soc.*, 63:461–477 (1773).
————Of torpedos found on the coast of England, *Phil. Trans. roy. Soc.*, 64:464–473 (1774).

[31]Michael Faraday (1791–1867). *Experimental Researches in Electricity*, Vol. 1, p. 99. Taylor, London, 1839. (And *Phil. Trans. roy. Soc.*)

[32]John Canton (1718–1772). Canton Manuscripts at the Royal Society. Vol. II.

[33]John Pringle (1707–1782). Discourse on the Torpedo delivered at the Royal Society, November 30, 1774. London, 1775.

[34]Carlo Matteucci (1811–1868). *Leçons sur les Phénomènes Physiques des Corps Vivants*. Masson, Paris, 1857.

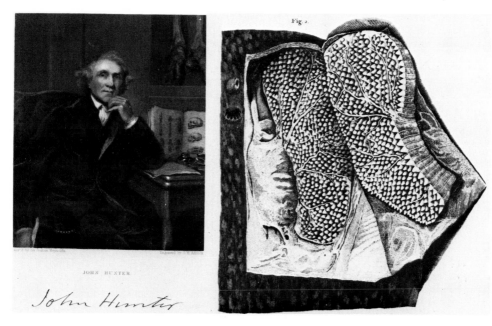

FIG. 89.   Left: John Hunter (1728–1793), surgeon and anatomist. (Portrait by Joshua Reynolds at the Royal College of Surgeons, London.)   **Right:** Hunter's dissection of the electric organs of the torpedo. Branching over the cut surface of these organs are the nerves which Hunter exposed. [From: *Phil. Trans. roy. Soc.*, 63:481–489 (1773).]

Walsh also took his results to a fellow member of the Royal Society, John Hunter. Hunter, a famous anatomist, provided a fine drawing not only of the columns of the electric organ, but of the nerves. These he described as consisting of three large branches on each side which entered into the electric organ. In proportion to its size, Hunter believed the torpedo to be extraordinarily well supplied with nerves. He felt they must be motor since he could conceive of no sensory function for the organs.[35] His conclusion was as follows.[36]

> If it be then probable, that those nerves are not necessary for the purposes of sensation, or action, may we not conclude that they are subservient to the formation, collection, or management of the electric fluid; especially as it appears evident, from Mr. Walsh's experiments, that the will of the animal does absolutely control the electric powers of its body; which must depend on the energy of the nerves.

John Hunter, Scottish born, had followed his brother to London, displaying the same interest in anatomy, which was to be the ruling one all his life, even after becoming a famous surgeon. His older brother, William, had preceded him as an instructor in anatomy, an interest he too followed throughout his life; his lectures and demonstrations in Windmill Street became legendary. John Hunter's special interest in the anatomy of marine animals was sparked by Walsh's description of the torpedo and he went on to dissect and examine another specimen, *Gymnotus Electricus*.[37]

All of Hunter's illustrations of the Torpedo and Gymnotus specimens in his communications to *Philosophical Transactions* have been preserved in spirits of wine at the Hunterian

[35]John Hunter (1728–1793). Anatomical observations on the torpedo. *Phil. Trans. roy. Soc.*, 63:481–488 (1773).

[36]John Hunter. An account of the Gymnotus Electricus. *Phil. Trans. roy. Soc.*, 65:395–407 (1775).

[37]John Hunter. An account of the Gymnotus Electricus. *Phil. Trans. roy. Soc.*, 65:395–407 (1775).

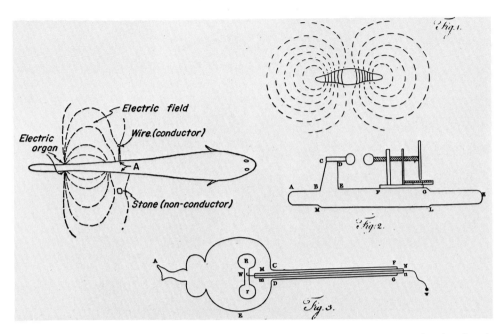

FIG. 90. **Above left:** A modern sketch of the fields of current around gymnotus, the electric eel. (Reproduced by permission from: R. Galambos. *Nerves and Muscles.* Science Study Series 1962.) **Above right:** *(Fig. 1)* Cavendish's sketch of electric fields around a torpedo; *(Fig. 2)* his apparatus to determine gap across which a spark will jump; and *(Fig. 3)* his sketch of the wooden model he made of the torpedo. *R* and *r* are pewter models of the electric organs of the fish. [From: *Phil. Trans. roy. Soc.*, 66:196–225 (1776).]

Museum, with several other unpublished drawings. Students of the nervous system regret his not printing an exceptionally fine drawing of a dissection of a torpedo with a large nerve trunk branching into the equivalent of the 7th, 9th, and 10th cranial nerves innervating the electric organ. In all but Malopterurus, in which the nerves invade glandular tissue, the terminus is a neuromuscular junction, the columns of the organ being pentagonal or hexagonal.

At the same time, an eccentric Englishman, Henry Cavendish, was making experiments in his home that convinced him that the variations in force of shock released by electric fish were understandable in terms of electric fields. The differences in severity of shock observed depended on the fish being in air or water, and on the distance from contact.

Henry Cavendish was an amateur scientist, born in 1731 a nobleman and of independent means; he set up a laboratory in his own home. In this laboratory he tested his theories on the electric fish. He made a model of the torpedo out of wood and on each surface inserted glass tubes into grooves cut in the wood (Figure 90). Through these tubes he inserted wires leading to "pieces of pewter" cut in the shape of the torpedo's electric organs; the whole model was covered with sheep skin. With the protruding wires, he charged the model "electric organs" by connecting them to batteries of varying strength as measured by an electrometer. The latter consisted of two gilded straws, 10 inches long, with cork balls on their ends. "The way," he said, "by which I estimated the divergence of these balls, was by feeling whether they appeared to coincide with parallel lines placed behind them at about ten inches distance." He looked for the critical strength of current and distance between the balls that would result in the spark that biologists had been unable to evoke from the fish. (He was working 50 years before Matteucci's successful demonstration.)

Later he changed his model to one made entirely of leather which he could soak in salt water to mimic the wet environment of the fish's tissues. He explained his results by plotting the fields of current, demonstrating that the nearer to the "fish" one placed one's hand, the stronger the shock. He concluded that there must indeed be a powerful "battery" in the fish and, though unable to satisfactorily account for the absence of the spark, he concluded that "on the whole, I think, there seems nothing in the phenomena of the torpedo at all incompatible with electricity" and that "the circumstance of their not having perceived any light is by no means repugnant to the supposition that the shock is produced by electricity." Henry Cavendish was introduced by his father, Lord Charles Cavendish, to the Royal Society, of which he was later made a Fellow. His unusual experiments are found in the Society's transactions.[38]

Interest in the electric fish persisted long into the next century for here indeed was an animal that could produce electricity. But two basic questions remained unsolved. Was this animal electricity to be equated with the electricity known to the physicists? Was it produced in the electric organs themselves, or did the trigger come from the brain and via the nerves? On the first question, even Faraday was ambivalent saying:[39]

> . . . though I am not yet convinced by the facts that the nervous fluid is only electricity, still I think that the agent in the nervous system may be an inorganic force, and if there be reasons for supposing that magnetism is a higher relation of force than electricity, so it may be well imagined that the nervous power may be of a still more exalted character, and yet within the reach of experiment.

Eighteenth century experimenters were unable to answer the second question, i.e., whether electricity came down the nerves to the electric organs, because they had no instrumentation that could detect the passage of small currents. As late as 1839, the Lecturer on Comparative Anatomy at the London Hospital, Henry Letherby, perceived the reason for this failure to detect electric current to be that "the brain and spinal cord are the seat of power." He went on to say "indeed, we can scarcely expect with our present means to be able to detect a current of such low tension as must be that of the nervous force."[40]

In the 19th century adequate instrumentation was invented and the electrical nature of nervous propagation was established by Emil Du Bois Reymond. But any understanding of how these strangely structured electric organs in the fish produced their electricity lay far in the future. Twentieth century understanding of membrane potentials shows that the myriad columns, depicted so clearly by Hunter, represent layers of nerve and muscle junctions which, on receipt of a nerve impulse with the consequent release of acetylcholine, discharge to produce a brief but powerful flow of current.

---

[38]Henry Cavendish (1731–1810). An account of some attempts to imitate the effects of the Torpedo by electricity. *Phil. Trans. roy. Soc.*, 66:196–225 (1776).

[39]Michael Faraday (1791–1867). Experimental researches in electricity. Fifteenth series. Notice of the character and direction of the electric force of Gymnotus. *Phil. Trans. roy. Soc.*, pp. 1–12 (1839).

[40]Henry Letheby (1816–1876). An account of the dissection of a Gymnotus Electricus—together with reasons for believing that it derives its electricity from the brain and spinal cord; and that the Electrical Forces are identical. *Proceedings of the London Electrical Society*, pp. 367–385 (1839).

SELECTED WRITINGS ON ELECTRIC FISH

Camerson Walker, W. Animal electricity before Galvani. *Ann. Sci.*, 2:84–113 (1937).

Cavendish, Henry (1731–1810). An attempt to explain some of the principal phenomena of electricity by means of an elastic fluid. *Phil. Trans. roy. Soc.*, 61:584–667 (1771).

Fritsch, G. T. (1838–1927). *Die elektrische Fische. I. Malopterurus.* 1887. *II. Torpede.* Leipzig, 1890.

Garten, S. In: *Winterstein's Handbuch d. verg. Physiol.*, Vol. 3, Part 2, pp. 106–224. Jena, 1910.

Geoffroy Saint-Hillaire, E. (1772–1844). Mémoire sur l'anatomie comparée des organes électriques de la raie torpille, du gymnote engourdissant, et du silure trembleur. *Ann. Mus. d'Hist. Nat.*, 1:392–407 (1803).

Humboldt, F. H. A. von (1769–1859). *Versuche über die electrischen Fische.* Erfurt, 1806.

Hunter, John (1728–1793). Anatomical observations on the Torpedo. *Phil. Trans. roy. Soc.*, 63:481–488 (1773).

Hunter, J. An account of the Gymnotus Electricus. *Phil. Trans. roy. Soc.*, 65:395–407 (1775).

Ibn Rushd [Averroes] (1125–1198). *Coliget*, Tract V, Leaf 10. Bonacosa, Padua, 1255. Arabic manuscripts in Yale University Library.

Kellaway, Peter. The part played by electric fish in the early history of bioelectricity and electrotherapy. *Bull. Hist. Med.*, 20:112–137 (1946).

Lacépède, B-G. le Compte de la Cépède (1756–1825). *Essai sur l'Électricité Naturelle et Artificielle*, 2 vols. Imprimerie de Monsieur, Paris, 1781.

Matteucci, Carlo (1811–1868). *Leçons sur les Phénomènes Physiques des Corps Vivants.* Masson, Paris, 1847.

Pliny (23–79 A.D.). *Libros Naturalis Historiae.* 35 books. Printed at Venice in 1469. (Translated into English. 6 vols. Bell, London 1855–1890.)

Pringle, J. (1707–1782). *Discourse on the torpedo.* (Privately printed, 1774.)

Pringle, J. Experiments on the Torpedo. *Phil. Trans. roy. Soc.*, 65:1–4 (1775).

Sirol, M. *Galvani et Galvanisme: l'Électricité Animale.* Vigot Frères, Paris.

Walsh, John (1725–1795). On the electric property of the torpedo. *Phil. Trans. roy. Soc.*, 63:461–477 (1773).

Walsh, J. Of Torpedos found on the coast of England. *Phil. Trans. roy. Soc.*, 64:464–473 (1774).

CHAPTER XVI

Animal Electricity Vindicated.
Galvani's Commentary

Luigi Galvani (1737–1798)

In the last decade of the 18th century one in the series of *Commentaries* that the Institute of Sciences in Bologna was publishing concerned work that had long-lasting influence on the fields of physics and physiology. This was a treatise, written in Latin by a professor at the University of Bologna, on the effects of electricity on muscular motion *(De Viribus Electricitatis in Motu Musculari: Commentarius)*. In this work, published locally in 1791, Galvani brought together his research on the mechanics of muscle contraction, experiments he had made over a period of ten years, and which he had recorded meticulously. Some of these had been reported to the Accademia but none were published in his lifetime. They were, however, preserved in the Archives of the Accademia delle Scienze which had merged with the Istituto in Bologna. Eventually these reports and his laboratory notes were published on the 200th anniversary of his birth.[1]

Luigi Galvani, a Bolognese by birth, spent his whole life there, taking degrees in medicine and philosophy at the age of 22. He was a life-long teacher at the Istituto delle Scienze and the University which, in his day, was housed in the beautiful Archiginnasio. There he taught anatomy, the subject of his first publications, many of which were on the structure of birds and focused on their kidneys and auditory systems. For his experiments with electricity, his chosen subject was the frog in which he had already examined the heart, and came close

[1]*Memorie ed Esperimenti Inediti di Luigi Galvani*, edited by Licinio Capelli. Bologna, 1937.

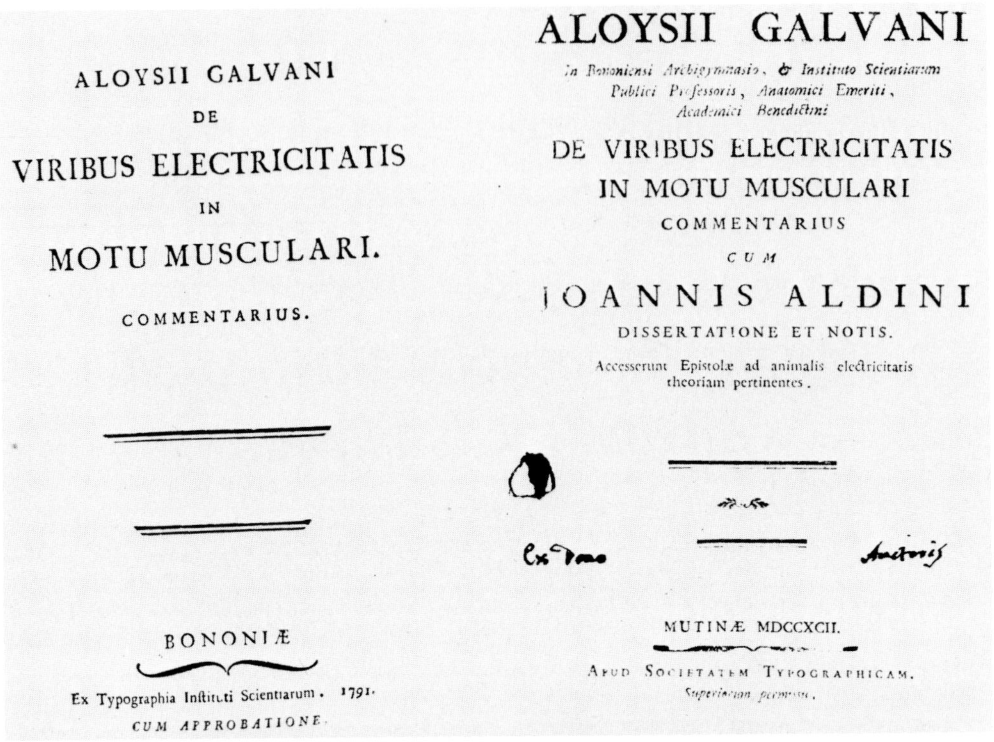

ALOYSII GALVANI

DE

VIRIBUS ELECTRICITATIS

IN

MOTU MUSCULARI.

COMMENTARIUS.

BONONIÆ

Ex Typographia Inftituti Scientiarum . 1791.

CUM APPROBATIONE.

ALOYSII GALVANI

In Bononiensi Archigymnasio , & Instituto Scientiarum Publici Professoris , Anatomici Emeriti , Academici Benedictini

DE VIRIBUS ELECTRICITATIS

IN MOTU MUSCULARI

COMMENTARIUS

C U M

IOANNIS ALDINI

DISSERTATIONE ET NOTIS.

Accesserunt Epistolæ ad animalis electricitatis theoriam pertinentes .

MUTINÆ MDCCXCII.

APUD SOCIETATEM TYPOGRAPHICAM.
Superiorum permissu .

FIG. 91. **Left:** Title page of the first reprint of the 1791 (Bologna) edition of Galvani's commentary. **Right:** Title page of the 1792 (Modena) edition inscribed "ex dono auctoris." This copy is in the Sylvanus R. Thompson Library at the Institution of Electrical Engineers, and in the folder in which it is preserved Sylvanus Thompson has entered a note that this is the copy Volta received from Galvani and that this is Volta's handwriting. (Photographs reproduced by courtesy of the Institution of Electrical Engineers, London.)

to discovering vagal inhibition by showing that localized puncture of the spinal cord could cause the heartbeat to stop.[2]

Galvani, in turning to muscle excitability, entered a field that was already being explored rather fitfully in his country even 30 years earlier. The Abbé Beccaria,[3] a physicist, correspondent of Franklin, and professor at the University of Turin, turned his interest briefly from his study of atmospheric electricity to demonstrating the contraction evoked by direct electrical stimulation of the leg of a live bird. And Galvani must have been familiar with his work and the work of Caldani and Fontana on the direct electrical stimulation of nerves.[4] Caldani promoted electricity as the most potent stimulus to animal tissues.[5] Galvani's first experiments on muscle contraction were in 1780, the year he acquired a frictional machine and a Leyden jar.[6] He tested the action of "fluido elettrico" applied in some cases to the

[2]Manuscript found by S. Gherardi, reported in 1839, and preserved in the Archives of the Accademia delle Scienze in Bologna. (Plico II. Fascicle II. *Experimente sulle rane*.)

[3]Giambatista Beccaria (1716–1781). *Dell'eletricismo artificiale e naturalae*, Vol. I. Campana, Turin, 1753.

[4]For the experiments of Caldani and Fontana see pages 138–149 in this volume.

[5]L. M. A. Caldani. Sull'insensitività ed irritabilità di alcune parti degli animali. Letter to Haller 1756. Published in: A. Haller. *Mémoires sur les parties sensibles et irritables du corps animal*, Vol. 3, pp. 143–144. D'Arnay, Lausanne, 1760.

[6]*Memorie ed Esperimenti Editi ed Inediti di Luigi Galvani*. Capelli, Bologna, 1937.

nerves or spinal cord, and in others to the muscles of the frog. He rarely used a live frog but a chosen preparation for which he frequently made a sketch in his notes, sometimes including himself.

At this time, when Galvani was trying to introduce the phenomenon of electricity into the nervous system, physicists were still floundering in their search for some practical explanation of this unseen but powerful agent. The many and somewhat haphazard demonstrations of other experimenters, which were described by Dufay[7] and by Stephen Gray,[8] led to recognition of the difference between conductors of electricity and insulators. It was also determined that the action of friction machines was to unbalance a pairing of opposite signs, producing a charge that would be delivered to other objects. The nomenclature used at the time was not "positive" and "negative" but "resinous" and "vitreous." The latter term derived from the discovery that glass could be charged, as demonstrated by Hawksbee.[9]

Illustrations in the first edition of *Commentary* show the frictional machine used by Galvani, and several Leyden jars. He wrote that it was by chance that he touched, with a scalpel, the exposed nerves of a frog preparation while one of his assistants was charging the frictional machine. A charge had been transferred to the insulated nerve-muscle preparation by induction from a distance. When the machine discharged by sparking, the nerve-muscle preparation also discharged through Galvani's scalpel to earth. It was the stimulus for contraction. Textbooks of the time named it the "returning stroke" but this was the first time it had been observed in a biological preparation.[10] The term had been devised to explain phenomena associated with lightning. Even the physicists could supply only a vague explanation of it, and it is not surprising that Galvani did not understand it.

Galvani did many experiments on this phenomenon, noting, for example, that if the scalpel had a bone handle no contraction resulted when the machine sparked. When he found that touching the nerves with iron or glass was as effective as using metal, he concluded that the failure of bone to elicit a response was due to its being a nonconductor of the "electric fluid." Galvani opened his *Commentary* with this experiment. His illustrations reflect the many ways in which he attempted to explore conduction. One of his most frequently used methods was to enclose a frog preparation in a glass jar placed on lead shot. A wire was strung across the ceiling to pick up the charge, and connected through the seal of the jar to the frog's spinal cord. When the machine sparked, the frog jumped—a clear demonstration that the frog's nerves conducted the electricity from the spinal cord to the muscles. His laboratory notes showed that this result was explored in 1781 with many variations of detail— some with a pair of jars (A, in Fig. 93), the lower one with the frog legs touching a layer of lead shot and its spinal cord hooked to a fine iron wire leading from the upper jar which in turn had its own layer of lead shot and, at the top, a wire to collect the charge. When the frictional machine discharged, a spark was seen in the upper jar (vividly depicted by Galvani in the sketches in his notebooks), and in the lower one movement of the frog legs

[7]Charles de Cisternai Dufay (1698–1739). Quatrième mémoire sur l'électricité. *Mém. Acad. Roy. Soc.*, pp. 457–476 (1733).

[8]Stephen Gray (?–1736). A letter to Cromwell Mortimer, MD, Secretary of the Royal Society, containing several experiments concerning electricity. *Phil. Trans. roy. Soc.*, 37:18–44 (1731).

[9]Francis Hawksbee (?–1713). Physico-mechanical experiments on various subjects, containing an account of several surprising phenomena touching light and electricity, producible on the attrition of bodies, together with the explanations of all machines and other apparatus used in making experiments. Printed for the author, London, 1709.

[10]In a volume published in 1779 entitled *Principles of Electricity* (Elmsly, London) the author, Lord Mahon, gave the name "returning stroke" to what he described as "that quantity of electric fluid which, by the vicinity of a cloud highly electrified, is driven away from certain bodies when the cloud happens to discharge its Electricity by a stroke of lightening to any other body."

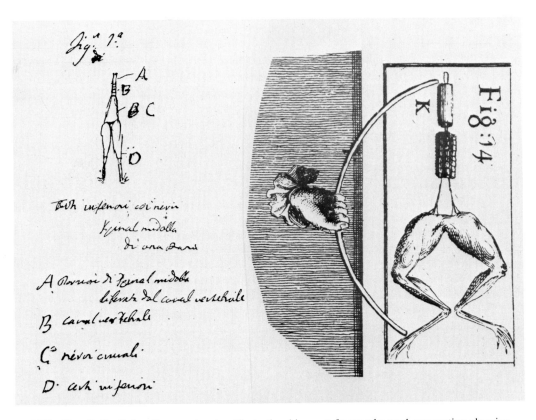

FIG. 92. **Left:** Galvani's own drawing illustrating his most frequently used preparation showing (C) the exposed crural (i.e., sciatic) nerves from the muscle (D) leading up through the vertebrae (B) to the exposed spinal cord (A). (From Cap III. Esp. I of Galvani's notes in the Archives of the Accademia delle Scienze in Bologna.)   **Right:** The artist's depiction of this favorite preparation of Galvani's published as part of the first illustration to the famous *Commentary* published in 1791.

was observed. The discharge from the machine could reach the wire of the upper jar but could not directly stimulate the frog insulated in the lower jar—only by passage of "electric fluid" down the spinal cord could the leg muscles be stimulated.

From his many experiments with "artificial electricity," Galvani concluded that there must be a nervous electric fluid, an opinion also confirmed by one of his rare experiments on a living frog. In this case the crural (sciatic) nerve of one leg was dissected and lifted above the surrounding tissue. On stimulation, only the leg muscles on that side gave contractions.

In the second part of his *Commentary*, Galvani studied "atmospheric" electricity, making use of lightning in a thunderstorm as the discharge to excite frog legs. He was disappointed that only negative results were obtained when he used sheet lightning, and he referred the explanation to the physicists. In the field of atmospheric electricity, important to the eventual clarification of nervous action, a major contribution was made by an American whose influence contributed to some of Galvani's findings. At the age of 40, while working as a printer, Benjamin Franklin became interested in the physical properties of electricity.[11] His

[11]Benjamin Franklin (1706–1790). *Experiments and Observations on Electricity, made at Philadelphia in America, by Mr. Benjamin Franklin, and Communicated in several Letters to P. Collinson, FRS.* Cave, London, 1751. (The work described in this publication was of four men: Franklin, Syng, Hopkinson, and Kumersky, but Franklin got all the credit.)

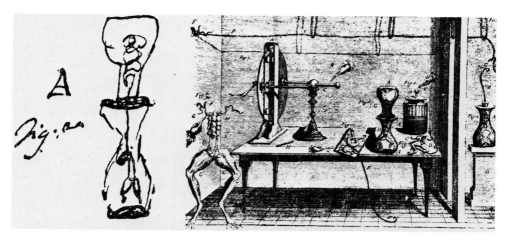

FIG. 93. Galvani's sketch of his preparation of inverted flasks containing the frog's nerve muscle preparation from an experiment dated December 10, 1781 *(Memorie ed Esperimenti Inediti)* and depicted again in the first illustration of his *Commentary*, 1791. This figure also shows his frictional machine, a Leyden jar, and the wire strung across the room to collect the charge (*Commentary*, 1791).

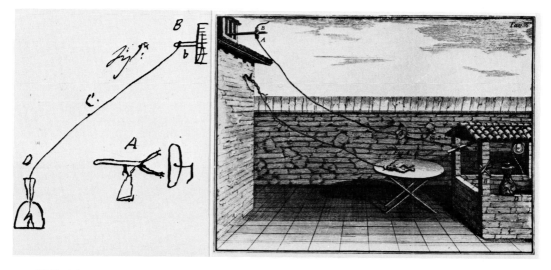

FIG. 94. **Left:** Galvani's experiments in capturing "atmospheric electricity" as a stimulus to his frog. He erected an iron post on the roof of his house from which he strung an iron wire. On this he hung the prepared frog legs and noted their contractions when lightning struck. An experiment dated December 16, 1781 *(Memorie ed Esperimenti Inediti)*. **Right:** Galvani's published figure on his success in stimulating frog legs exposed in this way during a thunderstorm (in 1st edition only of *Commentary*).

first hypothesis did not hold up. Using the concept of electric fluid, common at the time, he incorporated the 17th century notion of its corpuscular nature. He believed these corpuscular components were warring with each other and attracting other objects, thus establishing a kind of atmospheric influence. Galvani, when trying to establish the biological origin of electricity, ruled out this theory by insulating his frog legs within jars.

Franklin's concept of atmospheric electricity was attractive because there was a familiar phenomenon that appeared to support it: naturally occurring lightning. Franklin's famous experiment with a kite, confirming earlier work in France, gripped the imagination and demonstrated the similarity between lightning and an electric spark. Lightning caused the death of a Swedish experimenter, Richmann, working in St. Petersburg.[12] This event and Franklin's work had an impact on Galvani and led him to stimulate frog legs during a thunderstorm by connecting them by a high flung wire to a lightning stroke. He included illustrations of this in both editions of his *Commentary*.

To the biologists busy stimulating their animals—Caldani, Fontana, Galvani and his nephew, Aldini—the world of physicists only provided hypotheses and no data on the powerful "electric fluid" that was thought to hover in the atmosphere. Action at a distance seemed impossible and did not receive recognition for more than 200 years.[13] In order for one body to have action on another, earlier theorists felt that a material "something" must lie between the source and the detector. In the 17th century Descartes, for whom all phenomena were caused by matter in motion, had launched his scheme of a universe held together by celestial vortices.[14] In the 18th century, Newton dominated with his concept of an all-pervading ether. Newton speculated that this was the agent that we now call the nerve impulse. "I suppose," he wrote, "that the Capillamenta of the Nerves are each of them solid and uniform, that the vibrating Motion of the Aetherial Medium may be propagated along them from one end to the other uniformly, and without interruption...."[15] However, there is a partial retraction of his mechanistic view in *General Scholium*.[16] Newton was an intensely religious man and a vitalist, as revealed by his correspondence with John Locke. After he described "a most subtle spirit which pervades and lies hid in all gross bodies" and stated "electric bodies operate to greater distances" he added "the members of animal bodies move at the command of the will." Galvani held that they moved by animal electricity.

The observation of Galvani's that was, however, to become the cornerstone of the attacks on his theory of animal electricity was the one in which he hung prepared frog legs on the iron balcony outside the house in which he lived. Having succeeded so well with atmospheric electricity as a stimulus during a thunderstorm, Galvani proceeded to look for electrical effects of the atmosphere on clear days. In his notes of October 30, 1786 he wrote the following.

> Some frogs prepared in the usual way, with their spinal cords pierced, were one early evening in September suspended with iron hooks on the horizontal parapet. When a hook touched the iron railing quite often there were varied spontaneous movements in the frog. If the hook were pressed against the iron surface with a finger, the motionless frogs were excited, almost as often as this kind of pressure was exerted.[17]

Galvani also described these experiments in Part 3 of his *Commentary*, and his account reflects his puzzlement. He claimed that he tried "different metals" and noticed that each caused a different reaction. He called the metal "ferreo" (iron) in his notebooks and the railings "ringhiera di ferro."

In his *Commentary* he used "aereis" (bronze) for the hook and "ferreis cancellis" for the railings. It was the copper in the bronze that misled him and led to the explanation of the stimulus in this experiment being the current that flowed between two dissimilar metals.

[12]Georg Eilhelm Richmann (1711–1753).

[13]G. Burniston Brown. *Retarded Action-at-a-Distance*. Cortney, Luton, 1982.

[14]R. Descartes. *Principia Philosophiae*. Elzevir, Amsterdam, 1644.

[15]Isaac Newton. *Optics or a Treatise of the Reflections, Refractions, Inflections and Colours of Light*, 2nd edn, 24th Query. London, 1714.

[16]Isaac Newton. *General Scholium* (added to the 2nd edn of *Principia*). Elzevir, Amsterdam, 1714.

[17]*Memorie ed Esperimenti Inediti di Luigi Galvani*, p. 33. Capelli, Bologna, 1937.

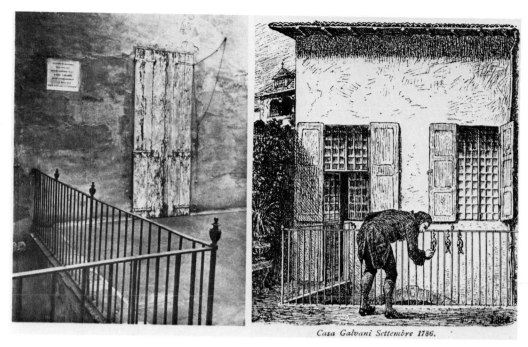

Casa Galvani Settembre 1786.

FIG. 95. Left: A house in Bologna (96 Strada San Felice, now demolished) with what was once thought to be the famous railings where Galvani hung his frog legs. More recent research on the dates of Galvani's residences makes this unlikely, for at the time of these first experiments he was living in the Via Tortoni. (From: *Nuove Ricerche Galvaniane*, by Candido Mesini. Bologna, 1971). **Right:** The picture that Du Bois Reymond had made by an artist from his own original sketch after a visit to the house in 1850. (From: *Reden von Emil Du Bois Reymond*, Vol. 2. Leipzig, 1887.)

The *Commentary* was reprinted three times, twice in Bologna in 1791 and again in Modena in the following year. The third edition reached scientists outside Italy and immediately attracted attention. One of the first to repeat Galvani's experiments was Volta whose immediate report confirmed Galvani's results.[18] Later he discounted "animal electricity," referring all his results to bimetallic electricity from which he produced his famous Voltaic Pile.[19]

Galvani was aware of bimetallic current. Many experiments described it in his notebooks.[20] In the *Commentary* he explicitly stated that if both the hook and the conducting surface were iron, no contractions resulted. These experiments, however, did not alter his conclusion that animal electricity was secreted in the brain and distributed by the nerves. Muscles, he held, were like Leyden jars, negative on the outside, positive on the inside. The oily outer layer of the nerves prevented the nervous fluid from dissipating so that it could flow down and trigger discharge of the irritable muscle. Haller had declared muscles were irritable and Galvani was schooled by the Hallerian group in Bologna where both Caldani and Fontana

[18]Alessandro Volta (1745–1827). Letter to Abbé Vassali April 1, 1792. In: *Opere di Alessandro Volta*, Edizione Nazionale sotto gli auspici della Reale Accademia dei Lincei e del Reale Istituto Lombardo di Scienze e Lettere, p. 36. Hoepli, Milan, 1918.

[19]A. Volta. Letter to Sir Joseph Banks, March 20, 1800, on electricity excited by the mere contact of conducting substances of different kinds. *Phil. Trans. roy. Soc.*, 90:403–431 (1800).

[20]For example, experiments of October 13, 1786, published in *Memorie ed Esperimenti Inediti*. Capelli, Bologna, 1937. And three manuscripts held in the Archives of the Accademia delle Scienze, Bologna.

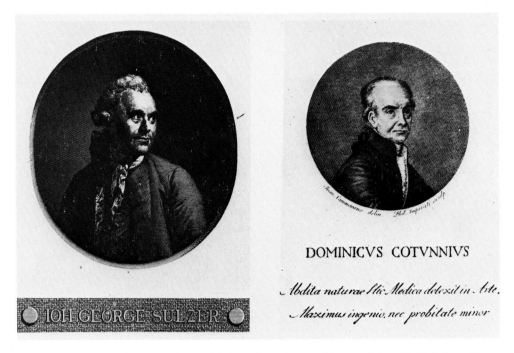

FIG. 96. Two experimenters who stumbled on effects they could not explain. **Left:** Johann Georg Sulzer (1720–1779) who first reported the tingling sensation when two different metals touched the tongue. **Right:** Domenico Cotugno (1736–1822) who described a shock felt when dissecting a mouse.

had worked. Early in his career, Galvani presented a report to the Academy entitled *Sull' irritabilità halleriana* (1772).

There was, however, an experiment published thirty years before the work of Galvani or Volta. It described a discovery of the generation of electricity by dissimilar metals. Johann Georg Sulzer, the 25th child of Swiss parents, gave a report on this to the Academy of Sciences in Berlin in 1752. He described the sensation produced by the contact of two different metals on the tongue. He described the taste as "assez approchant au gout de vitriol de fer"[21] and interpreted this with a current hypothesis that the sensation was produced by vibration. The junction of two different metals was all important.

Another report was unnoticed for many years. It came from a professor of anatomy in Naples, Domenico Cotugno, written in a letter to a friend.[22] In dissecting a mouse he had received a considerable shock which he presumed was electricity produced by the animal. This anecdote was recalled by Cavallo in the third edition of *Treatise on Electricity*[23] published four years after the appearance of Galvani's *Commentary*. However, insufficient detail was given to make this a supportive testimony, and it was dismissed by Volta. After his first reading of *Commentary*, Volta praised it, declaring Galvani's discoveries "great and brilliant."[24] Later he changed his opinion, denying the existence of animal electricity

[21]J. G. Sulzer (1720–1779). Recherches sur l'origine de sentiments agréables et desagréables. Troisième Partie. Des plaisirs des sens. *Histoire de l'Acad. Roy. Sci. Belles Lettres*, pp. 350–372. Berlin, 1754.

[22]Domenico Felice Antonio Cotugno (1736–1822). Reprinted by Magendie, *J. Physiol. Exper. Pathol.*, 7:85–96 (1827).

[23]Tiberius Cavallo (1749–1809). *Complete Treatise on Electricity*, 3rd edn, Vol. 3, pp. 7–8. Dilly and Bowen, London, 1795.

[24]Alessandro Giuseppe Antonio Anastasio Volta (1745–1827). Letter to Abbé Vassali, April 1, 1792. In: *Le Opere di Alessandro Volta*, Vol. 1, pp. 15–35. Hoepli, Milan, 1918.

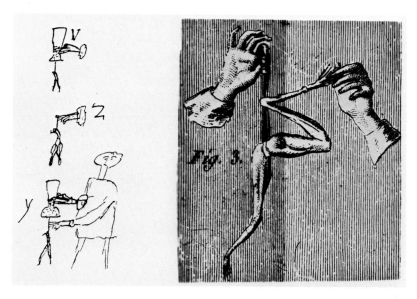

FIG. 97. **Left:** Galvani's sketch of himself making various experiments with his frog nerve-muscle preparation which he likened to a Leyden jar. (From notes he made December 10, 1781, preserved in the Archives of the University of Bologna.) **Right:** The critical experiment on muscle contraction in the absence of all metals. (From Aldini, G. *Essai Théorique et Expérimental sur le Galvanisme*, Vol. I. Fournier, Paris, 1804.)

in any creature but the electric fish. He believed all Galvani's results were based on the presence of dissimilar metals.[25]

Alessandro Volta (1745–1827)

Volta used bimetallic currents to explain all the frog experiments. He insisted that to produce electricity, three substances had to be present: two heterogeneous metals and between them a third conducting material to make a complete circuit. If the third material were frog muscle, it would, by virtue of its irritability, react to the flow of bimetallic electricity. Its role was solely that of an electroscope.[26] When Aldini, Galvani's nephew and Professor of Physics at the University of Bologna, demonstrated by dipping the ends of nerves and muscles into mercury that the same effect could be obtained with a single metal, Volta responded.[27] He pointed out that the surface of the mercury in contact with the air suffered a change that made it heterogeneous with the depth. This argument was later disproved by Humboldt.[28]

In the meantime an anonymous tract had been published, almost certainly with Galvani's collaboration, which included a description of the twitching of muscles in the absence of

[25]A. Volta. Account of some discoveries made by Mr. Galvani of Bologna, with experiments and observations on them. In two letters from Mr. Alexander Volta to Mr. Tiberius Cavallo. *Phil. Trans. roy. Soc.*, 83:10–44 (1793).

[26]A. Volta. Memoria prima sull'elettricità animale. *Giornale fisico-medico*, 2:146–187 (1792).

[27]Giovanni Aldini (1762–1834). *De Animali Electricitate. Dissertationes Duae.* Bologna, 1794.

[28]Frederick Alexander Humboldt (1769–1859). *Versuche über die gereizte Muskel und Nervenfasser.* Rottmann, Posen, and Decker, Berlin, 1797.

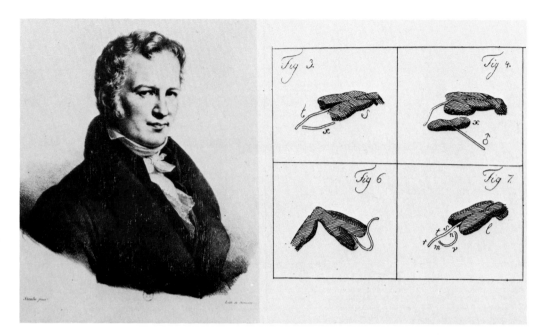

FIG. 98.   Left: Alexander von Humboldt (1769–1859) whose experiments confirmed Galvani (from the portrait by Karl von Steuben).   **Right:** Von Humboldt's experiments in which he demonstrated contraction of nerve-muscle preparations in the absence of any metals. His *Fig. 3* depicts a frog nerve-muscle preparation to which he applied a tube of glass *(x)*, producing a contraction. His *Fig. 6* shows an experiment in which he turned back the nerve against the muscle without interposing the glass rod. (From: *Versuche über die gereizte Muskel- und Nervenfasser nebst Vermuthungen über den chemischen Process des Lebens in der Thier und Pflanzenwelt.* Posen, 1797.)

any metals or external source of electricity.[29] A contraction was demonstrated when the cut end of a frog's spine fell over onto its muscle or when one limb was drawn up to touch the exposed nerves from the spinal column. In this case the source of electricity was what is now recognized as the current of injury. After this demonstration Volta tried to explain the current flow as being the result of heterogeneity of tissues (muscle and nerve). This specious argument was also disproved by Humboldt.

The design of Humboldt's experiments and the clarity of his reasoning are a pleasure to study in the welter of acrimonious controversy that greeted Galvani's findings. Without bias toward either protagonist, Humboldt repeated Volta's and Galvani's experiments. He examined their interpretations, designed new experiments to test their hypotheses, and concluded that Galvani had uncovered two genuine phenomena: bimetallic electricity and intrinsic animal electricity, and he felt these were not mutually exclusive. Humboldt demonstrated that both scientists had erred in interpreting their experiments; however, from these were to grow the science of electrophysiology, on the one hand and, on the other, the brilliant development of the electric battery.

Volta, for 40 years Professor of Physics at the University of Pavia, was born in Como in the period when Lombardy was under the rule of Austria, but during the height of his feud with Galvani, this duchy fell to the onslaught of Napoleon who created it the Cisalpine

[29]Anonymous. *Dell'uso e dell'attività dell'Arco conduttore nelle contrazioni dei muscoli. Supplemento*, Bologna, 1794.

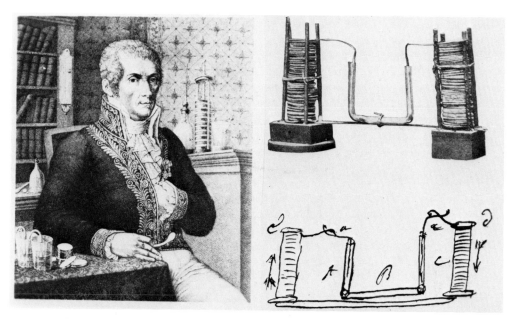

FIG. 99. Left: Alessandro Volta (1745–1827) from the portrait by Roberto Focasi. Volta was an admirer of and honored by Napoleon, one of whose gestures he seems to have caught. Behind him is a Voltaic pile. **Right:** Piles used by Volta preserved at the Temple to Volta in Como and his own sketch of the experiment. *Above:* Apparatus used by Volta to demonstrate that the pile makes the water alkaline in one arm and acid in the other. *Below:* A sketch drawing by Volta, regarding the above apparatus [*Edizione Nazionale*, 2:60–61 and 329 (1899)].

Republic with himself as President. Napoleon recognized the achievements of Volta, as well as his political support, and gave him medals, honors, and a title.[30] In 1802, Volta was elected a foreign member of the Académie des Sciences (bringing with him an example of a Voltaic Pile which is still preserved in the Conservatoire des Arts et Métiers).

On the south shore of the beautiful Lake Como a temple (the Tempio Voltano) was built in his honor. Intended to house his instruments and notebooks, it was destroyed by fire in 1899 and then pillaged. Within a few years certain items began to surface in pawnshops, among them a frictional electrical machine (now in the collection of the Wellcome Institute of the History of Medicine in London) which is thought to have come from that collection.

After his communication to the Royal Society on his invention of the Voltaic Pile, Volta made no further publications of great note although he lived to the age of eighty-two.[31]

Galvani died in 1798, at odds with Napoleon because he refused to take the oath of allegiance to the Cisalpine Republic, a stand which led to the loss of his positions at the University and the Istituto. He was buried unostentatiously in a monastery burial ground. Eventually, a special vault was built, for Galvani and his wife, in the Corpus Domini Church adjoining the burial ground. During World War II, a nun, fearing aerial bombing, moved the remains to safety at the Church of San Luca. On July 27, 1947 a bomb demolished the vault, but the famous bones were safe.[32] The city of Bologna had no statue to Galvani until

[30]Comte du Royaume Lombard.

[31]A. Volta. Letter to Sir Joseph Banks, March 20, 1800. On electricity excited by the mere contact of conducting substances of different kinds. *Phil. Trans. roy. Soc.*, 90:403–431 (1800).

[32]As told to the author by the late Professor G. C. Pupilli.

finally one was erected by the telephone company and stands in the square, now named for him, outside the famous old Archiginnasio where he taught for so long.

The arguments about electrical activity in the nervous system raged on until, in the century that followed, three great experimentalists gave it the final proof—Carlo Matteucci, Ludwig Hermann, and Emil Du Bois Reymond. Strangely, Galvani's name is still used in medical electricity, although the term "Galvanism" was originally restricted to bimetallic electricity. The name lives on to this day as galvanic current, and was used briefly in the form of "galvanoplastics" to the process we now call electroplating.[33]

Ironically, Galvani's name was given to a prize established by Napoleon to honor Volta. The prize was for the best work done in Galvanism or, in Bonaparte's words, "par ses expériences et ses découvertes, fera faire à l'électricité et au Galvanisme un pas comparable à celui qu'on a fait faire à ces sciences Franklin et Volta...."[34] Only in the 19th century do we find the successful recipients of this prize, the first being Ludimar Hermann from Königsburg and the second Humphrey Davy. Hermann's contributions[35] were directly related to animal electricity for he clarified the phenomenon of the current of injury (or demarcation current) in nerve. Davy's prize essay[36] was directed to an explanation of the chemistry of the Voltaic Pile.

BIBLIOGRAPHY

Luigi Galvani (1737–1798)

Selected Writings

Sull'irritabilita halleriana. The title and date (April 19, 1772) are recorded in the minutes of the Istituto delle Scienze. Bologna.

Aloysii Galvani de viribus electricitatis in motu musculari. Commentarius. De viribus electricitatis artificialis in motu musculari. *De Bononiensi Scientiarum et Artium Instituto atque Academia*, 7:363–418 (1791). (With 4 illustrations.) Reprinted twice in 1791. First commercial edition of the above with new engravings of 3 of original plates and with preface by J. Aldini. Societatum Typographicam, Modena, 1792. (English translation by R. M. Green. Licht, Cambridge, 1953.)

Letter to Carminati. *Giornale Fisicomedico* (Brugnatelli), 2:131–145 (1792).

Dell'Uso e dell' Attivita dell'Arco Conduttore nelle Contrazioni dei Muscoli con Supplemento (published anonymously). D'Aquino, Bologna, 1794.

Opere Edite ed Inedite. S. Gherardi, Bologna, 1841.

Memorie ed Esperimenti Inediti di Luigi Galvani. Capelli, Bologna, 1937.

Secondary Sources

Aldini, J. *Dissertationes Duae*. Istituto della Scienza, Bologna, 1794.

Aldini, J. *Essai Théorique et Experimental sur le Galvanisme*, 2 vols. Fournier, Paris, 1804.

[33]Hermann von Jacobi, Moritz (1801–1874). Berichte über die Entwicklung der Galvanoplastik. *Bull. Acad. Sci. Cl. Physico-Math., St. Petersburg*, 1:65–71 (1843).

[34]*Procès-verbaux des sceanes de l'Académie des Sciences*, 2:(1801).

[35]Ludimar Hermann (1833–1914). Über sogenannten secondär-electromotrische Erscheinungen an Muskeln und Nerve. *Pflüg. Arch. ges. Physiol.*, 33:103–168 (1884).

[36]Humphrey Davy (1778–1829). Le mode d'action chimique de l'électricité. Bakerian lecture. Mémoire couronne par l'Académie des Sciences de Paris, 1807, and the Bakerian lecture on some chemical agencies. *Phil. Trans. roy. Soc.*, 97:1–56 (1807).

Foley, M. G. *Galvani's Commentary on the Effects of Electricity on Muscular Motion* (Translation with notes). Burndy Library, Norwalk, Conn. 1958.

Fulton, J. F., and Cushing, H. A bibliographical study of the Galvani and the Aldini writings on animal electricity. *Ann. Sci.*, 1:239–268 (1936).

Hoff, H. E. Galvani and the pre-Galvanian electrophysiologists. *Ann. Sci.*, 1:66–100 (1936).

Home, F. W. Electricity and the nervous fluid. *J. Hist. Biol.*, 3:235–251 (1970).

Mauro, A. The role of the Voltaic Pile in the Galvani-Volta Controversy concerning animal versus metallic electricity. *J. Hist. Med.*, 140–150 (1969).

Mesini, Candido. *Nuovo Ricerche Galvaniane*. Tamari Editori, Bologna, 1971.

Pupilli, G. C. *Luigi Galvani. Studi et memorie per la Storia dell'Universita di Bologna*, Vol. I (of new series), pp. 445–459. 1956.

Pupilli, G. C., and Fadiga, E. The origins of electrophysiology. Studies on Italian History. *J. World History*, 7:547–589 (1963).

Sirol, M. *Galvani et le Galvanisme. Electricité Animale*. Vigot, Paris, 1938.

Walker, W. C. The detection and estimation of electric charges in the eighteenth century. *Ann. Sci.*, 1:66–100 (1936).

Motu Musculari Commentarius. Licht, Cambridge, 1953.

CHAPTER XVII

Dissemination of Knowledge in the 18th Century

For the interchange of scientific information the 17th century had had to rely heavily on personal correspondence because there were few academies and even fewer journals, but it had laid the ground for the great academies to follow the examples of the Royal Society and the Académie Royale des Sciences.[1]

In 1700, the German Academy opened in Berlin, the capital of the Principality of Brandenburg, the culmination of the work of Leibniz. The academy had great backing from the Elector, Frederick the Great, when he succeeded his father, Friedrich Wilhelm I. He was a man of broad opinions, drawing to his group men who had caused offence elsewhere with their free thinking—for example, Voltaire, Maupertius, and La Mettrie. (One of the most outstanding scientists in the academy was the Swiss mathematician Leonard Euler who later left the Berlin Academy for St. Petersburg.) But his was what became known as an enlightened despotism for all decisions were made by Frederick himself. He focused on the sciences that would develop the country and the military armory to defend it.

Just as the groundwork for the Berlin Academy had been laid by Leibniz in the 17th century, so had that for St. Petersburg Academy been laid by Peter the Great. However, he did not live to see its opening in 1725. Peter, himself a physician, had traveled to the Netherlands, France, and England to study their universities, hospitals, and academic institutions. In all of these western countries, universities had been established long before the creation of an academy. In his own country, Peter reversed the order, pushing his plans

---

[1] *Journal des Scavans* (1663). *Philosophical Transactions* (1665). *Mémoires de l'Académie Royale des Sciences* (1699).

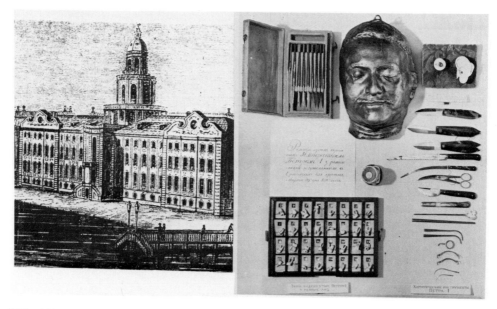

FIG. 100. **Left:** An early print of the first building of the Russian Academy of Science and the Kunstcamera built by Peter the Great on the banks of the Neva and opened in 1725, the year after his death. **Right:** The death mask of Peter, and his surgical instruments preserved in the Kunstcamera.

for an academy ahead of those for a university. He also established a hospital (patterned on Greenwich Hospital on the Thames) and a Medical-Surgical School in Moscow in 1706. As he was to do repeatedly and as another monarch, Christina, had done for Sweden, he recruited the ablest men he could from the west. He appointed Nicolaus Bidloo, from the school of Boerhaave in Leyden, to direct the teaching of medicine. Bidloo was the son of the anatomist whose atlas, with Winslow's classic text, was the principal teaching source.[2] As scientific terminology did not exist in the Russian language, courses were taught in Latin. Only at the end of the 18th century did instruction in Russian commence.

Peter planned his Academy for his new city, St. Petersburg. He recruited scientists and materials, and arranged for the printing of Russian translations from Latin texts. One of Peter's purchases was the anatomical collection of the Dutch anatomist Frederic Ruysch, an amazing display which can still be seen in the Kunstcamera in Leningrad. Among those whose aid was sought in establishing the Academy was Christian von Wolf from Marburg, a prominent German philosopher.[3] A war with Sweden delayed the completion of Peter's plans until 1725, a year after his death, but then, with the opening of a port on the Baltic, the Academy buildings and the Kunstcamera were erected on the banks of the Neva. Other distinguished scientists drawn from the west were Leonard von Euler,[4] the two sons of the famous Swiss mathematician, Jean Bernouilli, and, by invitation of Peter's successor, Catherine II, the nephews of Boerhaave and Denis Diderot (who stayed only briefly to organize her library). Others, such as d'Alembert, Maupertius, and Voltaire, were sought but would not come. But the persistent Catherine obtained their libraries after their deaths. Diderot's

[2]J-B. Winslow. *L'Exposition Anatomique de la Structure du Corps Humain.* Duprez & Dessartz, Paris, 1732.
[3]Christian von Wolf (1679–1754).
[4]Leonard von Euler (1707–1783).

library unfortunately disappeared but Voltaire's is honored with its own building in Leningrad, in the Saltykov-Scheidrin State Public Library.

In the middle of the 18th century, Russia produced its own scientist of great distinction: Mikhael Vasilyevich Lomononosov (1711–1765). He was a pupil of Christian Wolf at the Academy in St. Petersburg, and later in Marburg. A talented chemist, poet, and dramatist, he was influential in founding the University of Moscow in 1755, with chairs in philosophy, law, and medicine. His statue stands outside the new buildings of the University of Moscow in the Lenin Hills. Studies of the nervous system at the Moscow University and the Academy in St. Petersburg were made in terms of anatomy and its application to medical problems. In 1726 Bernouilli published papers on muscular movements and the optic nerve—both subjects fascinating to a mathematician.[5]

The University of Moscow was not the first in Russia. Two others had been won as spoils of war. On the defeat of the Swedes, at the Treaty of Nystadt in 1721, the ancient University of Dorpat[6] (in Estonia) founded by Queen Christina's father, Gustavus Adolphus, in 1632, became a Russian possession. The Academy of Wilno[7] (in Lithuania) was also taken by Russia during the division of Poland. Founded by the Jesuits in 1578, and aided by the Pope, this "academy" in Wilno was essentially a university. In the early 19th century both of these institutions were enlarged and made into official Russian Universities, specializing in medical training. In the 19th century there was a great expansion of teaching in Russia and universities were founded in Kazan, Kharkov, and Kiev. At the end of the century universities were also opened at Tomsk, in 1888 (to serve Siberia), and at Odessa, in 1896 (to serve the south). Both essentially provided instruction in medicine. The Congress of Vienna in 1815 brought the University of Warsaw onto Russian soil for a few years before being dissolved. The varied origins of the centers for learning under Russian rule caused a language problem for teaching. For this reason we find Peter's Academy using French, as did the Berlin Academy on its opening.

The planning of Peter's Academy continued while Russia was in a long drawn out war with Sweden. This was not the only great academy to arise in a time of war. During the American Revolution the people of the American colonies were planning for an academy and in 1780 succeeded "although involved in all the calamities and distresses of a severe war" in getting a charter passed by the Massachusetts House of Representatives for the establishment of "a body politic and corporate, by the name of the American Academy of Arts and Sciences." The prime mover was John Adams who became the second president of the United States. This academy was intended primarily to "promote and encourage the knowledge" of America but in the more than 200 years of its existence it has become a leading institution with strong international ties.

Before the close of the 18th century many provincial Academies had opened in western Europe, mostly medically or philosophically oriented. For pursuit of studies of the nervous system those in Montpellier and Bordeaux were outstanding. All in France were closed in 1793 but reopened with new vigor before the end of the century.

The 18th century saw the emergence of textbooks on physiology as distinct from clinical treatises or anatomical texts. In these, one could find sections on the nervous system with the study of function being far more complex than the study of structure. The first book on

---

[5]D. Bernouilli. *Testamenta novae de motu musculorum.* 1726. Published in Russian in the commentaries of the Academy of Sciences, St. Petersburg, 1728.

[6]Now named Tartu.

[7]Now named Vilnius.

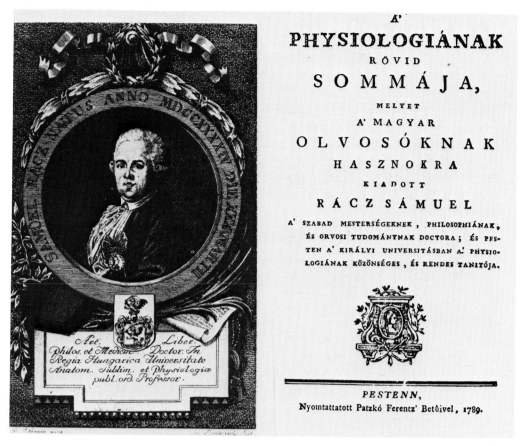

FIG. 101. Left: Samuel Racz (1744–1807), who produced the first textbook of physiology in the Hungarian language, entitled modestly, *A Short Summary of Physiology.* **Right:** The original title page.

physiology from the North American continent was the work of Marcos Jose Salgado, born in 1671, in New Spain, now Mexico.[8] The Spaniards had founded no less than thirty universities during their colonial period in the New World, including Mexico's University in 1551. It was at this university that Salgado taught and published his book, *Cursus medicus Mexicanus.* The first volume is dedicated to Physiology and dated 1727. Nothing was published in the Colonies, or the States, until nearly the end of the 19th century. Medical practitioners from Europe settled and practiced in the Colonies (the first was Richard Townshend who came to Virginia in 1621) but no one from the great schools of physiological research in England, Holland, France, Germany, or Italy left their laboratories to come and work in the new found land. The flow was in the opposite direction. Americans went to Europe to study and then returned to create centers of research. The first chair in physiology went to Henry Bowditch at Harvard in 1871.

In 1789 the first Hungarian textbook of physiology, written by Samuel Racz, a professor at the University in Pest, gave prominence to the then current problems of irritability and contractility and their bearing on the seat of the soul.[9] And in spite of wars, revolutions,

[8]M. J. Salgado. *Cursus medicus Mexicanus: para Prima Physiologica*. Michaelis de Rivera, Mexico, 1727.

[9]Samuel Racz (1744–1807). *Lehrbuch der Physiologie*. Pest. 1789. (Translated into English by C. Kovach, and McC. Brooks. *A Short Symmary of Physiology*. Akademiai Kiado, Pergamon, 1980.)

and disasters, the 18th century ended having earned the title of "le Siècle des Lumières" in France, and "the Age of Reason" in England.

SELECTED WRITINGS FOR THE DISSEMINATION OF KNOWLEDGE IN THE 18TH CENTURY

Bertrand, J. *L'Académie des Sciences et des Académiciens de 1606 à 1793*. Paris, 1869.

Butterfield, H. *The Origins of Modern Science*. London, 1949.

Calinger, R. S. Frederick the Great and the Berlin Academy of Sciences (1740–1766). *Ann. Sci.*, 24:239–249 (1968).

Hall, A. R. *The Scientific Revolution*. Longman, London, 1954.

Nicolson, H. *The Age of Reason*. Constable, London, 1960.

Rothschuh, K. E. *History of Physiology* (translated by G. B. Riese). Krieger, New York, 1973.

Taton, R. *Enseignement et Diffusion des Sciences en France au XVIIIᵉ Siècle*. Hermann, Paris, 1964.

Voltaire, F. M. A. Histoire de l'Empire de Russie sous Pierre le Grand. In: *Oeuvres Complètes de Voltaire*, pp. 371–648. Garnier, Paris, 1878.

Wolf, A. *History of Science, Technology and Philosophy in the Sixteenth, Seventeenth and Eighteenth Centuries*, 2 vols. Harper, New York, 1959.

Indexes

Name Index

Pages that contain illustrations and portraits are indicated by italicized page numbers.

Subject Index